Case Studies in Nephrology

Case Studies in Nephrology

Editor: Ivor Morrison

AMERICAN
MEDICAL PUBLISHERS
www.americanmedicalpublishers.com

AMERICAN
MEDICAL PUBLISHERS
www.americanmedicalpublishers.com

Cataloging-in-Publication Data

Case studies in nephrology / edited by Ivor Morrison.
p. cm.
Includes bibliographical references and index.
ISBN 979-8-88740-607-7
1. Nephrology. 2. Kidneys--Diseases. I. Morrison, Ivor.
RC902 .N47 2023
616.61--dc23

© American Medical Publishers, 2023

American Medical Publishers,
41 Flatbush Avenue,
1st Floor, New York,
NY 11217, USA

ISBN 979-8-88740-607-7 (Hardback)

This book contains information obtained from authentic and highly regarded sources. Copyright for all individual chapters remain with the respective authors as indicated. All chapters are published with permission under the Creative Commons Attribution License or equivalent. A wide variety of references are listed. Permission and sources are indicated; for detailed attributions, please refer to the permissions page and list of contributors. Reasonable efforts have been made to publish reliable data and information, but the authors, editors and publisher cannot assume any responsibility for the validity of all materials or the consequences of their use.

Trademark Notice: Registered trademark of products or corporate names are used only for explanation and identification without intent to infringe.

Contents

Preface

Nephrology is a specialized branch of internal medicine that deals with the physiology, diagnosis, and treatment of kidney-related diseases. Kidneys are bean-shaped organs located on either side in the retroperitoneal space and are a part of the urinary system. They are responsible for filtering blood and removing the waste products, excess water and electrolytes from the body. Some of the various conditions and diseases that can affect the kidneys include kidney/bladder cancer, excess excretion of protein in urine, glomerular diseases, kidney/bladder stones, acute or chronic kidney failure, and nephritis. A few symptoms that are associated with kidney diseases include swelling in the legs and feet, unexplained blood pressure changes, gradual loss of sense of taste and appetite, problem sleeping at night, and reduced urine output. Apart from medications, advanced treatments available for kidney diseases include continuous renal replacement therapy (CRRT), plasmapheresis, liver dialysis (MARS therapy), peritoneal dialysis (CPD), kidney biopsy, and kidney transplant. In this book, using case studies, constant effort has been made to make the understanding of the difficult concepts of nephrology as easy and informative as possible, for the readers. It will provide comprehensive knowledge to the readers.

This book has been the outcome of endless efforts put in by authors and researchers on various issues and topics within the field. The book is a comprehensive collection of significant researches that are addressed in a variety of chapters. It will surely enhance the knowledge of the field among readers across the globe.

It gives us an immense pleasure to thank our researchers and authors for their efforts to submit their piece of writing before the deadlines. Finally in the end, I would like to thank my family and colleagues who have been a great source of inspiration and support.

Editor

1

Acute Uric Acid Nephropathy following Epileptic Seizures: Case Report and Review

Chinmay Patel,[1] Caitlin P. Wilson,[2] Naveed Ahmed,[3] and Yousef Hattab[4]

[1] *University of Pikeville, Kentucky College of Osteopathic Medicine, Division of Nephrology, Pikeville Medical Center, USA*
[2] *Family Practice Residency Program, Pikeville Medical Center, USA*
[3] *Neurology Program, University of Pikeville, Kentucky College of Osteopathic Medicine, Pikeville Medical Center, USA*
[4] *Division of Pulmonary and Critical Care Medicine, Pikeville Medical Center, USA*

Correspondence should be addressed to Chinmay Patel; chinmay.patel@pikevillehospital.org

Academic Editor: Yoshihide Fujigaki

Acute hyperuricemia most commonly occurs in patients who experience tumor lysis syndrome. Hyperuricemia along with other electrolyte abnormalities like hyperkalemia, hypocalcemia, and hyperphosphatemia leads to acute kidney injury (AKI) due to acute uric acid nephropathy which is associated with significant morbidity. High risk patients are thus closely monitored for signs of these laboratory abnormalities. Extreme exercise, rhabdomyolysis, and seizures are rare causes of acute hyperuricemia. Serum uric acid level is not routinely monitored as a part of postictal labs. We report an unusual case of AKI in a young male with recurrent seizures and no associated rhabdomyolysis who was found to have acute uric acid nephropathy. Timely administration of Rasburicase prevented the need for dialysis in this patient and led to complete renal recovery. This case illustrates the importance of doing a urine microscopy and checking uric acid level in patients with recurrent seizures who develop unexplainable AKI, as timely management helps improve outcome. We also briefly review the pathophysiology of seizure related hyperuricemia and acute uric acid nephropathy.

1. Introduction

Uric acid is the final end product of purine metabolism. Acute hyperuricemia is caused by the increase of purine metabolism, which is the result of the increased cellular turnover or the aggressive cancer chemotherapy regimens which cause cell lysis and release of purine metabolites [1]. The deposition and accumulation of uric acid in renal tubules leads to acute uric acid nephropathy typically characterized by oliguric AKI, elevated serum uric acid concentration (usually more than 10-15 mg/dL), presence of uric acid crystals in the urinary sediment, and an elevated urine uric acid to creatinine ratio of greater than 1 [2]. Acute uric acid nephropathy is readily recognized when acute kidney injury (AKI) develops in cancer patients either due to spontaneous tumor lysis or following chemotherapy. Seizures seldom cause acute hyperuricemia and acute uric acid nephropathy and thus its diagnosis may be missed or delayed in this uncommon presentation. With timely recognition and management, the pathologic features of acute uric acid nephropathy are reversible. We report a patient who developed AKI due to acute uric acid nephropathy following recurrent seizures. Timely therapy with Rasburicase prevented the need for renal replacement therapy in our patient and resulted in complete renal recovery.

2. Case Presentation

A 28-year-old white male with past medical history of epilepsy and asthma was referred to us from an outside hospital for recurrent seizures and higher level of care. EMS was called to his home after family reported him having two or three episodes of generalized tonic clonic (GTC) seizure like activity for an undocumented duration of time. EMS noted the patient was in a postictal phase and he was then taken to the nearest hospital where patient had another episode of GTC seizures lasting about 5-10 mins. Patient also became apneic and cyanotic and was subsequently sedated and intubated for airway protection. Levetiracetam loading dose was given. Brain CT done was unremarkable. Vitals signs showed elevated blood pressure of 170/90 and heart rate in 120s. Initial labs showed mild leukocytosis and a normal renal function with serum creatinine (scr) of 1.3 mg/dL. Urine drug screen was negative. He was then transferred to our hospital for neurology consultation and ICU admission. Laboratory test results are shown in Table 1. Repeat labs showed mild elevation in scr of 1.7mg/dL. Initial serum electrolytes and lactic acid were within normal limits. Serum creatine kinase (CK) level was mildly elevated at 297 U/L. Pt was started on iv hydration with ringers lactate (LR) at 100 ml/hr along with antiseizure medications, namely, iv Midazolam, Levetiracetam, and Lacosamide. He remained seizure free. Labs on day 2 showed worsening AKI with scr of 4.9 mg/dL and bicarbonate of 18 mEq/L with CK level of 663 U/L. Repeat scr was noted to be 5.2mg/dL with lactic acid of 3.6 mmol/L and phosphorus of 5.4 mg/dL. Patient had remained nonoliguric with urine output of about 40-60 ml/hr. Urgent urine microscopy was performed which showed numerous uric acid crystals and occasional granular casts [Figures 1, 2, and 3]. A stat serum uric acid level was noted to be significantly elevated at 15 mg/dL. Urinalysis showed clear urine with ph 5.5, specific gravity of 1.005, 0-5 RBCs, 0-5 WBCs, no proteins, and 1+ blood. A spot urine uric acid to creatinine ratio was found to be elevated at 1.2. Based on the above findings a diagnosis of acute uric acid nephropathy was made. IV fluids were changed from LR to iv sodium bicarbonate at 150ml/hr. Patient was given a dose of iv Rasburicase 0.2 mg/ kg. Repeat labs done about 4 hrs after Rasburicase administration showed that serum uric acid level had dropped to 4 mg/dL. Scr however continued to rise to 6.1mg/dL with CK level of 464 U/L. A significant increase in urine output of about 100-150 ml/hr was however noted soon after Rasburicase administration. Day 3 scr started trending down to 6 mg/dL and serum uric acid had further dropped to 0.8. There was continued renal recovery with scr of 5.5 and CK level of 792 U/L on day 4. Patient remained seizure free throughout his hospital stay and his renal function completely recovered to normal by day 7.

3. Discussion

Uric acid is the final oxidation product of dietary and endogenous purine metabolism. Uric acid must be continuously excreted to prevent its toxic accumulation in human tissues in which it is poorly soluble, especially in the acidic environment of the distal nephron. Approximately 75% of daily uric acid is excreted by the kidney [2]. Hyperuricemia is caused by states of enhanced purine catabolism which increases the urate load on the kidney leading to their intrarenal precipitation. Tumor lysis syndrome (TLS) is one such potentially life-threatening complication that occurs in high risk cancer patients with highly proliferative malignancies and large tumor burdens receiving cytotoxic chemotherapy. Lysed cancer cells release phosphorus, potassium, and nucleic acids which are metabolized to xanthine and then oxidized to uric acid. Patients at the highest risk of TLS are thus closely monitored for these laboratory abnormalities and started on appropriate preventive measures to reduce risk of acute uric acid nephropathy.

Acute hyperuricemia plays a major role in the pathogenesis of uric acid nephropathy. Supersaturation of urine and precipitation of uric acid crystals cause intraluminal obstruction of the distal nephron. This in turn leads to dilatation, inflammation, and obstruction of the proximal tubules [3]. Ejaz et al. have also described at least five crystal independent mechanisms by which uric acid contributes to AKI [4]. It induces renal vasoconstriction through direct inhibition of the endothelial nitric oxide synthase causing reduction in nitric oxide through stimulation of the renin-angiotensin system. Inflammatory pathways by which uric acid causes AKI include activation of proinflammatory mediators like monocyte chemoattractant protein-1, C reactive protein, and mitogen-activated protein kinase. In addition, uric acid also stimulates the production of oxidants via an increase in nicotinamide adenine dinucleotide phosphatase oxidase in both adipocytes and endothelial cells. Uric acid also has been found to have antiangiogenic properties by causing inhibition of endothelial migration and proliferation and inducing endothelial cell apoptosis. Finally, hyperuricemia leads to development of preglomerular arteriolar disease which impairs the renal autoregulatory response. Uric acid has also been reported to have antioxidant properties and it is possible that, in conditions of severe oxidative stress, a rise in uric acid might provide some antioxidant benefit [4, 5]. Ejaz el al. proposed that although the antioxidant properties of uric acid may be beneficial under certain conditions, the net effect of hyperuricemia, particularly if marked and persistent, will affect the renal outcome adversely.

Acute uric acid nephropathy should be suspected in high risk patients who develop oliguric AKI with significantly elevated serum uric acid concentration of more than 10-15 mg/dL and presence of copious uric acid crystals in the urinary sediment [3]. The urinalysis however may be normal if there is no output from the obstructed nephrons [4]. As renal failure is also associated with a rise in serum uric acid as a result of decreased excretion, it may be difficult to determine if hyperuricemia or AKI developed first. Kelton J et al. have proposed that, in adults, a urine uric acid to creatinine ratio of more than 1 is highly suggestive of acute uric acid nephropathy [6]. Some researchers also report that the calculation of uric acid excretion corrected for creatinine greater than 0.57 mg/dL GFR is suggestive of uric acid nephropathy since other forms of AKI would have reduced uric acid excretion [3].

Seizures lead to distinctive metabolic changes depending on the type, length, and intensity of the seizures as well as the patients preexisting condition. Whole body muscle contractions and the activation of the neuroendocrine system to secrete catecholamines increase the cerebral, muscular, and cardiac oxygen demands, while impaired breathing impedes the compensatory mechanisms to satisfy this demand. This causes the irritated muscles to release CK and myoglobin and hypoxic tissues to leak lactate, ammonia, and urea. Afterwards, an inflammatory reaction with cytokine release

Table 1: Laboratory data of the patient.

Time after admission (time after Rasburicase administration)	Day1	Day2	Day2 (0 hrs)	Day2 (4 hrs)	Day3 (12 hrs)	Day4 (24 hrs)	Day5 (48 hrs)	Day6	Day7
BUN (mg/dL)	14	29		39	43	55	65	47	29
Creatinine (mg/dL)	1.7	4.9	5.2	6.1	6	5.5	3.1	1.8	1.2
Sodium (mEq/L)	141	140		139	140	139	143	140	
Potassium (mEq/L)	3.7	3.8		3.7	3.5	4.6	4.5	4.4	
CK (U/L)	297	663		464	501	792			
Uric acid (mg/dL)	NA	NA	15	4	0.8	<0.2	<0.2		

Abbreviations. BUN: blood urea nitrogen; CK: creatine kinase; NA: not available.

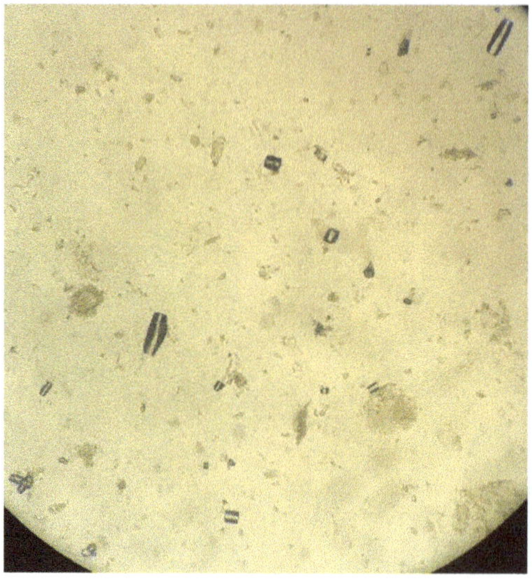

Figure 1: Urine microscopy under low power magnification showing uric acid crystals.

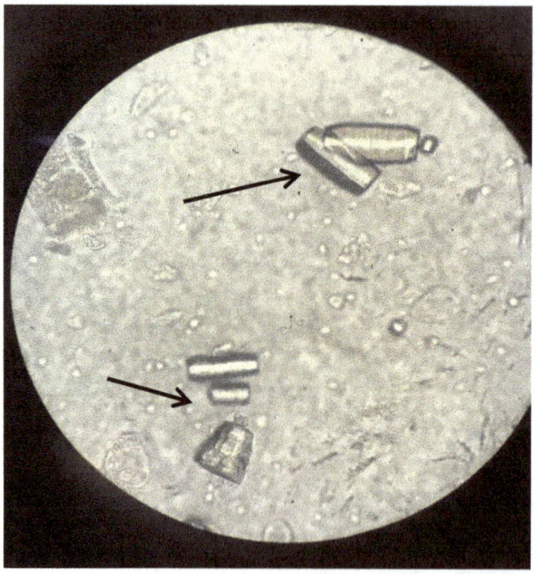

Figure 2: Barrel shaped uric acid crystals under high power magnification.

and leukocytosis occurs [7]. Seizure induced rhabdomyolysis and AKI have been reported [7, 8]. However, seizures have rarely been reported as cause of hyperuricemia and acute uric acid nephropathy.

Acute severe hyperuricemia following recurrent episodes of grand mal seizures or status epilepticus was first reported by Warren et al. in 1975 [9]. None of the patients had significant myoglobinuria nor pigmented granular casts in the urine. All the seven patients reported in the study developed reversible renal failure with two requiring hemodialysis. In 1978, Luhdorf et al. found a significant increase in serum uric acid level in seventeen patients, within 24 hours of two or more grand mal seizures [10]. Of the six patients with severe hyperuricemia only two had developed

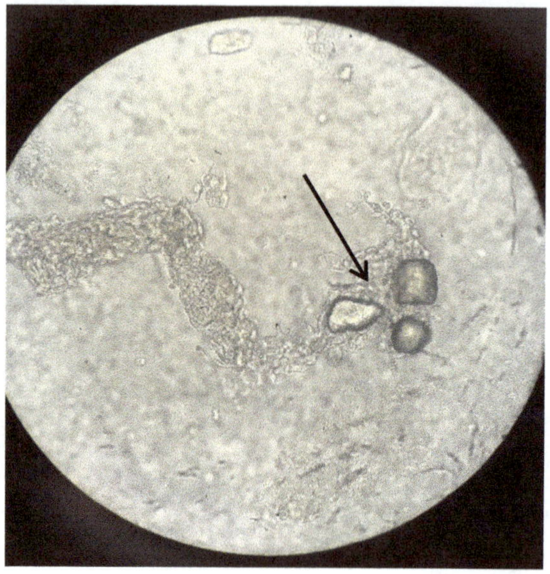

Figure 3: Diamond shaped uric acid crystals embedded in granular cast under high power magnification.

impaired renal function. A case of seizure induced acute urate nephropathy has been reported in a young male following status epilepticus. This patient developed rhabdomyolysis and anuric renal failure requiring renal replacement therapy despite allopurinol and Rasburicase administration [11]. A case of rhabdomyolysis following status epilepticus with hyperuricemia was also recently reported in young male who developed oliguric renal failure requiring hemodialysis [12].

Increased uric acid production and increased serum uric acid have been noted in people undergoing hard physical exercise in hot climates, largely due to breakdown of endogenous muscle protein. It is possible that similar mechanisms would operate in patients experiencing prolonged or recurrent episodes of seizures [9]. Our patient however developed severe hyperuricemia and acute uric acid nephropathy following recurrent seizures without a dramatic rise in the serum CK level. A possible explanation is that seizures can also cause direct nucleotide breakdown, producing increased levels of adenosine which is then converted by xanthine oxidase in the liver to uric acid [13]. In addition, Grosso et al. found the serum nucleotidase activity to be elevated in patients for several hours after seizures, possibly leading to increased systemic breakdown of adenosine triphosphate and generation of urate [14].

Hypoxia and seizure induced lactic acidosis also impairs the renal tubular secretion of uric acid. Warren et al. postulate that seizure induced hyperuricemia could be due to a combination of overproduction and impaired tubular secretion of uric acid. Saugstad [15] has also proposed that excessive release of hypoxanthine by hypoxic tissues after seizures could be transformed to uric acid by xanthine oxidase thus causing hyperuricemia. As uric acid is also considered an effective antioxidant, it is possible that an elevation in uric acid would be to counteract the oxidative stress during epileptic seizure [16]. Metabolic acidosis which accompanies seizures creates an acidic urine in which uric acid is less soluble causing precipitation of uric acid in the tubular lumen [10]. Dehydration due to profuse sweating and hyperthermia during seizures causes increased tubular water resorption and increased urine uric acid concentration. Renal ischemia due to shunting of blood flow from visceral organs to muscles during seizures may also contribute to the kidney injury [10]. Urine microscopy in our patient also showed occasional granular casts suggesting that uric acid also caused mild tubular injury. Early markers of renal tubular injury like urinary $\beta 2$ microglobulin and N-acetyl-beta-D-glucosaminidase (NAG) were however not measured in our patient.

The pathologic features of acute uric acid nephropathy are reversible [2]. The most efficient therapy for dramatically lowering uric acid is Rasburicase, a recombinant form of urate oxidase, a nonhuman proteolytic enzyme that oxidizes uric acid to allantoin, and a metabolite that is far more soluble than uric acid. Rasburicase is contraindicated in patients with G6PD deficiency (G6PDD) due to risk of drug induced hemolytic anemia [17]. G6PD level was however not checked before administering Rasburicase in our patient. He had a low risk for developing hemolytic anemia due to him being from an ethnicity with low prevalence of G6PDD and absence of any prior history of anemia. He was however closely monitored after Rasburicase administration and tolerated it well. Rasburicase therapy is efficacious in reducing serum uric acid levels with associated diuresis much faster and more effectively than allopurinol, a xanthine oxidase inhibitor [18]. Allopurinol prevents the formation of new uric acid; however, it does not remove the existing uric acid. Moreover, allopurinol also increases the urinary excretion of xanthine which can crystallize and cause kidney injury [2]. Urinary alkalization to pH>6 helps uric acid solubility; however it has not been proven to be an effective therapy in TLS with acute uric acid nephropathy, due to increased calcium phosphate precipitation [2]. Hemodialysis is also quite effective in rapidly reducing uric acid concentrations. Kjellstrand et al. found that oliguria due to acute uric acid nephropathy responds quickly to hemodialysis with initiation of diuresis when serum uric acid concentration falls below 10 mg/dL. Peritoneal dialysis is much less efficient in reducing uric acid concentration [19].

In our patient urine microscopic findings of uric acid crystals lead to early diagnosis of uric acid nephropathy. Timely administration of Rasburicase prevented the need for hemodialysis in this patient and led to complete renal recovery. Our case illustrates the importance of urine microscopy and of monitoring uric acid levels in patients with prolonged seizures and AKI without rhabdomyolysis, as uric acid could be the likely culprit.

Acknowledgments

Funding for this case report was provided by the Education Department of Pikeville Medical Center.

References

[1] C. Giordano, O. Karasik, K. King-Morris, and A. Asmar, "Uric acid as a marker of kidney disease: review of the current literature," *Disease Markers*, vol. 2015, Article ID 382918, 6 pages, 2015.

[2] S. A. Fathallah-Shaykh and M. T. Cramer, "Uric acid and the kidney," *Pediatric Nephrology*, vol. 29, no. 6, pp. 999–1008, 2014.

[3] L. A. Baldree and F. B. Stapleton, "Uric acid metabolism in children," *Pediatric Clinics of North America*, vol. 37, no. 2, pp. 391–418, 1990.

[4] A. A. Ejaz, W. Mu, D.-H. Kang et al., "Could uric acid have a role in acute renal failure?" *Clinical Journal of the American Society of Nephrology*, vol. 2, no. 1, pp. 16–21, 2007.

[5] B. N. Ames, R. Cathcart, E. Schwiers, and P. Hochstein, "Uric acid provides an antioxidant defense in humans against oxidant- and radical-caused aging and cancer: a hypothesis," *Proceedings of the National Acadamy of Sciences of the United States of America*, vol. 78, no. 11, pp. 6858–6862, 1981.

[6] J. Kelton, W. N. Kelley, and E. W. Holmes, "A Rapid Method for the Diagnosis of Acute Uric Acid Nephropathy," *JAMA Internal Medicine*, vol. 138, no. 4, pp. 612–615, 1978.

[7] R. D. Nass, R. Sassen, C. E. Elger, and R. Surges, "The role of postictal laboratory blood analyses in the diagnosis and prognosis of seizures," *Seizure*, vol. 47, pp. 51–65, 2017.

[8] P. Gupta, V. P. Singh, S. Chatterjee, and A. K. Agarwal, "Acute renal failure resulting from rhabdomyolysis following a seizure," *Singapore Medical Journal*, vol. 51, no. 4, pp. e79–e80, 2010.

[9] D. Warren, A. G. Leitch, and Leggett R. J., "Hyperuricqmic acute renal failure after epileptic seizures," *The Lancet*, vol. 306, no. 7931, pp. 385–387, 1975.

[10] K. Luuhdorf, H. Petersson, and K. Pedersen, "Grand mal-provoked hyperuricemia," *Acta Neurologica Scandinavica*, vol. 58, no. 5, pp. 280–287, 1978.

[11] N. Makki, G. Hajj, and G. A. Schmidt, "Seizure-induced acute urate nephropathy: Case report and review," *CHEST*, vol. 144, no. 2, pp. 666–669, 2013.

[12] L. Wang, S. Hong, H. Huang, and M. Yang, "Rhabdomyolysis following status epilepticus with hyperuricemia," *Medicine*, vol. 97, no. 26, p. e11281, 2018.

[13] R. W. Greene, "Adenosine: Front and center in linking nutrition and metabolism to neuronal activity," *The Journal of Clinical Investigation*, vol. 121, no. 7, pp. 2548–2550, 2011.

[14] S. Grosso, R. Rocchi, M. Margollicci et al., "Postictal serum nucleotidases activities in patients with epilepsy," *Epilepsy Research*, vol. 84, no. 1, pp. 15–20, 2009.

[15] O. D. Saugstad, "Hyperuricaemia and epileptic seizures: a possible explanation," *The Lancet*, vol. 2, no. 7936, p. 665, 1975.

[16] S. A. Hamed, M. M. Abdellah, and N. El-Melegy, "Blood levels of trace elements, electrolytes, and oxidative stress/antioxidant systems in epileptic patients," *Journal of Pharmacological Sciences*, vol. 96, no. 4, pp. 465–473, 2004.

[17] M. Akande, A. N. Audino, and J. D. Tobias, "Rasburicase-induced hemolytic anemia in an adolescent with unknown glucose-6-phosphate dehydrogenase deficiency," *The Journal of Pediatric Pharmacology and Therapeutics*, vol. 22, no. 6, pp. 471–475, 2017.

[18] C. Ronco, P. Inguaggiato, V. Bordoni et al., "Rasburicase therapy in acute hyperuricemia and renal dysfunction," *Contributions to Nephrology*, vol. 147, pp. 115–123, 2005.

2

Atypical Causes of Urinary Tract Obstruction

Ernie Yap, Moro Salifu, Tahir Ahmad, A. Sanusi, Anthony Joseph, and Mary Mallappallil

State University of New York, Downstate Medical Center, Brooklyn, NY 11203, USA

Correspondence should be addressed to Ernie Yap; ernie.yap@downstate.edu

Academic Editor: Władysław Sułowicz

Acute kidney injury due to urinary tract obstruction invariably suggests lower urinary tract obstruction or bilateral ureteric obstruction since obstruction of a single kidney while the contralateral kidney is normal and not obstructed would not cause a perceptible rise in creatinine. Assuming a total body volume of 42 L, 70 kg male that generates approximately 1400 mg of creatinine daily (20 mg/kg/day) who has complete urinary tract obstruction would experience a 3.33 mg/dL per day increase in serum creatinine. Thus, for an individual who had prior normal renal function and who presents with a creatinine of 30 mg/dL, one could surmise that the obstructive pathology had lasted at least 10 days. However, the rise in serum creatinine is a poor marker of renal injury and subsequent prognosis. Urinary tract obstruction leading to AKI can be due to a variety of causes, and its management is tailored to the underlying etiology. This case series describes the varied clinical course of four patients at our center who experienced AKI from atypical causes of obstructive uropathy. Current and future diagnostic modalities and caveats in the treatment of this disease entity are also discussed.

1. Introduction

Acute kidney injury (AKI) is one of the commonest reasons for nephrology consultation. Of these, 5-10% of cases are due to urinary tract obstruction (UTO). UTO may result from stones or external compression from tumors, adenopathy, or retroperitoneal fibrosis. Early diagnosis of UTO is important since most cases can be corrected and delay in therapy can lead to irreversible renal injury. The degree of azotemia at time of presentation does not reflect the extent of kidney injury and subsequent prognosis. Herein we present a series of four cases of obstructive uropathy that had various atypical causes and natural histories.

2. Patient 1. Multi-Pronged Assault by Plasma Cell Dyscrasias

A 40-year-old man of West African origin was diagnosed with IgG lambda multiple myeloma with urinary free lambda light chains of 0.34 mg/L (normal range: 0.24-6.66 mg/L)) and plasmacytomas involving the pleura and bone marrow. He was treated with bortezomib-based chemotherapy with no response. Salvage chemotherapy resulted in tumor lysis syndrome (K 7.4 mmol/L; uric acid 12.9 mg/dL, serum creatinine 2.0 mg/dL) that resolved with chemotherapy de-escalation, rasburicase, and a single hemodialysis session. His renal function then returned to normal and the patient continued salvage chemotherapy as an outpatient. Eight months later, he presented to the Emergency Department (ED) with abdominal discomfort and AKI (serum creatinine 18.2 mg/dL) and was found to have bilateral severe hydronephrosis, due to upper ureteral obstruction caused by retroperitoneal adenopathy. Upon relief with percutaneous nephrostomy, his renal function normalized (serum creatinine 1.1 mg/dL), with suppression of monoclonal protein (M-spike 1.4 g/dL). Two months later, the patient was admitted to hospital for another episode of AKI that progressed despite supportive care. His M-spike was 5.3 g/dL and urinary free lambda light chain was 5080 mg/dL, consistent with myeloma kidney. He ultimately required hemodialysis support. The patient succumbed to complications of multiple myeloma and sepsis soon after, 14 months after diagnosis.

Table 1: Characteristics of patients with UTO.

Patient #	1	2	3	4
Peak creatinine (mg/dL)	18.2	35.92	31.4	17.3
BUN (mg/dL)	85	148	187	86
Lowest creatinine at recovery (mg/dL)	0.92	1.06	1.31	1.6
Cause	Bilateral ureteral obstruction	Urethral obstruction	Bladder outlet obstruction	Endometriosis
Pathology findings	Plasmacytomas	Prostate adenocarcinoma	Benign prostatic hyperplasia	Endometriosis
Management	Percutaneous nephrostomy and chemotherapy	Bladder catheterization	Bladder catheterization	Hysterectomy, hormonal therapy, hemodialysis
DDAVP given	Y	N	N	N/A
Days to lowest creatinine	51	1	5	44
Peak serum potassium (mmol/L)	6.4	7.9	7.4	6.0
pH	7.25	7.12	7.18	7.33
Bicarbonate (mmol/L)	17.1	10.4	10	17
pCO2 (mmHg)	42.7	33.5	20.8	32.8

3. Patient 2. Extreme Elevation of Serum Creatinine with Prostate Adenocarcinoma from Urethral Obstruction with Full Recovery of Renal Function

A 66-year-old man presented to the ED for a 3-week history of bilateral leg edema, distended abdomen, dysuria, and anorexia. He was recently treated for a urinary tract infection. Physical examination disclosed a distended bladder. Initial laboratory data revealed AKI with hyperkalemia (K 7.9 mEq/L, blood urea nitrogen (BUN) was 148 mg/dL and serum creatinine of 35.92 mg/dL); an urgent nephrology consultation was requested for emergency hemodialysis. In the meantime, a bladder catheter was placed with approximately 9 liters of urine output. Over the next 30 hours the patient's laboratory data improved dramatically (Table 1). His BUN dropped to 36 mg/dL within one day. The cause of AKI was later found to be UTO secondary to prostatic adenocarcinoma. His renal function improved spontaneously without the need for hemodialysis.

4. Patient 3. Extreme Elevation of Serum Creatinine with Benign Prostatic Hypertrophy with Full Recovery of Renal Function

A 58-year-old man with mild mental retardation and diabetes mellitus was brought to the ED for vomiting, diarrhea, and progressive weakness for several days. He had significant azotemia with serum creatinine of 31 mg/dL and BUN of 187 mg/dL with hyperkalemia and high anion gap metabolic acidosis (Table 1). Computed tomography (CT) of the abdomen showed moderate to severe bilateral hydronephrosis and a very large prostate gland protruding into the bladder, which is significantly distended. Renal ultrasonography showed mild bilateral hydronephrosis. The patient was treated medically for hyperkalemia, and a Foley catheter was placed with resultant good urinary flow, followed by rapid resolution of his azotemia and electrolyte derangements. His BUN decreased to 41 mg/dL in 2 days. A prostate biopsy performed later revealed benign prostatic hyperplasia.

5. Patient 4. Endometriosis Presenting as an Intraluminal Colon Mass Causing Chronic Ureteral Obstruction

A 40-year-old woman with a past medical history of hypertension and severe endometriosis presented to the ED with a serum creatinine of 17 mg/dL and BUN of 86 mg/dL. Renal sonogram disclosed moderate hydronephrosis with hydroureter compressed by a large myomatous uterus. A hysterectomy was performed which resulted in renal function improvement but did not normalize. However, the patient continued to develop multiple bouts of AKI and progressive chronic kidney disease (CKD) for the next several years. An episode of lower gastrointestinal bleeding prompted a colonoscopy that revealed a mass at the rectosigmoid junction which was resected and confirmed to be colonic endometriosis and leuprolide was started. By this time, the patient's CKD had progressed to end-stage renal disease and she was placed on maintenance hemodialysis.

6. Discussion

We present these four cases to illustrate atypical causes of UTO leading to AKI. A thorough history-taking and physical examination is imperative in the approach of a patient with AKI from any cause. Other nonobstructive causes of AKI such as ischemia, tubulointerstitial injury, glomerular diseases, tubular nephritis, or CKD from systemic illnesses ought to be considered as part of the differential diagnosis.

There are no pathognomonic findings attributed to UTO-related AKI. Palpation of the abdomen may reveal a suprapubic mass that typically represents a distended bladder. If UTO is suspected, the initial imaging modality of choice is ultrasonography, which has a high sensitivity and specificity even when performed and interpreted by nonradiologists [1]. It does not require radiocontrast and the detection of hydronephrosis is a sensitive marker for urinary tract obstruction [2–4]. In addition, ultrasonography can determine the size and shape of the kidneys. However, it is noteworthy that sonographic demonstration of significant renal parenchymal loss does not necessarily predict an irreversible cause for renal failure [2]. Patient 3 has renal sonographic findings that were discordant with clinical features and CT imaging. Renal ultrasonography can be negative in early obstruction, when the pyelocalyceal system is not yet dilated [5]. In such cases, CT scanning is useful. Also, scintigraphy with use of technetium 99m labeled mercaptoacetyltriglycine (MAG3) or diethylenetriaminepentaacetic acid (DTPA) can evaluate renal perfusion, glomerular function, and gross renal structure as well as excretory function.

Following relief of UTO, there is usually a resultant increase in sodium and water excretion even with the temporary decrease in glomerular filtration rate, as exemplified by Patient 2. This is because the volume expansion that occurs during UTO suppresses antidiuretic hormone (ADH) and aldosterone, leading to minimal reabsorption at the distal and collecting duct level until volume depletion sets in to re-establish reabsorption. It is usually self-limiting and can be a composite of both solute (urea and sodium) and water diuresis. Nevertheless, some patients will continue to eliminate salt and water even after homeostasis has been reached [6], a condition referred to as pathologic postobstructive diuresis (POD). These patients are at risk of severe dehydration, electrolyte imbalances, hypovolemic shock, and even death if not recognized and treated promptly. Patients with pathologic POD require strict monitoring of fluid status and serum electrolyte levels. Intravenous fluid replacement is often warranted and the type and amount of fluids should be tailored to the patient's serum electrolyte levels and clinical hydration status.

Pathologic POD is estimated to occur in 0.5% to 52% of patients who underwent relief of obstruction [7]. Animal experiments have shown that, in POD, solute and water dynamics alone are inadequate to fully account for the natriuresis and diuresis that follows obstruction relief [8]. Using micro puncture and microinjection methods, McDougal et al. demonstrated that there are defects in both proximal and distal sodium reabsorption that persist for 2-3 days after obstruction relief [9]. In addition, the decrease in water reabsorption in POD has been postulated to be due to a decrease in sodium chloride (NaCl) gradient in the thin ascending loop of Henle. This in turn is brought on by decreased NaCl reabsorption in the medullary ascending limb, caused by increased prostaglandin synthesis. Prostaglandins increase blood flow within the vasa recta, thus facilitating solute washout from the medulla, diluting the countercurrent effect. The increased medullary prostaglandins also antagonize the effect of ADH, thereby reducing the water permeability of the collecting tubule, contributing to the decrease in urine osmolality [10].

Another important cause of morbidity in the patient whose UTO has been relieved is rapid lowering of plasma osmolality, leading to rapid water transfer into the central nervous system, resulting in cerebral edema. Symptoms of this disequilibrium syndrome can range from lethargy, headache, drowsiness, and confusion to serious complications such as seizures, cardiac arrhythmias, coma, and pulmonary edema [11] and are well described in patients undergoing hemodialysis for the first time but have been reported in nondialysis patients as well [12]. In our series, Patient 2 and Patient 3 demonstrated rapid improvement in BUN but did not develop any neurological sequelae. Risk factors for development of disequilibrium syndrome include markedly elevated BUN, concurrent CKD, hyponatremia, hepatic encephalopathy, malignant hypertension, pediatric age, or conditions that compromise the blood-brain barrier such as sepsis or thrombotic thrombocytopenic purpura [13].

Our experience with Patient 4 is a rare but growing body of literature describing an unusual presentation of UTO [14–17]. The ureters are rarely involved in endometriosis; however, the close anatomical proximity of the distal ureter to the female reproductive organs makes it a plausible target for the development of UTO. In addition to external compression, intrinsic renal involvement is also a consideration in the evaluation of a renal mass in a patient without traditional risk factors for malignancy, as a biopsy that confirms endometriosis may obviate an unnecessary nephrectomy [18].

The biochemical findings of AKI due to UTO are indistinguishable from AKI from other causes. The rapid normalization of serum creatinine upon obstruction relief shows that serum creatinine is poor marker of severity of injury. The observation that certain proteins are differentially expressed in nephropathy from obstructive causes and can be measured in whole urine and in urine exosomes suggests that more definitive biomarkers for UTO-related AKI such as KIM-1 may be feasible [19–22].

Battle et al. studied 13 patients with UTO with resultant AKI and found that they were associated with hyperkalemic hyperchloremic metabolic acidosis with features of impaired urinary acidification and mineralocorticoid deficiency [23]. This phenomenon was observed in most of our patients (Table 1) and we agree that the otherwise asymptomatic patient who presents with AKI and hyperkalemic hyperchloremic metabolic acidosis should undergo evaluation for UTO.

The treatment of relieving obstruction includes percutaneous nephrostomy, an invasive procedure that carries bleeding risk. It can be argued that this risk is augmented in patients with AKI, although this has not been clearly demonstrated. Desmopressin (1-deamino-8-D-arginine vasopressin, DDAVP) is a synthetic analogue of the antidiuretic hormone vasopressin that increases plasma concentrations of von Willebrand factor and factor VIII, which underlies its hemostatic effect [24]. Kim et al. prospectively investigated the potential of desmopressin to improve platelet dysfunction and lower bleeding risk after emergent invasive procedures in 23 patients who were uremic and who were infused with DDAVP before their invasive procedures (7 of which are percutaneous nephrostomy) and found that collagen/epinephrine-closure time was significantly shortened from 252.7±40.7 to 144.6±51.0 s with no severe bleeding event observed [25]. Also, DDAVP is used to treat diabetes insipidus due to its antidiuretic effect and has been used successfully to ameliorate pathologic POD [26].

A Pertinent Question That Confronts Clinicians Is Does This Patient with UTO-AKI Require Hemodialysis? The roles of hemodialysis in UTO-AKI are no different from AKI from other causes: correction of electrolyte derangements, acidosis, and fluid management. Our cases above illustrate that recovery of renal function invariably occurs as soon prompt corrective measures were undertaken, emphasizing the need for a systematic and global approach to the patient with unexplained AKI. However, prognosis is variable and some patients may progress to chronic kidney disease even after obstruction has been relieved, as interstitial fibrosis and inflammation may have supervened. The prolonged recovery seen in Patients 1 and 3 was associated with concomitant infection that resulted in acute tubular necrosis. Once a diagnosis is confirmed, it is sometimes not fully reversible such as malignancy and discussion of treatments including percutaneous nephrostomies, ureteral stents, resection of malignancy, or hemodialysis which should be undertaken with the goal of providing comfort and improving quality of life.

In summary, we have described a series of patients with UTO-related AKI that presented with significantly elevated creatinine, most of whom regained renal function after relief of obstruction without requiring urgent hemodialysis. There is an unmet medical need for the development of more specific biomarkers of AKI from UTO. The utility of DDAVP in patients with AKI undergoing invasive procedures merits further study.

References

[1] V. E. Noble and D. F. Brown, "Renal ultrasound," *Emergency Medicine Clinics of North America*, vol. 22, no. 3, pp. 641–659, 2004.

[2] R. H. Gottlieb, E. P. Weinberg, D. J. Rubens, R. D. Monk, and E. B. Grossman, "Renal sonography: can it be used more selectively in the setting of an elevated serum creatinine level?" *American Journal of Kidney Diseases*, vol. 29, no. 3, pp. 362–367, 1997.

[3] P. H. Ellenbogen, F. W. Scheible, L. B. Talner, and G. R. Leopold, "Sensitivity of gray scale ultrasound in detecting urinary tract obstruction," *American Journal of Roentgenology*, vol. 130, no. 4, pp. 731–733, 1978.

[4] R. G. Kamholtz, J. J. Cronan, and G. S. Dorfman, "Obstruction and the minimally dilated renal collecting system: US evaluation," *Radiology*, vol. 170, no. 1 Pt 1, pp. 51–53, 1989.

[5] E. S. Amis Jr., J. J. Cronan, R. C. Pfister, and I. C. Yoder, "Ultrasonic inaccuracies in diagnosing renal obstruction," *Urology*, vol. 19, no. 1, pp. 101–105, 1982.

[6] J. F. Maher, G. E. Schreiner, and T. J. Waters, "Osmotic diuresis due to retained urea after release of obstructive uropathy," *The New England Journal of Medicine*, vol. 268, no. 20, pp. 1099–1104, 1963.

[7] M. A. Nyman, N. M. Schwenk, and M. D. Silverstein, "Management of urinary retention: rapid versus gradual decompression and risk of complications," *Mayo Clinic Proceedings*, vol. 72, no. 10, pp. 951–956, 1997.

[8] R. H. Harris and W. E. Yarger, "The pathogenesis of post obstructive diuresis. The role of circulating natriuretic and diuretic factors, including urea," *The Journal of Clinical Investigation*, vol. 56, no. 4, pp. 880–887, 1975.

[9] W. S. McDougal and F. S. Wright, "Defect in proximal and distal sodium transport in post-obstructive diuresis.," *Kidney International*, vol. 2, no. 6, pp. 304–317, 1972.

[10] L. B. Kinter, M. J. Dunn, T. R. Beck, R. Beeuwkes, and A. Hassid, "The interactions of prostaglandins and vasopressin in the kidney," *Annals of the New York Academy of Sciences*, vol. 372, no. 1, pp. 163–179, 1981.

[11] S. M. Rosen, K. O'Connor, and S. Shaldon, "Haemodialysis disequilibrium," *British Medical Journal*, vol. 2, no. 5410, pp. 672–675, 1964.

[12] F. K. Luni, A. R. Khan, Y. Yoon, D. Malhotra, and S. Vetteth, "Disequilibrium syndrome and prevention in nonhemodialysis patients," *The American Journal of the Medical Sciences*, vol. 349, no. 5, pp. 438–441, 2015.

[13] N. Patel, P. Dalal, and M. Panesar, "Dialysis disequilibrium syndrome: a narrative review," *Seminars in Dialysis*, vol. 21, no. 5, pp. 493–498, 2008.

[14] D. W. Laube, G. W. Calderwood, and J. A. Benda, "Endometriosis causing ureteral obstruction," *Obstetrics & Gynecology*, vol. 65, no. 3, pp. 69s–71s, 1985.

[15] P. Dutta, M. H. Bhat, A. Bhansali, and V. Kumar, "A young woman with endometriosis of kidney," *Saudi Medical Journal*, vol. 27, no. 2, pp. 244–246, 2006.

[16] F. Rousselot and M. E. Liard-Meillon, "Renal endometriosis. Report of a case," *Progrès en Urologie*, vol. 6, no. 6, pp. 936–939, 1996.

[17] R. G. Uzzo, D. P. Poppas, R. W. Schuman, and E. Darracott Vaughan Jr., "An unusual cause of duodenal obstruction: ureteropelvic junction obstruction and the renoalimentary relationship," *Urology*, vol. 44, no. 3, pp. 433–436, 1994.

[18] J. Yang, R.-J. Song, C. Xu, S.-Q. Zhang, and W. Zhang, "Renal endometriosis tends to be misdiagnosed as renal tumor: a rare case report," *International Surgery*, vol. 100, no. 2, pp. 376–380, 2015.

[19] P. Trnka, L. Ivanova, M. J. Hiatt, and D. G. Matsell, "Urinary biomarkers in obstructive nephropathy," *Clinical Journal of the American Society of Nephrology*, vol. 7, no. 10, pp. 1567–1575, 2012.

[20] G. Lucarelli, V. Mancini, V. Galleggiante et al., "Emerging urinary markers of renal injury in obstructive nephropathy," *BioMed Research International*, vol. 2014, Article ID 303298, 7 pages, 2014.

[21] D. Olvera-Posada, T. Dayarathna, M. Dion et al., "KIM-1 is a potential urinary biomarker of obstruction: results from a

prospective cohort study," *Journal of Endourology*, vol. 31, no. 2, pp. 111–118, 2017.

[22] Y. Xie, W. Xue, X. Shao et al., "Analysis of a urinary biomarker panel for obstructive nephropathy and clinical outcomes," *Plos One*, vol. 9, no. 11, Article ID e112865, 2014.

[23] D. C. Batlle, J. A. L. Arruda, and N. A. Kurtzman, "Hyperkalemic distal renal tubular acidosis associated with obstructive uropathy," *The New England Journal of Medicine*, vol. 304, no. 7, pp. 373–380, 1981.

[24] P. M. Mannucci, G. Remuzzi, F. Pusineri et al., "Deamino-8-D-arginine vasopressin shortens the bleeding time in uremia," *The New England Journal of Medicine*, vol. 308, no. 1, pp. 8–12, 1983.

[25] J. H. Kim, C. H. Baek, J. Y. Min, J.-S. Kim, S. B. Kim, and H. Kim, "Desmopressin improves platelet function in uremic patients taking antiplatelet agents who require emergent invasive procedures," *Annals of Hematology*, vol. 94, no. 9, pp. 1457–1461, 2015.

[26] E. Cimentepe, A. Unsal, Z. Akbulut, and M. D. Balbay, "Prolonged urinary drainage from nephrostomy tract after percutaneous nephrolithotomy can be treated with oral desmopressin," *Scandinavian Journal of Urology*, vol. 38, no. 3, pp. 266-267, 2004.

3

Dialysis Disequilibrium: Is Acidosis More Important than Urea?

Akshay Athavale[1,2] **Kate R Wyburn**[1,2] **Paul L Snelling,**[1,2] **and Steven J Chadban**[1,2]

[1]*Department of Renal Medicine, Royal Prince Alfred Hospital, Sydney, New South Wales, Australia*
[2]*Central Clinical School, Faculty of Medicine and Health, University of Sydney, Sydney, New South Wales, Australia*

Correspondence should be addressed to Akshay Athavale; akshay.athavale@health.nsw.gov.au

Academic Editor: David Mudge

Dialysis disequilibrium syndrome is a severe complication associated with dialysis treatment. Manifestations may range from mild such as headache to severe such as seizures and coma. Risk factors for development include initial dialysis treatment, uraemia, metabolic acidosis, and extremes of age. We report a case of dialysis disequilibrium in a patient with a failing kidney transplant secondary to the recurrence of IgA nephropathy. Disturbance in cognition and neurologic functioning occurred six hours after the completion of initiation of intermittent haemodialysis. During two sessions of intermittent haemodialysis of 3 and 4 hours, urea was reduced by 21.9 and 17.2 mmol/L and measured serum osmolality was reduced by 25 and 14 mOsm/kg, respectively. Subsequent admission to the intensive care unit and initiation of continuous renal replacement therapy for 48 hours resulted in complete resolution of symptoms. In this case report, we discuss atypical clinical and radiologic features of dialysis disequilibrium occurring with modest reductions in urea and serum osmolality.

1. Introduction

Severe dialysis disequilibrium syndrome (DDS) is an increasingly rare complication following the initiation of dialysis treatment [1]. The clinical syndrome is defined by neurological symptoms occurring in close association with haemodialysis and can range from very mild, such that they go unnoticed, to severe (shown in Table 1) [2, 3]. There are numerous risk factors associated with the development of DDS (shown in Table 1) which most commonly present during or immediately following dialysis in treatment naïve patients [4]. Dialysis disequilibrium syndrome is a diagnosis of exclusion and is difficult to make due to the nonspecific nature of signs and symptoms, all of which may be present in alternative diagnoses such as encephalopathy (shown in Table 1) [3, 4].

There are three hypotheses considered to underpin the pathophysiology of DDS, and they likely do not exist in isolation. The "reverse osmosis effect" suggests that rapid removal of urea during haemodialysis establishes an osmotic gradient favouring movement of water into cells, resulting in cerebral oedema [5]. Secondly, "paradoxical brain acidosis" suggests that rapid correction of pH during haemodialysis results in a rise in the partial pressure of CO_2 which forms carbonic acid in the brain and cerebrospinal fluid. The resulting reduction in pH displaces bound sodium and potassium, which increases intracellular osmolality and promotes cerebral oedema [1]. Finally, unidentified solutes generated in the cerebral cortex known as "idiogenic osmoles" may preserve intracerebral osmolality when haemodialysis and urea clearance are instituted, resulting in cerebral oedema [1, 6].

2. Case Report

A 35-year-old man presented with a 2-week history of progressively worsening fatigue, anorexia, vomiting and diarrhoea, exertional dyspnoea, and worsening oedema. Initial physical examination revealed a blood pressure of 144/94 mmHg and gross peripheral oedema of the upper and lower limbs and sacrum. Pulmonary auscultation demonstrated no features of pulmonary oedema. Background medical history was significant for living donor kidney transplantation 15 years earlier, with recurrence of IgA

Table 1: Signs, symptoms, risk factors, and differential diagnoses for dialysis disequilibrium syndrome.

Signs	Symptoms	Risk factors	Differential diagnoses
Asterixis	Headache	New dialysis initiation	Malignant hypertension
Altered mental status	Nausea	Chronic kidney disease	Posterior reversible encephalopathy syndrome (PRES)
Seizures	Vomiting	Urea >60 mmol/L	Cerebrovascular accident
Coma	Muscle cramps	Metabolic acidosis	Hyponatraemia
	Confusion	Extremes of age	Uraemia
	Tremor	Preexisting neurologic disorder	Intracranial haemorrhage
	Visual disturbance	Conditions associated with cerebral oedema	Hypoglycaemia
			Meningoencephalitis
			Seizure disorder
			Uraemic encephalopathy

nephropathy and consequent nephrotic syndrome. Two months prior to the hospital admission, biochemistry demonstrated a serum creatinine (sCr) of 572 umol/L, urea of 30 mmol/L, potassium of 4.7 mmol/L, bicarbonate of 16 mmol/L, corrected calcium of 1.96 mmol/L, and phosphate of 2.82 mmol/L.

Following admission to the hospital, acute on chronic kidney injury was noted with an sCr of 1439 umol/L and urea of 53.2 mmol/L. Serum potassium was raised at 6.1 mmol/L and bicarbonate was critically low at 6 mmol/L with a pH of 7.06. Corrected calcium had reduced further to 1.67 mmol/L, and phosphate had increased to 5.97 mmol/L. Serum sodium and blood glucose were normal, and measured serum osmolality was 337 mOsm/kg. A complete blood count demonstrated anaemia with a haemoglobin of 98 g/L.

Initial medical management was instituted over the first 36 hours and involved parenteral loop diuretic therapy for fluid overload, oral bicarbonate replacement for acidosis, and both insulin dextrose treatment and oral potassium exchange resins for hyperkalaemia. Oral calcitriol and calcium carbonate were administered for hypocalcaemia. Despite medical management, bicarbonate remained unchanged at 6 mmol/L with a pH of 7.13, and phosphate worsened to 6.03 mmol/L. Serum potassium and corrected calcium both improved to 5.1 mmol/L and 1.72 mmol/L, respectively. Measured serum osmolality increased to 341 mOsm/kg. The patient deteriorated further, developing uraemic encephalopathy as evidenced by delirium, fluctuating levels of consciousness, dysarthria, and asterixis. A widespread tremor was also present. The patient was urgently initiated on haemodialysis treatment.

The first haemodialysis treatment was 3 hours in duration, with an ultrafiltration volume of 3000 mL. The dialysis membrane used was Polyflux 140H, and the dialysate was Baxter CX265G. The dialysate flow rate was 500 mL/min and the blood flow rate was 200 mL/min. The patient demonstrated a significant improvement in symptoms within 24 hours following dialysis, with complete resolution of cognitive and speech deficits but persisting tremor. Twenty-four hours later, he underwent a second session of haemodialysis of 4 hours' duration with an ultrafiltration volume of 4000 mL. The dialysis membrane used was Polyflux 140H, and the dialysate was Baxter CX275G. The dialysate flow rate was 500 mL/min and the blood flow rate was 250 mL/min. Immediately following the second session of dialysis, complete resolution of all symptoms was achieved, and the patient was planned for discharge home. Dialysis prescription and biochemistry before and after both dialysis sessions are summarised in Table 2.

Six hours after completing the second session of haemodialysis, the patient developed severe hypertension with a blood pressure of 187/102 mmHg (143/92 mmHg following dialysis) and was found to be stuporous with hyperreflexia and sustained clonus. There was no response to visual threat bilaterally; however, he was able to follow commands. As a result of this marked deterioration, he was intubated and transferred to the intensive care unit (ICU) for further evaluation.

Contrast computed tomography of the brain showed no abnormality, and magnetic resonance imaging of the brain revealed bilateral symmetric diffusion restriction in the supratentorial white matter of both cerebral hemispheres without evidence of overt cerebral oedema or features of posterior reversible encephalopathy syndrome (PRES; shown in Figure 1). Lumbar puncture demonstrated no evidence of meningoencephalitis or autoimmune encephalitis, and an electroencephalogram (EEG) had no features of seizure activity. Ammonia concentrations were not elevated and cryptococcal testing was negative.

The patient was diagnosed with dialysis disequilibrium syndrome and commenced on continuous venovenous haemodiafiltration (CVVHDF) to manage severe fluid overload and hypertension, which was continued for a total of 48 hours. During this time, urea was slowly reduced from 27.8 mmol/L to 11 mmol/L, bicarbonate was increased from 18 mmol/L to 28 mmol/L, and corrected calcium increased from 2.11 mmol/L to 2.54 mmol/L. The ultrafiltration volume achieved was 6300 mL, and he was subsequently extubated and demonstrated complete resolution of all signs and symptoms. Forty-eight hours after leaving the ICU, he was discharged home on maintenance intermittent haemodialysis.

Written informed consent was obtained from the patient for the publication of this case report and any accompanying images.

Table 2: Dialysis prescription, before and after haemodialysis biochemistry.

	Before HD (1)	After HD (1)	Before HD (2)	After HD (2)
Dialysis membrane	Polyflux 140H		Polyflux 140H	
Dialysate (mmol/L)	Baxter CX265G (K^+ 2, Ca^{2+} 1.65, Mg^{2+} 0.5, Na^+ 140, HCO_3^- 34)		Baxter CX275G (K^+ 2, Ca^{2+} 1.75, Mg^{2+} 0.5, Na^+ 140, HCO_3^- 34)	
DFR/BFR (mL/min)	500/200		500/250	
Creatinine (umol/L)	1535	929	1201	858
Urea (mmol/L)	55.9	34.0	41.8	24.6
Sodium (mmol/L)	139	142	140	143
Potassium (mmol/L)	5.1	3.3	3.9	3.6
Bicarbonate (mmol/L)	6	12	14	20
Corrected calcium (mmol/L)	1.72	2.11	1.82	2.20
Phosphate (mmol/L)	6.03	3.72	5.40	3.48
Osmolality (mOsm/kg)	341	316	324	310
Ultrafiltration (mL)	N/A	3000	N/A	4000

HD: haemodialysis; DFR: dialysate flow rate; BFR: blood flow rate; mmol/L: millimoles per litre; K^+: potassium; Ca^{2+}: calcium; Mg^{2+}: magnesium; Na^+: sodium; HCO_3^-: bicarbonate.

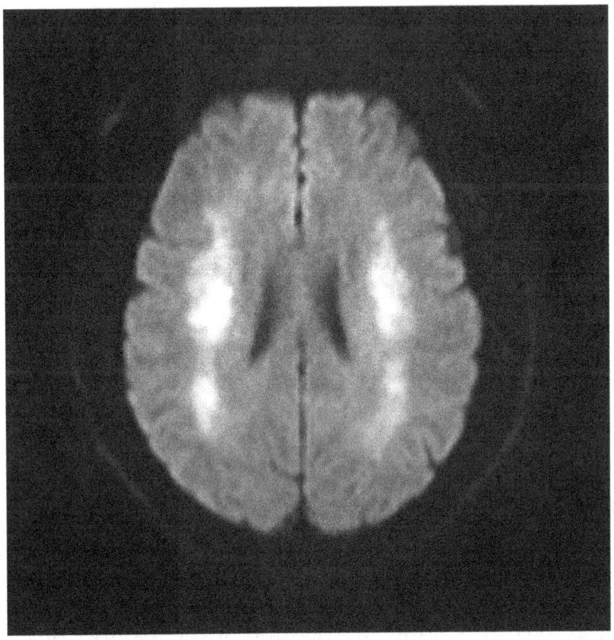

Figure 1: Magnetic resonance imaging findings demonstrating symmetrical bilateral supratentorial restriction in keeping with leukoencephalopathy.

3. Discussion

We report a case of dialysis disequilibrium syndrome manifesting six hours after the completion of the second haemodialysis session in a patient with a failing kidney transplant. The dialysis disequilibrium was the most likely diagnosis as other differentials including meningoencephalitis, autoimmune encephalitis, PRES, and seizure disorder were excluded. Most commonly, dialysis disequilibrium occurs during or immediately after haemodialysis, and late presentations such as in our case are less common [1, 7].

Dialysis disequilibrium syndrome is a rare and potentially fatal complication of dialysis treatment [8, 9]. Signs and symptoms range from mild such as nausea and vomiting to severe and life-threatening such as seizures and coma [1]. While DDS is most commonly associated with first haemodialysis treatment, there are reports of DDS in patients treated with continuous renal replacement therapies (RRTs) such as continuous venovenous haemodialysis (CVVHD) and continuous venovenous haemofiltration (CVVH) [2].

Development of DDS is variable and dependent on both the extent and rate of change of osmotically active solutes such as urea [2]. Central to the underlying pathogenesis of DDS is the establishment of an osmotic gradient between the blood compartment and the brain and cerebrospinal fluid (CSF) [3]. In states of chronic uraemia, a steady state is established between compartments, preventing significant fluid shifts. Dialysis treatment, both intermittent and continuous, will remove urea from the central blood compartment, resulting in a net movement of fluid into the brain, causing cerebral oedema [10, 11]. Rodent models have demonstrated an upregulation of aquaporin channels and downregulation of rapid urea transporters in the brain as a result of uraemia, and these phenomena may also contribute to the development of cerebral oedema seen in DDS [12].

The "paradoxical brain acidosis" hypothesis suggests that the rapid correction of pH by dialysis results in a rise in the partial pressure of carbon dioxide which forms carbonic acid in the brain. The reduced intracerebral pH causes displacement of bound cations such as sodium and potassium, thereby causing a rise in intracerebral osmolality. This situation favours the movement of water into the brain, further compounding cerebral oedema [13]. Finally, "idiogenic osmoles" which are intracellular osmoles generated as a compensatory mechanism to maintain intracerebral osmolality in states of hyperosmolality (e.g., hyperglycaemia and uraemia) may drive movement of water into the brain during dialysis [14].

Autopsy and neuroimaging data in both animals and humans have demonstrated evidence of cerebral oedema in DDS [15, 16]. Importantly, however, while cerebral oedema is frequently seen in DDS, other patterns of injury including demyelination and leukoencephalopathy have been demonstrated [17, 18]. Leukoencephalopathy has many causes including cerebral oedema, immunosuppressive medications, central nervous system infections, and impaired cellular immunity [17]. In our case, imaging findings did not demonstrate overt cerebral oedema, but were suggestive of an acute leukoencephalopathy, which was likely a consequence of diffuse interstitial cerebral oedema that may be seen in DDS [18].

There is a lack of data demonstrating the optimal parameters to reduce the risk of DDS. It is generally accepted that reducing urea by approximately 40% over a 2-hour haemodialysis session is reasonable, though this is not evidence-based [9]. In our case, urea was reduced by 39% over the initial 3-hour haemodialysis session and by 41% over the following 4-hour session. Further, ensuring that the reduction in plasma osmolality does not significantly exceed 24 mOsm/kg may be of benefit in preventing DDS [3]. In our case, serum osmolality was reduced by 25 mOsm/kg and 14 mOsm/kg after the first and second haemodialysis sessions, respectively. This suggests that perhaps in our case, rapid correction of metabolic acidosis rather than urea reduction may have contributed more significantly to the development of DDS.

While DDS has been reported to occur up to 24 hours following dialysis, most commonly, it presents towards the end or immediately after completing dialysis. In our case, signs and symptoms manifested 6 hours after completion of dialysis. Given that the rate of reduction of urea was in line with accepted recommendations, it is unclear as to why signs and symptoms were delayed. It is likely that development of DDS in our case was more in keeping with the "paradoxical brain hypothesis" as bicarbonate increased by 14 mmol/L over 7 hours of dialysis. Therefore, as blood bicarbonate increased, carbon dioxide diffused slowly into the brain, reducing pH and slowly displacing tissue-bound cations. This would likely be a slower process than simply establishing an osmotic gradient secondary to urea removal and may explain the delayed onset of signs and symptoms.

Treatment of DDS is supportive and may involve discontinuation of dialysis [3]. In cases such as ours, where neither urea nor osmolality were reduced at rates significantly greater than recommended [9], consideration should be given to the use of a lower bicarbonate dialysate, to limit the rate of correction of metabolic acidosis. Dialysate solutions vary globally, but solutions containing less than 30 mmol/L of bicarbonate are available [19] and may represent a safer choice in cases such as ours. Continuous RRT may also represent a reasonable approach, but DDS occurring with this treatment has also been reported [2]. Furthermore, in patients at high risk of developing DDS, shorter dialysis sessions of 2 hours with slower blood flow rates of 150–250 mL/min, a smaller dialyzer, and both a lower target for urea reduction and a slower rate of urea reduction during the initial dialysis may be appropriate [9, 20].

Additionally, in patients considered high risk of DDS, such as those with risk factors shown in Table 1, antiepileptic drugs (AED) have been used as both a preventative and a therapeutic treatment [21]. Currently, there are no randomised data to support the use of prophylactic AEDs in DDS, and their use does little to address the underlying pathophysiology of cerebral oedema, which is central to DDS [20, 21]. Data from neurological literature suggest that newer AEDs, such as levetiracetam, may be preferred due to fewer drug interactions, but the dose and duration of treatment remain unclear [22]. Acute seizures occurring as a consequence of DDS may be terminated using benzodiazepines or other AEDs [21].

Finally, the use of exogenous solutes such as intravenous mannitol (1 mg/kg), higher dialysate urea, or glucose can be administered to counteract the reduction in urea and serum osmolality associated with dialysis [21]. While there are no randomised data on this approach, current evidence suggests that it may reduce the incidence of symptoms of DDS [4] and could be considered in patients at high risk of DDS.

4. Conclusion

We have presented a unique case of dialysis disequilibrium syndrome where the classic precipitant of extensive urea reduction on dialysis was absent. We propose that the 6-hour delay to the onset of signs and symptoms was due to the correction of metabolic acidosis, in keeping with the "paradoxical brain acidosis" hypothesis. Dialysis disequilibrium is an increasingly rare complication of treatment, but awareness of risk factors, timing, spectrum of severity, and treatment are important to all physicians prescribing dialysis.

Consent

Written informed consent was obtained from the patient for the publication of this case report and any accompanying images.

Authors' Contributions

All authors were involved in the preparation of this work. AA contributed to obtaining consent, collection of data, and writing and revision of the manuscript. KRW, PLS, and SJC contributed to writing and revision of the manuscript.

References

[1] M. Ali and U. Bakhsh, "A vanishing complication of haemodialysis: dialysis disequilibrium syndrome," *Journal of the Intensive Care Society*, vol. 21, no. 1, pp. 92–95, 2020.

[2] S. Tuchman, Z. P. Khademian, and K. Mistry, "Dialysis disequilibrium syndrome occurring during continuous renal replacement therapy," *Clinical Kidney Journal*, vol. 6, no. 5, pp. 526–529, 2013.

[3] K. Mistry, "Dialysis disequilibrium syndrome prevention and management," *International Journal of Nephrology and Renovascular Disease*, vol. 12, pp. 69–77, 2019.

[4] D. Zepeda-Orozco and R. Quigley, "Dialysis disequilibrium syndrome," *Pediatric Nephrology*, vol. 27, no. 12, pp. 2205–2211, 2012.

[5] S. M. Silver, J. A. DeSimone, D. A. Smith, and R. H. Sterns, "Dialysis disequilibrium syndrome (DDS) in the rat: role of the "reverse urea effect"," *Kidney International*, vol. 42, no. 1, pp. 161–166, 1992.

[6] S. M. Silver, R. H. Sterns, and M. L. Halperin, "Brain swelling

after dialysis: old urea or new osmoles?" *American Journal of Kidney Diseases*, vol. 28, no. 1, pp. 1–13, 1996.

[7] S. Adapa, V. M. Konala, N. R. Aeddula, V. Gayam, and S. Naramala, "Dialysis disequilibrium syndrome: rare serious complication of hemodialysis and effective management," *Cureus*, vol. 11, no. 6, Article ID e5000, 2019.

[8] A. I. Arieff, "Dialysis disequilibrium syndrome: current concepts on pathogenesis and prevention," *Kidney International*, vol. 45, no. 3, pp. 629–635, 1994.

[9] N. Patel, P. Dalal, and M. Panesar, "Fellows' forum fellows' forum in dialysis edited by mark A. Perazella: dialysis disequilibrium syndrome: a narrative review," *Seminars in Dialysis*, vol. 21, no. 5, pp. 493–498, 2008.

[10] S. M. Rosen, K. O'Connor, and S. Shaldon, "Haemodialysis disequilibrium," *BMJ*, vol. 2, no. 5410, pp. 672–675, 1964.

[11] C. R. Kleeman, H. Davson, and E. Levin, "Urea transport in the central nervous system," *American Journal of Physiology-Legacy Content*, vol. 203, no. 4, pp. 739–747, 1962.

[12] M.-M. Trinh-Trang-Tan, J.-P. Cartron, and L. Bankir, "Molecular basis for the dialysis disequilibrium syndrome: altered aquaporin and urea transporter expression in the brain," *Nephrology Dialysis Transplantation*, vol. 20, no. 9, pp. 1984–1988, 2005.

[13] A. I. Arieff, R. Guisado, S. G. Massry, and V. C. Lazarowitz, "Central nervous system pH in uremia and the effects of hemodialysis," *Journal of Clinical Investigation*, vol. 58, no. 2, pp. 306–311, 1976.

[14] A. I. Arieff, S. G. Massry, A. Barrientos, and C. R. Kleeman, "Brain water and electrolyte metabolism in uremia: effects of slow and rapid hemodialysis," *Kidney International*, vol. 4, no. 3, pp. 177–187, 1973.

[15] C. P. Harris and J. J. Townsend, "Dialysis disequilibrium syndrome. West," *Journal of Medicine*, vol. 151, no. 1, pp. 52–55, 1989.

[16] S. M. Bagshaw, A. D. Peets, M. Hameed, P. J. Boiteau, K. B. Laupland, and C. J. Doig, "Dialysis Disequilibrium Syndrome: brain death following hemodialysis for metabolic acidosis and acute renal failure-a case report," *BMC Nephrology*, vol. 5, no. 1, Article ID 9, 2004.

[17] C.-H. Chang, K.-T. Hsu, C.-H. Lee et al., "Leukoencephalopathy associated with dialysis disequilibrium syndrome," *Renal Failure*, vol. 29, no. 5, pp. 631–634, 2007.

[18] R. Hayashi, K. Kitazawa, D. Sanada et al., "Diffuse leukoencephalopathy associated with dialysis disequilibrium syndrome," *Internal Medicine*, vol. 54, no. 21, pp. 2753–2758, 2015.

[19] M. K. Abramowitz, "Bicarbonate balance and prescription in ESRD," *Journal of the American Society of Nephrology*, vol. 28, no. 3, pp. 726–734, 2017.

[20] C. Wirawan, I. K. Sumada, D. Yuliani, N. K. C. Wiratmi, and R. Sukiandra, "Dialysis disequilibrium syndrome induced seizure following hemodialysis," *Cureus*, vol. 13, no. 9, Article ID e17821, 2021.

[21] M. M. Sahani, T. M. Daoud, R. Sam et al., "Dialysis disequilibrium syndrome revisited," *Hemodialysis International*, vol. 5, no. 1, pp. 92–96, 2001.

[22] P. S. Bhattathiri, A. Hegde, and A. Kumar, "Anti-epileptic drug prophylaxis in neurosurgery–what we know and what we do," *Current Practices in Neurosciences*, vol. 3, no. 4, pp. 1–12, 2021.

4

Pericardial Tamponade: An Uncommon Clinical Presentation in cANCA Related Vasculitis and Glomerulonephritis in Association with Very High Titres of ANA

Amaresh Vanga,[1] Amna Z. Rana,[2] Jolanta Kowalewska,[3] and Harlan Rust[1]

[1]*Nephrology, Eastern Virginia Medical School, 855 W Brambelton Ave, Norfolk, VA 23510, USA*
[2]*Eastern Virginia Medical School, Norfolk, VA, USA*
[3]*Pathology, Eastern Virginia Medical School, 855 W Brambelton Ave, Norfolk, VA 23510, USA*

Correspondence should be addressed to Amaresh Vanga; amareshvanga@yahoo.com

Academic Editor: Yoshihide Fujigaki

ANCA (anti-neutrophil cytoplasmic antibody) vasculitides are systemic autoimmune diseases in which anti-neutrophilic cytoplasmic antibodies activate primed neutrophils, thereby generating an inflammatory cascade resulting in the damage of small sized blood vessels in various organs of the body, including the heart. Pleuropericardial involvement is underrecognized as a complication of ANCA vasculitis and is highlighted in this case report of a 51-year-old male who presented with an initial symptomatic presentation of pleuropericardial effusion progressing to pericardial tamponade in the setting of a later renal biopsy proven pauci-immune crescentic glomerulonephritis with high ANA titres along with positive cANCA (cytoplasmic ANCA) and PR3 (proteinase 3) antibodies. He was found to have acute renal failure which progressively got better with cyclophosphamide.

1. Introduction

ANCA (anti-neutrophil cytoplasmic autoantibody) vasculitis consists of multiorgan related small vessel pathology due to the generation of autoantibodies that activate neutrophils and generate an inflammatory cascade. There are two major groups of ANCA vasculitis based on the target antigens: proteinase-3 (PR-3) and myeloperoxidase (MPO) [1]. PR-3 is associated with cytoplasmic neutrophilic staining (c-ANCA) and MPO is associated with perinuclear neutrophilic staining (p-ANCA). PR-3+ c-ANCA vasculitis generally presents with granulomatosis with polyangiitis (GPA), formerly known as Wegener's vasculitis, whereas p-ANCA has traditionally been related to microscopic polyangiitis (MPA) and eosinophilic granulomatosis with polyangiitis (EGPA), formerly known as Churg-Strauss syndrome [2]. The various clinical and pathologic manifestations of ANCA vasculitis include glomerulonephritis, respiratory complications including interstitial lung disease and upper respiratory tract ulcer formation, and dermatologic pathology such as palpable purpura and urticarial vasculitis [1, 2]. In this case report of a 51-year-old male with ANCA positive serology, we discuss the rarely associated ANCA related pleural and pericardial involvement with progression to pericardial effusion.

2. Case Presentation

A 51-year-old white male, with a past medical history of hypertension and hypothyroidism, presented with a 12-day history of shortness of breath, cough, and fever with new onset lower extremity swelling, orthopnea, paroxysmal nocturnal dyspnea, and dyspnea on exertion. He was seen by his primary care physician approximately one week ago and started on azithromycin, but did not improve. He had also been taking 5 mg of motrin and had used 30 tablets of motrin in the past week. His other medications included amlodipine 10 mg once daily and levothyroxine 50 mcg once daily. He was afebrile on initial presentation. Physical exam was pertinent for rales auscultated in the left lower lung base. EKG only pertinent for sinus tachycardia with no ST segment changes. His initial labs were pertinent for findings of new onset acute

TABLE 1: Laboratory workup.

Labs	Reference Values	Values
White Blood Count	*4.0 - 11.0 K/uL*	*20.7*
ANA Screen by IFA	*Negative*	*Positive*
ANA Speckled	*Negative Titer*	*> = 1:1280*
Anti-dsDNA	Negative	Negative
Anti-GBM	0-20 units	5
C3 Complement	83 - 177 mg/dL	162
C4 Complement	10 - 40 mg/dL	16
Cytoplasmic ANCA	*Neg: <1:20 titer*	*1:160*
PR-3 Antibody EIA	*0.0-3.5 U/mL*	*> 100*
MPO Antibody, EIA	0.0-9.0 U/mL	< 9.0
Perinuclear ANCA	Neg: <1:20 titer	<1:20 titer
Urine Protein	*Negative*	*100*
Urine RBC	*0-2/hpf*	*50-100*
Urine WBC	*0-2/hpf*	*20-50*
Urine Protein: Creatinine	*< .2*	*1.34*

TABLE 2: Pericardial studies.

Pericardiocentesis	Results
Pericardial LDH	*1784 U/L*
Serum LDH	208 U/L
Pericardial Protein	*5 g/L*
Serum Protein	6.7 g/L
Culture and Gram Stain.	No bacterial growth noted. No anaerobes cultured. No acid fast bacteria seen at 200x magnification. No organisms seen on gram stain.
Cytology	Negative for malignancy. Marked acute inflammation present.
Pericardial Glucose	< 19 mg/dL
Pericardial Triglycerides	87 mg/dL
Serum Triglycerides	152 mg/dL
Pericardial Cholesterol	85 mg/dL
Serum Cholesterol	96 mg/dL

renal failure with a creatinine (Cr) of 3.4 mg/dL, microscopic hematuria and proteinuria on urinalysis, with urine protein: creatinine ratio of 1.34 g/gCr. He had appreciable leukocytosis with white blood cell count of approximately 20k. CT chest revealed small to moderate sized bilateral pleural effusions and moderate to large sized pericardial effusion. He was admitted to the inpatient service. Over the next 48 hours, he developed worsening shortness of breath, hypoxemia, and pericardial tamponade with echocardiogram (ECHO) revealing a worsening large circumferential pericardial tamponade in comparison to an ECHO done the previous day. ECHO also noted paradoxical septal motion during cardiac cycles with diastolic collapse of the right ventricle and right atrium. Pericardiocentesis was performed and approximately 500 mL of serosanguinous fluid was drained from the pericardial space with noted improvement in the patient's blood pressure and heart rate (see Tables 2 and 3 for pericardial studies).

Further workup revealed positive autoantibodies for c-ANCA (1:160), ANA (1:1280) and PR-3 (>100). Anti-SSA (Sjogren's Syndrome–A), anti-SSB (Sjogren's Syndrome–B), anti-dsDNA (double stranded-DNA), anti-Smith, anti-RNP (ribonucleoproteins), and anti-GBM (glomerular basement membrane) were reported negative (Table 1). This prompted a renal biopsy which revealed fibrinoid necrosis, capillary wall rupture, fibrin formation, and cellular crescents consistent with rapidly progressive crescentic glomerulonephritis (Figure 1). Examination of provided electron microscopy images showed 2 glomeruli which revealed no evidence of immune type electron dense deposits in the glomeruli, tubular basement membranes, or the interstitium (Figure 2).

Normal findings on electron microscopy were thought to be related to sampling error. Immunofluorescence revealed pauci-immune pattern. Based on the renal biopsy, he was diagnosed with PR3-ANCA related pauci-immune glomerulonephritis with extra renal manifestation of pleuropericardial disease progressing to pericardial tamponade. Patient then received pulse steroids and a dose of rituximab. BUN and Cr were 91 mg/dL and 3.2 mg/dL after getting this

TABLE 3: Pericardial studies.

Appearance Fluid	Latest Ref Range: Clear	Bloody (A)
Condition Fluid	Latest Ref Range: No clot present	No clot present
WBC Fluid	Latest Units: /cumm	34,295
Neutrophils Fluid	Latest Units: %	90
Lymphocytes Fluid	Latest Units: %	1
Macrophages Fluid	Latest Units: %	9
LDH FLUID	Latest Units: U/L	
AMYLASE FLUID	Latest Units: U/L	56
SPECIFIC GRAVITY FLUID	Unknown	1.033
pH Fluid	Latest Units: pH	6.53

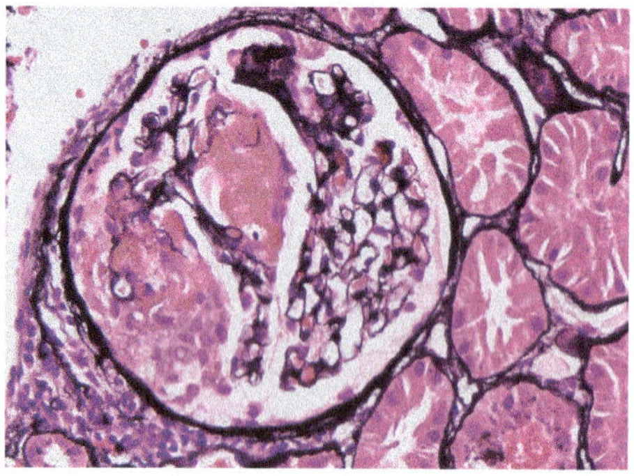

FIGURE 1: Glomerulus with segmental necrosis characterized by rupture of capillary wall and accumulation of fibrin and a segmental cellular crescent (by periodic acid-methenamine silver (PAM) with hematoxylin and eosin staining, original magnification 200x).

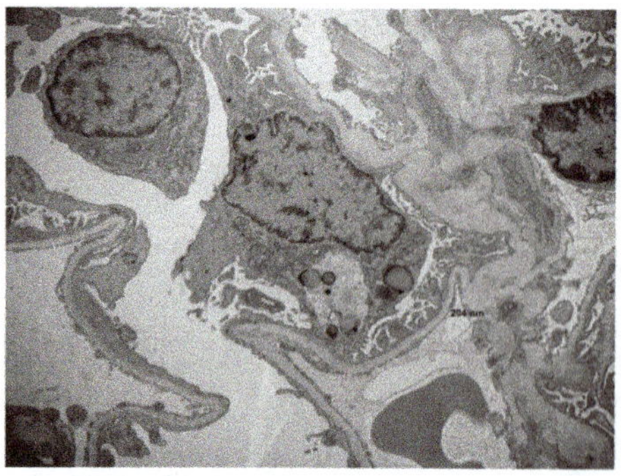

FIGURE 2: No abnormal deposits found on sampled glomerulus.

treatment. He was then discharged after one week of inpatient stay with plans to slowly taper steroids and to continue with weekly rituximab injections.

However, BUN/Cr worsened over the course of the next week to 176 mg/dL and 8.6 mg/dL, and thus he was concluded as rituximab failure and started on cyclophosphamide and plasmapheresis in the inpatient setting.

An ECHO done on readmission showed a small fibrin filled pericardial effusion which required no clinical intervention. Chest X-ray (CXR) on readmission showed stable opacity consistent with prior pleural effusion. Pericardial effusion remained stable in size and patient remained asymptomatic when ECHO was repeated 10 days after readmission. After 7 sessions of plasmapheresis and treatment with 1200 mg IV cyclophosphamide, his creatinine stabilized at 1.7 mg/dL (Figure 3).

3. Discussion

The underlying pathophysiology of ANCA vasculitis is thought to be secondary to the formation of antibodies against key neutrophil antigens which are typically sequestered within the neutrophil and have migrated to the cell membrane of the neutrophil. This migration of typically sequestered antigens is thought to be secondary to cytokine release due to previous or concurrent inflammatory insult and is referred to as "priming" of neutrophils. Antibodies, such as anti-PR3 or anti-MPO, thus activate the neutrophil via interaction with their respective antigens and cause a respiratory burst with degranulation and release of complement activating factors with proinflammatory enzymes. This autoimmune process goes on to affect small-medium sized vessels with organ selectivity depending on the type of ANCA process [1]. Various case reports in the past have reported an association between ANCA vasculitides and pleuropericardial involvement [3–7]. However, cardiac involvement is more common in p-ANCA associated vasculitis including EGPA and it is reported that 13-47% of patients with EGPA have been found to have a myocardial, endocardial, or pericardial lesion with another source reporting 8-32% incidence of pericardial involvement in patients with EGPA [8–10]. Nonetheless, c-ANCA vasculitides have also been associated with cardiac involvement with a reported 19% incidence of pericardial involvement in GPA patients [9].

In this case report, the patient presented with an initial predominant presentation of pericardial tamponade and was then discovered to have renal biopsy proven PR3 pauci-immune glomerulonephritis. Pericardial effusions can be secondary to a wide range of etiologies, including idiopathic, malignancy, infectious, and systemic conditions such as hypothyroidism and autoimmune disorders [11]. In this case, pericardiocentesis yielded an exudative effusion, per Light's criteria, with a fluid protein: serum protein ratio of .75. Furthermore, cytology was pertinent for no malignant cells but indicated acute inflammation. Pericardial fluid gram stain and culture were negative. Blood, respiratory, and

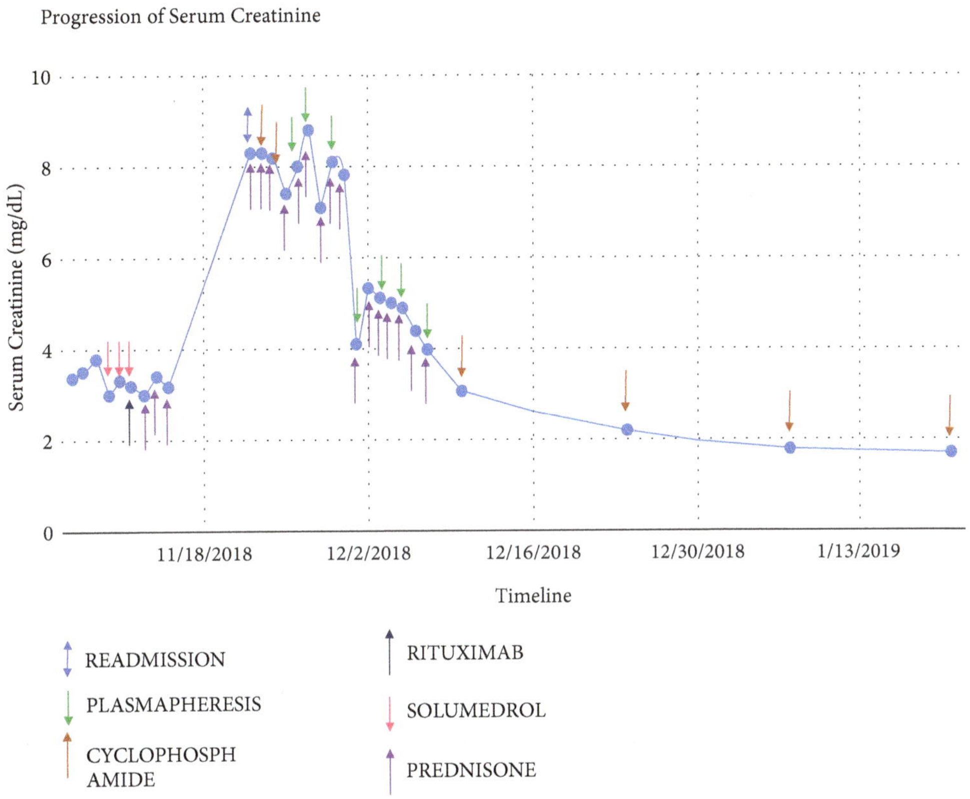

FIGURE 3: Creatinine response to treatment regimen.

urine cultures were also negative. Workup lowered suspicion for infectious or malignant etiologies. Normal complement levels with an autoimmune workup negative for all other antibodies, including dsDNA, SS-A, SS-B, anti-Jo 1, and anti-Scl, lowered the suspicion for lupus or other autoimmune pathologies. Hence, the remarkable ANA titres, positive PR-3, and cANCA antibodies with biopsy proven pauci-immune crescentic glomerulonephritis created the case for vasculitis associated pericardial involvement with progression to pericardial tamponade. Of note, a biopsy of the heart could have further elucidated the role of vasculitis induced pericardial effusion. However, it was felt to be unnecessary given the timeline, presentation, and associated positive findings in laboratory workup and renal biopsy.

This case report is significant as it highlights the importance of considering a pericardial effusion as the initial presenting sign of a vasculitis. It certainly underscores the point that ANCA vasculitides are systemic diseases which may go on to affect various organs in the body, aside from the pathognomonic presentations.

References

[1] J. C. Jennette, R. J. Falk, P. Hu, and H. Xiao, "Pathogenesis of antineutrophil cytoplasmic autoantibody–associated small-vessel vasculitis," *Annual Review of Pathology: Mechanisms of Disease*, vol. 8, no. 1, pp. 139–160, 2013.

[2] A. Radice and R. Sinico, "Antineutrophil cytoplasmic antibodies (ANCA)," *Autoimmunity*, vol. 38, no. 1, pp. 93–103, 2009.

[3] A. C. Keefe, J. C. Hymas, L. L. Emerson, and J. J. Ryan, "An atypical presentation of cardiac tamponade and periorbital swelling in a patient with eosinophilic granulomatosis with polyangiitis: A case report," *Journal of Medical Case Reports*, vol. 11, no. 1, Article ID 271, 2017.

[4] N. E. Goodfield, S. Bhandari, W. D. Plant, A. Morley-Davies, and G. R. Sutherland, "Cardiac involvement in Wegener's granulomatosis," *Heart*, vol. 73, no. 2, pp. 110–115, 1995.

[5] A. G. Blundell and S. Roe, "Wegener's granulomatosis presenting as a pleural effusion," *British Medical Journal*, vol. 327, no. 7406, pp. 95-96, 2003.

[6] K. Yıldızer, S. Paydaş, E. Serin, and Y. Sağlıker, "Wegener's granulomatosis complicated by pericardial tamponade and renal failure," *Nephron*, vol. 72, no. 2, pp. 339-340, 1996.

[7] R. M. Robert Dennert, P. van Paassen, S. Schalla et al., "Cardiac involvement in Churg-Strauss syndrome," *Arthritis & Rheumatism: Official Journal of the American College of Rheumatology*, vol. 62, no. 2, pp. 627–634, 2010.

[8] C. Pagnoux and L. Guillevin, "Cardiac involvement in small and medium-sized vessel vasculitides," *Lupus*, vol. 14, no. 9, pp. 718–722, 2005.

[9] A. M. S. Laurés, L. Quiñones, A. Torres et al., "Un caso de vasculitis p-ANCA positivo con derrame pericárdico asociado," *Nefrología (Madrid)*, vol. 30, no. 2, pp. 268-269, 2010.

[10] G. Thompson, B. Michael, M. Moura et al., "prevalence of pleuritis and peri- carditis in anca-associated vasculitis," *Chest*, vol. 154, no. 4, 2018.

[11] M. Imazio and Y. Adler, "Management of pericardial effusion," *European Heart Journal*, vol. 34, no. 16, pp. 1186–1197, 2013.

5

The Black Esophagus in the Renal Transplant Patient

Michael Andrew Yu,[1] Ramzi Mulki,[2] and Julia Massaad[2]

[1]*Emory University, Department of Internal Medicine, USA*
[2]*Emory University, Division of Digestive Diseases, USA*

Correspondence should be addressed to Michael Andrew Yu; michael.yu@emory.edu

Academic Editor: Anja Haase-Fielitz

Acute esophageal necrosis (AEN) is an uncommon disease characterized by gastrointestinal bleeding and endoscopic findings of circumferential black-colored necrosis of the distal esophagus. Patients at risk include elderly males over the age of 65, who typically have multiple chronic medical issues including vascular disease and diabetes. Mortality is reported to be 32%. Here, we present a case of AEN in a renal transplant patient and describe potential inciting factors such as immunosuppression and opportunistic diseases.

1. Introduction

Black esophagus, commonly known as acute esophageal necrosis (AEN), is a rare clinical condition typically resulting from a combination of ischemic insult, caustic injury from gastric contents, and impaired mucosal protection [1–3]. It is most commonly observed in older males with multiple comorbidities, and has a reported overall mortality of 32% [1]. Patients classically present with hematemesis or melena, with esophagogastroduodenoscopy (EGD) findings of circumferential, black-colored diffuse necrosis at the distal esophagus terminating sharply at the gastroesophageal junction [1, 2]. Treatment includes maintaining hemodynamic stability, antimicrobial therapy, and proton pump inhibition [1, 2].

Interestingly, several reports of AEN have been described in renal transplant patients [4–9]. This particular group is especially vulnerable to gastrointestinal complications from opportunistic infections and mucosal injury due to immunosuppression [10, 11]. CMV esophagitis has been shown to be source of AEN and responds well to antiviral treatment [4, 5]. Transplant patients are often on chronic corticosteroids which increases the risk of peptic ulcer disease, or mycophenolate mofetil (MMF) which has been linked to increased GI bleeding by slowing intestinal cell turnover; this effect is heightened with concomitant NSAID use [10, 12, 13]. AEN has also been diagnosed in the immediate posttransplant period in the setting of hypoperfusion states from hemodynamic compromise and delayed graft function [6, 7]. In the literature, graft versus host disease and graft rejection have also been described as a culprit for AEN [8, 9]. Here, we describe a renal transplant patient on immunosuppression who developed AEN following vascular bypass surgery for limb ischemia.

2. Case Report

A 35-year-old male with history of end stage renal disease from hypertensive nephrosclerosis status post kidney transplant complicated by a right external iliac artery dissection, recurrent acute cellular rejection, and recurrent parvovirus infection presented with worsening chronic right foot pain. He was found to have right lower extremity limb ischemia due to right external iliac artery pseudoaneurysm with distal thromboembolism. He was started on heparin and on hospital day 3, underwent successful revascularization of his R lower extremity. No blood products were needed. Upon completion, heparin was continued. Notably, of his transplant immunosuppression regimen of MMF, tacrolimus, and prednisone, he had only been receiving tacrolimus from admission to his procedure, and was subsequently started on IV methylprednisolone and MMF. Post-procedural white blood cell count and hemoglobin were 20,000/mL and 12.5 g/dL, respectively.

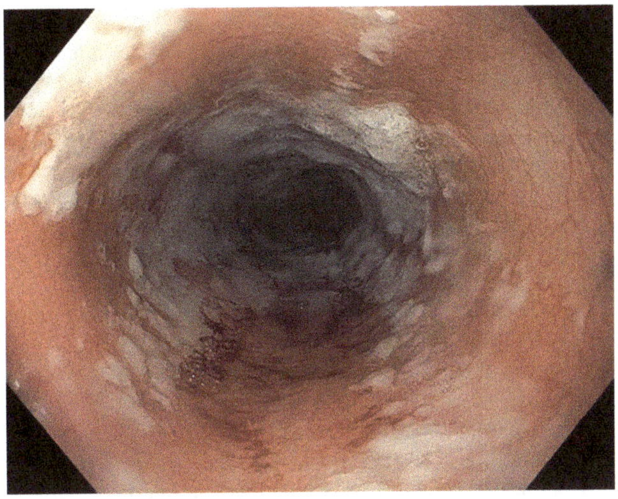

FIGURE 1: LA Grade D esophagitis extending to the middle esophagus.

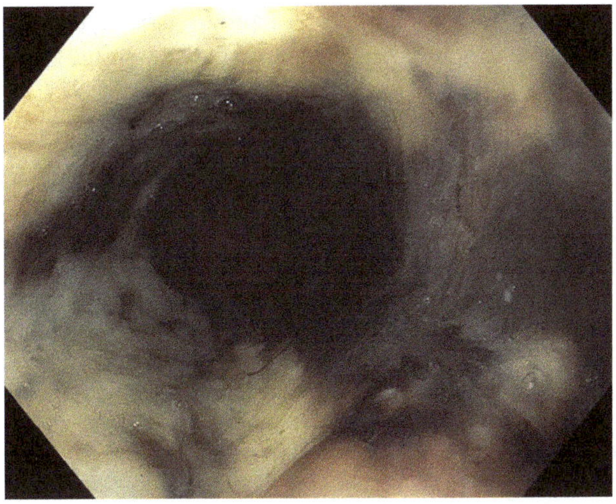

FIGURE 2: Necrotic appearing mucosa of distal esophagus.

Starting postop day (POD) 2, patient developed persistent nausea and hiccups and was made nil-per-os. He was tachycardic but afebrile and normotensive, and was started on broad spectrum antibiotics. By POD3, patient complained of abdominal pain and was without bowel movements since prior to surgery. Leukocytosis worsened to 25,400/mL and hemoglobin decreased to 9.6 g/dL. A CT abdomen/pelvis showed expected postsurgical changes without acute abnormalities. Patient received an aggressive bowel regimen and on POD4, had 3 episodes of melena. A hemoglobin checked afterwards was 7.3 g/dL. Heparin was discontinued and 1 unit of packed red blood cells was transfused with subsequent hemoglobin of 9.0 g/dL. Intravenous pantoprazole was started. On POD5, he underwent EGD, which showed LA Grade D esophagitis in the mid and distal esophagus. (Figure 1) There was necrotic appearing mucosa in the distal esophagus. (Figures 2 and 3) The mid esophagus was friable and bled on contact with the gastroscope. Endoscopic biopsy was deferred. Anticoagulation was resumed and patient was treated with sucralfate for 8 weeks and pantoprazole twice per day for 8 weeks. CMV level on PCR was undetectable. A later CT chest/abdomen showed circumferential thickening of the distal esophagus. (Figure 4). Melena resolved and patient tolerated a clear liquid diet. He completed a 7-day course of antibiotics and was bridged to coumadin. He was discharged following an unremarkable remaining hospital course. Notably, patient reported taking aspirin 81 daily and a prior ibuprofen use. On one-month follow up, patient was well with white blood cell count of 5,900/mL and hemoglobin of 10.9 g/dL.

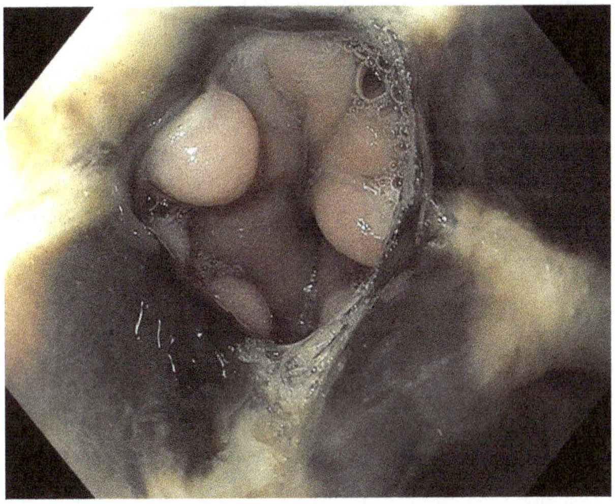

FIGURE 3: Necrotic appearing mucosa of distal esophagus.

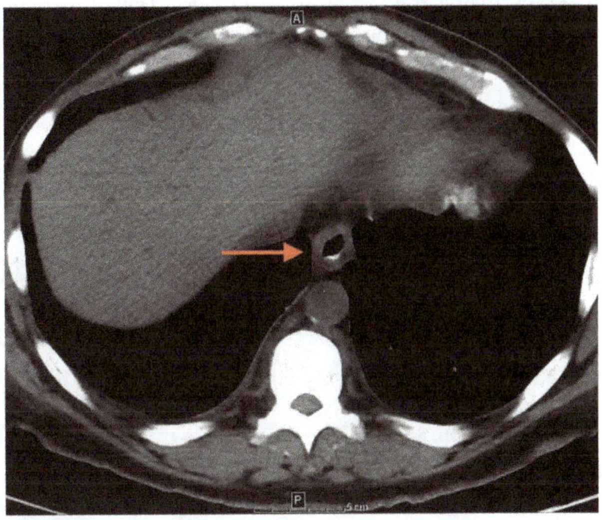

FIGURE 4: CT scan showing circumferential thickening of the distal esophagus.

3. Discussion

Black esophagus or AEN is a rare disease often seen in frail elderly males with multiple comorbidities including alcohol use disorder, peripheral vascular disease, diabetes, atherosclerosis, and cardiovascular and renal disease [1, 2]. It is thought to be multifactorial, likely caused from a mix of hemodynamic compromise leading to tissue hypoperfusion, corrosive injury from stomach contents, and impaired mucosal defense [1, 2]. Classically, the diagnosis is made based on signs and symptoms of GI bleeding, leukocytosis, and EGD findings of diffuse, circumferential necrosis at the distal esophagus [1, 2]. Accepted treatment include making the patient nil-per-os, maintaining optimal organ perfusion, treating any infection with antibiotics, and starting adequate acid suppressing agents such as a PPI or antihistamines [1, 2].

This renal transplant patient has multiple issues making him especially vulnerable to AEN. First, patients with kidney disease have a higher chance of developing peripheral vascular disease, another risk factor for AEN [14]. In patients undergoing renal transplants, there is increased risk of ischemic injury from circulatory instability, and AEN has been described as a complication in the immediate post-transplant period [6, 7]. Next, these patients are prescribed various immunosuppressing agents like corticosteroids and MMF which compromise the gastrointestinal mucosa ability to maintain effective barrier function and give risk to opportunistic infections such as CMV esophagitis [4, 5, 10]. Finally, graft rejection has also been described to cause AEN, likely through hemodynamic compromise [8, 9].

Our case highlights the various risk factors a renal transplantation patient possesses for developing AEN. The patient was admitted for limb ischemia due to complication of the right external iliac artery dissection from renal transplant but was likely aggravated by peripheral vascular disease of renal disease. He underwent revascularization of his right lower limb which added a component of hemodynamic compromise. Gastrointestinal mucosal barrier compromise from chronic steroids, MMF, and NSAIDs probably also exacerbated his risk of AEN. It is unlikely that the patient's history of acute cellular rejection played a role.

Extra vigilance is needed when caring for renal transplant patients. Certain immunosuppression agents have gastrointestinal complications and should be carefully selected and coupled with acid suppressing agents. If AEN is considered, esophagitis from opportunistic infections must be ruled out. EGD during the post-transplant period or after major procedures may also be considered, especially if there was significant hemodynamic insult.

References

[1] G. E. Gurvits, "Black esophagus: acute esophageal necrosis syndrome," *World Journal of Gastroenterology*, vol. 16, no. 26, pp. 3219–3225, 2010.

[2] G. E. Gurvits, K. Cherian, M. N. Shami et al., "Black esophagus: new insights and multicenter international experience in 2014," *Digestive Diseases and Sciences*, vol. 60, no. 2, pp. 444–453, 2015.

[3] S. Shafa, N. Sharma, J. Keshishian, and E. S. Dellon, "The black esophagus: a rare but deadly disease," *ACG Case Reports Journal*, vol. 3, no. 2, pp. 88–91, 2016.

[4] R. Trappe, H. Pohl, A. Forberger, R. Schindler, and P. Reinke, "Acute esophageal necrosis (black esophagus) in the renal transplant recipient: manifestation of primary cytomegalovirus infection," *Transplant Infectious Disease*, vol. 9, no. 1, pp. 42–45, 2007.

[5] A. Mena Lora, J. Khine, N. Khosrodad, and V. Yeldandi, "Unusual manifestations of acute cytomegalovirus infection in solid organ transplant hosts: a report of two cases," *Case Reports in Transplantation*, vol. 2017, Article ID 4916973, 4 pages, 2017.

[6] D. Mealiea, D. Greenhouse, M. Velez, P. Moses, and C. Marroquin, "Acute esophageal necrosis in an immunosuppressed kidney transplant recipient: a case report," *Transplantation Proceedings*, vol. 50, no. 10, pp. 3968–3972, 2018.

[7] F. Caravaca-Fontan, S. Jimenez, A. Fernandez-Rodriguez, R. Marcen, and C. Quereda, "Black esophagus in the early kidney post-transplant period," *Clinical Kidney Journal*, vol. 7, no. 6, pp. 613-614, 2014.

[8] D. Singh, R. Singh, and A. S. Laya, "Acute esophageal necrosis: A case series of five patients presenting with 'Black esophagus,'" *Indian Journal of Gastroenterology*, vol. 30, no. 1, pp. 41–45, 2011.

[9] I. A. N. Grover, "Acute esophageal necrosis in an end-stage renal disease patient: Endoscopic images," *Edorium Journal of Gastroenterology*, vol. 1, pp. 1–3, 2014.

[10] J. H. Helderman and S. Goral, "Gastrointestinal complications of transplant immunosuppression," *Journal of the American Society of Nephrology*, vol. 13, no. 1, pp. 277–287, 2002.

[11] A. C. Steger, A. S. Timoney, S. Griffen, R. R. Salem, and G. Williams, "The influence of immunosuppression on peptic ulceration following renal transplantation and the role of endoscopy," *Nephrology Dialysis Transplantation*, vol. 5, no. 4, pp. 289–292, 1990.

[12] M. Ardalan, J. Etemadi, M. Somi, A. Ghafari, and M. Ghojazadeh, "Upper gastrointestinal bleeding during the first month after renal transplantation in the mycophenolate mofetil era," *Transplantation Proceedings*, vol. 41, no. 7, pp. 2845–2847, 2009.

[13] R. M. Ali, M. Ali, O. Grandes et al., "Mycophenolate mofetil-associated gastrointestinal hemorrhage in renal transplant recipients, a 3 year prospective evaluation of clinical and endoscopic findings at a large community transplant center," *American Journal of Gastroenterology*, vol. 95, no. 9, p. 2492, 2000.

[14] F. Lüders, H. Bunzemeier, C. Engelbertz et al., "CKD and acute and long-term outcome of patients with peripheral artery disease and critical limb ischemia," *Clinical Journal of the American Society of Nephrology*, vol. 11, no. 2, pp. 216–222, 2016.

6

Two Cases of the *MYH9* Disorder Fechtner Syndrome Diagnosed from Observation of Peripheral Blood Cells before End-Stage Renal Failure

Shin Teshirogi,[1] Jun Muratsu ,[1] Hidenori Kasahara,[1] Ken Terashima,[1] Sho Miki,[1] Tomohiro Minami,[1] Yujiro Okute,[1] Suguru Yoneda,[1] Atsuyuki Morishima ,[1] Shinji Kunishima,[2] and Katsuhiko Sakaguchi [1]

[1]*Department of Nephrology and Hypertension, Sumitomo Hospital, 5-3-20 Nakanoshima, Kita-ku, Osaka 530-0005, Japan*
[2]*Department of Advanced Diagnosis, Clinical Research Center, National Hospital Organization Nagoya Medical Center, Nagoya, Japan*

Correspondence should be addressed to Jun Muratsu; jm27252725@yahoo.co.jp

Academic Editor: Yoshihide Fujigaki

As a *MYH9* disorder, Fechtner syndrome is characterized by nephritis, giant platelets, granulocyte inclusion bodies (Döhle-like bodies), cataract, and sensorineural deafness. Observation of peripheral blood smear for the presence of thrombocytopenia, giant platelets, and granulocyte inclusion bodies (Döhle-like bodies) is highly important for the early diagnosis of *MYH9* disorders. In our two cases, sequencing analysis of the *MYH9* gene indicated mutations in exon 24. Both cases were diagnosed as the *MYH9* disorders Fechtner syndrome before end-stage renal failure on the basis of the observation of peripheral blood smear.

1. Introduction

MYH9 mutations cause the autosomal dominant macrothrombocytopenic syndrome of May-Hegglin anomaly, Fechtner syndrome, Sebastian syndrome, and Epstein syndrome. Recently, these diseases are being referred to as *MYH9* disorders. The MYH9 gene encodes the nonmuscle myosin heavy chain -IIA (NMMHC-IIA). *MYH9* disorders are characterized by giant platelets, thrombocytopenia, and characteristic Döhle-like bodies in granulocytes. Among these diseases, the involvement of Alport syndrome symptoms, namely nephritis, cataract, and sensorineural deafness, is associated with the mutation site of the *MYH9* gene. Fechtner syndrome, a *MYH9* disorder, develops nephritis and end-stage renal failure. In most previous reports of *MYH9* disorders in Japan, Fechtner syndrome was diagnosed after end-stage renal failure. Here, our two cases were diagnosed before end-stage renal failure on the basis of the observation of peripheral blood smear, neutrophil inclusion bodies (Döhle-like bodies), and giant platelets.

In the management of chronic kidney disease, the findings from peripheral blood smear, presence of the Döhle-like bodies in neutrophils, and giant platelets are important for the early diagnosis of *MYH9* disorders, especially if the symptoms are not evident.

2. Case Presentation

2.1. Case 1. A 56-year-old male was referred to our hospital for the management of chronic kidney disease. At the age of 17 years, hematuria and proteinuria were observed. At the age of 30 years, he presented with thrombocytopenia, sensorineural deafness, and cataract. At the age of 56 years, he was referred to our hospital for the management of hypertension and elevated serum creatinine level. His blood and urinary analysis results are shown in Table 1. In the peripheral blood smear, thrombocytopenia, giant platelets, and neutrophil inclusion bodies (Döhle-like bodies) were observed with May-Giemsa staining (Figure 1). We identified a relevant family history

Table 1: Clinical characteristics, blood and urinary analysis of these cases.

	Case 1	Case 2	Reference range
Height (cm)	173	164	
Weight (kg)	79.2	64.1	
BMI (kg/m^2)	26.5	23.8	
Urinary analysis			
pH	6.0	5.0	5.0–7.5
Specific gravity	1.003	1.019	1.005–1.030
Protein (g/day)	1.5	0.02	negative
Urine occult blood reaction Cast	1+ fatty cast, epithelial cast and granular cast	Negative hyaline cast, epithelial cast and granular cast	Negative negative
Blood analysis			
White blood cell (/μL)	4,300	4,000	3,300–8,600
Red blood cell ($\times 10^6/\mu$L)	3.00	4.38	4.30–5.60
Hemoglobin (g/dL)	9.8	13.6	13.5–17.0
Hematocrit (%)	29.9	40.9	40.0–51.0
Platelet counts ($\times 10^4/\mu$L)	8.2	8.7	15.0–35.0
Mean platelet volume (fL)	11.5	13.2	6.8–9.4
Bleeding time (minutes)	1	1	1–5
Sodium (mEq/L)	141	143	143
Potassium (mEq/L)	4.7	4.2	3.6–5.0
Chloride (mEq/L)	109	109	98–108
Calcium (mg/dL)	8.7	8.9	8.2–10.2
Phosphorus (mg/dL)	6.2	2.8	2.7–4.4
Total protein (g/dL)	7.0	6.4	6.7–8.3
Albumin (g/dL)	4.1	4.4	3.8–5.3
Blood urea nitrogen (mg/dL)	78	17	8–20
Creatinine (mg/dL)	5.91	1.24	0.36–1.06
estimate glomerular filtration rate (eGFR) (mL/min/1.73m^2)	8.8	47.6	
Hemoglobin A1c (NGSP) (%)	5.7	5.3	4.6–6.2
Antinuclear antibody	×40	<×40	<×40

(Figure 2(a)). His son had thrombocytopenia. His mother died of subarachnoid hemorrhage at the age of 61 years, and his younger brother had thrombocytopenia and renal dysfunction.

From these findings, we considered the possibility of *MYH9* disorders and performed immunofluorescence analysis for neutrophil NMMHC-IIA localization [1, 2]. We found a few large NMMHC-IIA aggregates in the neutrophils (Figure 1). Mutational analysis of the *MYH9* gene revealed a heterozygous duplication of 21 nucleotides in exon 24 (p.E1066_A1072dup, c.3195_3215dup; Figure 2(a)).

We started a nutritional therapy and an angiotensin receptor II; antagonist (olemsartan 20 mg/day) to reduce proteinuria.

2.2. Case 2. A 59-year-old male was referred to our hospital because elevated serum creatinine level was indicated in his medical examinations. Renal dysfunction was only recognized at the age of 59 years, when he presented with cataract and sensorineural deafness. In his family history, his father had sensorineural deafness from the age of 20 years and died of cerebral infarction at the age of 84 years. His mother had hypertension from the age of 50 years (Figure 2(b)). Blood and urinary analysis results are shown in Table 1. In the peripheral blood smear, thrombocytopenia, giant platelets, and neutrophil inclusion bodies (Döhle-like bodies) were observed using May-Giemsa staining (Figure 1). We suspected the possibility of a *MYH9* gene abnormality. Immunofluorescence micrographs of neutrophils showed granular accumulation of NMMHC-IIA in the neutrophils (Figure 1). Subsequent genetic mutation analysis revealed p.E1084del mutation (c.3250_3252delGAG) in *MYH9* exon 24 (Figure 2(b)). To determine other factors of renal dysfunction, we performed renal biopsy by percutaneous needle aspiration. In the histological analysis, no significant changes were observed in the mesangium and tubulointerstitial lesions on light microscopy. However, on electron microscopy, focal effacement of podocytes and loss of the interpodocyte slit diaphragm were observed (Figure 3). From these findings, he was diagnosed with Fechtner syndrome, a *MYH9* disorder. Hypertension and additional risk factors of renal failure had been managed mainly with dietary intervention. Even at 5 years after the diagnosis, his creatinine level remained at 1.3 mg/dL.

The institutional review boards of Sumitomo Hospital and Nagoya Medical Center approved this study. Written informed consent was obtained from all the patients in accordance with the principles of the Declaration of Helsinki.

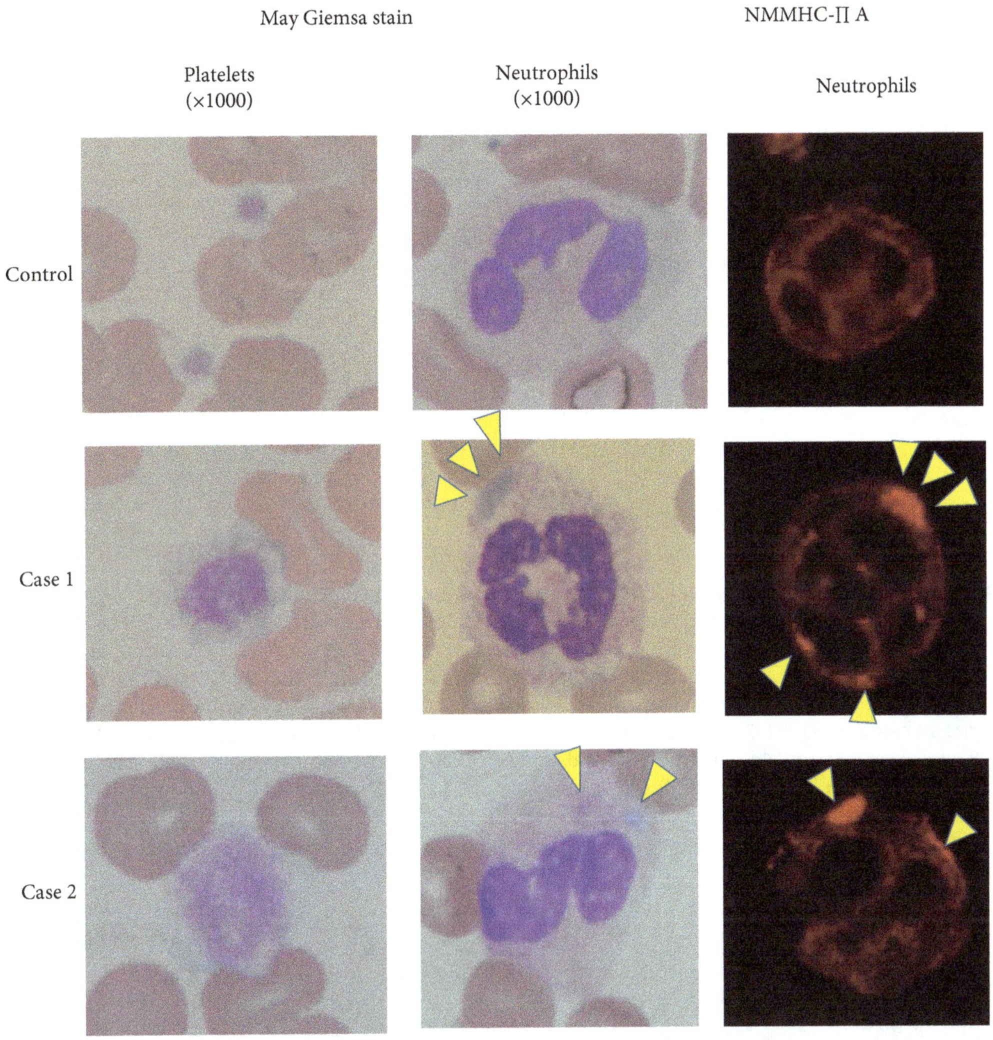

FIGURE 1: Upper panels present the control samples; middle panels, case 1 samples; and lower panels, case 2 samples. The May-Giemsa-stained platelets (in the left: original magnification ×1000) show giant platelets from the case 1 and 2 samples. In the May-Giemsa-stained neutrophils (in the middle: original magnification ×1000), the cytoplasmic inclusion bodies (Döhle-like bodies) in the case 1 and case 2 samples are indicated with arrowheads. The nonmuscle myosin heavy chain-II A (NMMHC-II A) distribution in neutrophils is shown in the immunofluorescence micrographs of the neutrophils (in the right). NMMHC-II A is diffusely distributed in the control neutrophils. Arrowheads represent the accumulation of granular NMMHC-II A in neutrophils of cases 1 and 2.

3. Discussion

MYH9 disorders include May-Hegglin anomaly, Sebastian syndrome, Fechtner syndrome, and Epstein syndrome. These are classified according to the presence of giant platelets, granulocyte inclusion bodies (Döhle-like bodies), nephritis, sensorineural deafness, and cataract [1–3] (Table 2). Here, we describe two cases of Fechtner syndrome before end-stage renal failure. In case 1, a large amount of proteinuria was observed. Owing to renal atrophy, we did not perform a renal biopsy. In contrast, in case 2, mild proteinuria was observed. However, electron microscopy revealed focal and segmental effacement of podocytes and loss of the interpodocyte slit diaphragm. The *MYH9* gene encodes the nonmuscle myosin heavy chain -IIA (NMMHC-IIA). NMMHC-II A is an actin-binding protein that also plays an important role in cell adhesion and maintenance of tissue architecture [4]. It forms myosin II A with myosin light chain and is responsible for the contractile mechanism in the foot process of podocytes [5]. In previous studies, these changes were reported to be associated with the loss of NMMHC-II A expression [6]. This falling out of the foot process is responsible for proteinuria [7]. In many previous reports of *MYH9* disorders, cases of Fechtner syndrome complicated with renal failure were diagnosed after end-stage renal failure [8, 9]. Here, our two cases could be diagnosed before end-stage renal failure on the basis of the main findings, including giant platelets and granulocyte inclusion bodies (Döhle-like bodies). As an advantage of diagnosis before end-stage renal failure, erroneous treatment such as immunosuppressive therapy can be prevented. In addition, antihypertensive therapy can be started early, as done in our cases. In previous studies, administration of an angiotensin II receptor blocker or an angiotensin-converting enzyme inhibitor for renal injury associated with *MYH9* disorders was

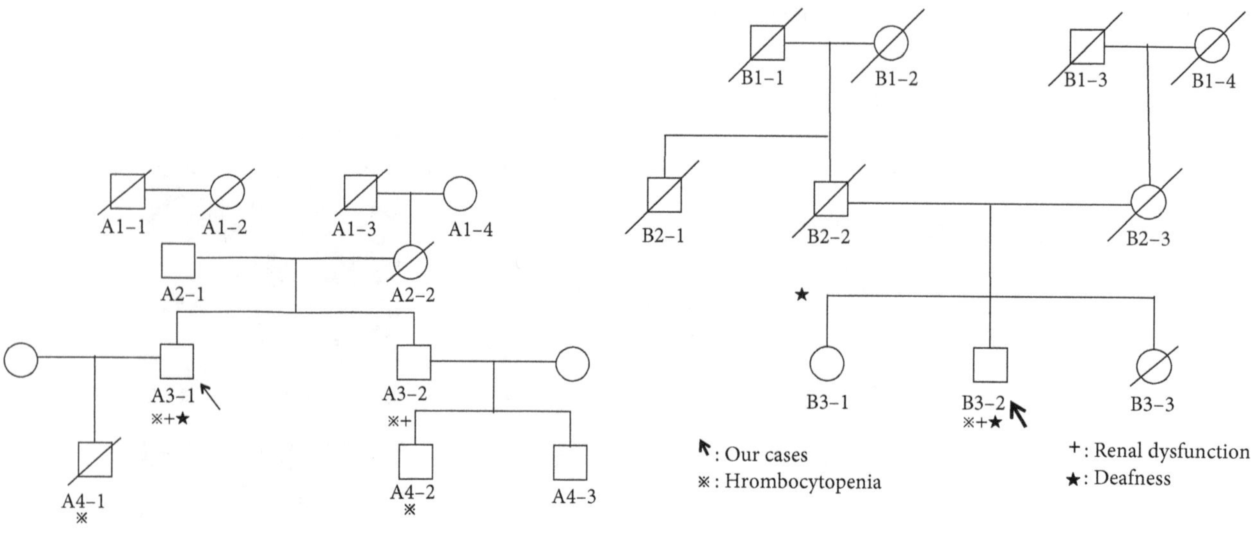

(a) (b)

FIGURE 2: Family pedigree of our cases and sequence electropherogram of the complementary strand of the *MYH9* gene. (a: case 1) Family pedigree of case 1: A1-1 died of tuberculosis at 40 years old. A1-2 died of senility at 90 years old. A1-3 died of gastric cancer at 60 years old. A1-4 had blindness and died of senility at 80 years old. A2-1 had diabetes and was 87 years old. A2-2 died of subarachnoid hemorrhage at 61 years old. A3-1 was case 1. A3-2 was 56 years old. He had thrombocytopenia and renal dysfunction. A4-1 had thrombocytopenia. He died of colon cancer at 29 years old. A4-2 had thrombocytopenia. He was 24 years old. A4-3 had no significant findings. He was 22 years old. (b: case 2) Family pedigree of case 2. B1-1, B1-2, and B1-3 died from senility at around 80 years old. B1-4 died at 60 years old. The cause of her death was unclear. B2-1 died at 62 years old. The cause of his death was unclear. B2-2 had hearing loss. He died of cerebral infarction at 84 years old. B2-3 had hypertension and died from senility at 90 years old. B3-1 was 65 years old. He had no significant findings. B3-2 was case 2. B3-3 had a gallstone. He was 62 years old.

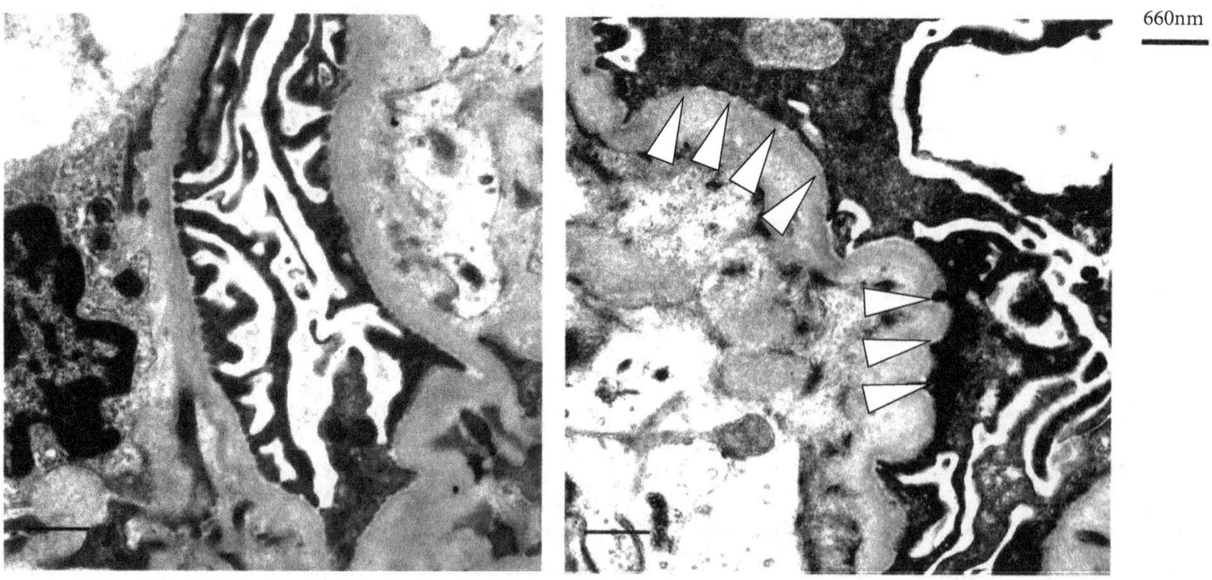

(a) (b)

FIGURE 3: Electron microscopy image of a renal history obtained by percutaneous needle biopsy from case 2 (original magnification ×12000). Normal podocytes and a slit diaphragm are shown (a). In the other field, focal effacement of podocytes and loss of the interpodocyte slit diaphragm are indicated by arrowheads (b).

identified to be effective to reduce proteinuria and suppress the development of renal dysfunction [10]. Diagnosis before end-stage renal failure is necessary for the management around the perioperative period, such as hemostasis during maintenance hemodialysis or tube insertion for peritoneal dialysis. Finally, because *MYH9* disorders are genetic diseases, early detection of patients based on family history is also important. We can offer a genetic consultation to patients' families and other relatives. In fact, in the younger brother of case 1, therapeutic intervention started to suppress the

TABLE 2: *MYH9* disorders; May-Hegglin syndrome, Sebastian syndrome, Epstein syndrome and Fechtner syndrome and clinical features. Clinical features of our cases and previous reported cases with the same mutations of the *MYH9* gene in exon 24.

MYH9 disorders		Giant platelets	Granulocyte inclusion bodies	Nephritis	Sensorineural deafness	Cataract
May-Hegglin syndrome		+	+ (large)	−	−	−
Sebastian syndrome		+	+ (small)	−	−	−
Epstein syndrome		+	−	+	+	−
Fechtner syndrome		+	+	+	+	+
MYH9 gene mutations	Age and sex	Giant platelets and platelet count (reference range: $15.0–35.0\times10^4/\mu L$)	Granulocyte inclusion bodies	Nephritis	Sensorineural deafness	Cataract
Case 1 p.E1066_A1072dup	56 Male	+ ($8.2\times10^4/\mu$)	+	+	+	+
N. Pujol-Moix et al. [12], De Rocco D et al. [13] p.E1066_A1072dup	50 Female	+ ($1.7–8.3\times10^4/\mu$)	+	−	−	−
De Rocco D et al. [13] p.E1066_A1072dup	23 Male	+ ($3.0–8.0\times10^4/\mu$)	+	−	−	+
De Rocco D et al. [13] p.E1066_A1072dup	25 Female	+ ($3.0–8.0\times10^4/\mu$)	+	−	−	−
Case 2 p.E1084del	59 Male	+ ($8.7\times10^4/\mu$)	+	+	−~±	+
Miyazaki et al. [14] p.E1084del	21 Male	+ ($8.5\times10^4/\mu$)	+	−	−	−

development of renal failure. As mentioned earlier, the diagnosis of *MYH9* disorders before end-stage renal failure is meaningful; therefore, careful observation of giant platelets and Döhle-like bodies in patients with chronic kidney disease (CKD) is important. However, in Epstein syndrome, inclusion bodies are difficult to recognize in granulocytes.

Cases with *MYH9* mutations in exon 24 might clearly show Döhle-like bodies and giant platelets. Previously, about 30 mutations of the *MYH9* gene were reported. However, among the 40 exons in the *MYH9* gene, mutations are concentrated in the specific codons of exons 1, 16, 26, 30, 38, and 40 [11]. Both our cases had mutations in exon 24. In previous studies, cases with mutations in exon 24 were very rare [12–14]. Even among the same genetic mutations, the phenotype can vary [15]. Kidney damage occurs in approximately 25% of patients with *MYH9* disorders as progressive proteinuric nephropathy. In most cases, nephropathy occurs before the age of 35 years and presents an aggressive course. In some cases, proteinuria may appear later and/or show a slower progression [16]. Hearing loss occurred in approximately 50% of cases at a mean age of 33 years [17]. As indicated in Table 2, thrombocytopenia is common, but the occurrence of symptoms such as renal disorder, deafness, and cataract differed from each other even in the same genetic mutation. These findings indicate that other factors such as age or sex might be required for the onset and progression of symptoms. Therefore, in cases with thrombocytopenia, attention should be paid to the possibility of *MYH9* disorders.

There still remain many unknown points regarding the pathophysiology of *MYH9* disorders, particularly Fechtner syndrome. Further investigation is required to assess the incidence and mechanism of renal failure in *MYH9* disorders, especially Fechtner syndrome.

In conclusion, in patients with chronic kidney disease, findings of giant platelets and granulocyte inclusion bodies (Döhle-like bodies) are important for the diagnosis of *MYH9* disorders, particularly Fechtner syndrome.

Disclosure

Shinji Kunishima, Department of Medical Technology, School of Health Sciences, Gifu University of Medical Science, Seki, Gifu, Japan.

Authors' Contributions

Shin Teshirogi and Jun Muratsu contributed equally to this work.

References

[1] S. Kunishima, T. Kojima, T. Matsushita et al., "Mutations in the NMMHC-A gene cause autosomal dominant macrothrombocytopenia with leukocyte inclusions (May-Hegglin anomaly/Sebastian syndrome)," *Blood*, vol. 97, no. 4, pp. 1147–1149, 2001.

[2] S. Kunishima, T. Matsushita, T. Kojima et al., "Identification of six novel *MYH9* mutations and genotype-phenotype relationships in autosomal dominant macrothrombocytopenia with leukocyte inclusions," *Journal of Human Genetics*, vol. 46, no. 12, pp. 722–729, 2001.

[3] S. Kunishima, T. Matsushita, T. Kojima et al., "Immunofluorescence analysis of neutrophil nonmuscle myosin heavy chain-A in *MYH9* disorders: association of subcellular localization with *MYH9* mutations," *Laboratory Investigation*, vol. 83, no. 1, pp. 115–122, 2003.

[4] M. Vicente-Manzanares, X. Ma, R. S. Adelstein, and A. R. Horwitz, "Nonmuscle myosin II takes centre stage in cell adhesion and migration," *Nature Reviews Molecular Cell Biology*, vol. 10, no. 11, pp. 778–790, 2009.

[5] T. Sekine, M. Konno, S. Sasaki et al., "Patients with Epstein-Fechtner syndromes owing to *MYH9* R702 mutations develop progressive proteinuric renal disease," *Kidney International*, vol. 78, no. 2, pp. 207–214, 2010.

[6] K. Miura, H. Kurihara, S. Horita et al., "Podocyte expression of nonmuscle myosin heavy chain-IIA decreases in idiopathic nephrotic syndrome, especially in focal segmental glomerulosclerosis," *Nephrology Dialysis Transplantation*, vol. 28, no. 12, pp. 2993–3003, 2013.

[7] G. M. Ghiggeri, G. Caridi, U. Magrini et al., "Genetics, clinical and pathological features of glomerulonephritis associated with mutations of nonmuscle myosin IIA (Fechtner syndrome)," *American Journal of Kidney Diseases*, vol. 41, no. 1, pp. 95–104, 2003.

[8] R. Ishida, T. Kusaba, Y. Kirita et al., "A case of a hemodialysis patient with *MYH9* disorders," *Japan Journal of Nephrology*, vol. 53, no. 2, pp. 195–199, 2011.

[9] J. Shibuya, A. Kiya, and T. Kuroda, "The start of hemodialysis in a patient with May-Hegglin anomaly complicated by Alport-like symptoms," *Journal of Japanese Society for Dialysis Therapy*, vol. 44, no. 8, pp. 689–694, 2011.

[10] A. Pecci, A. Granata, C. E. Fiore, and C. L. Balduini, "Renin-angiotensin system blockade is effective in reducing proteinuria of patients with progressive nephropathy caused by *MYH9* mutations (Fechtner-Epstein syndrome)," *Nephrology Dialysis Transplantation*, vol. 23, no. 8, pp. 2690–2692, 2008.

[11] S. Kunishima and H. Saito, "Advances in the understanding of *MYH9* disorders," *Current Opinion in Hematology*, vol. 17, no. 5, pp. 405–410, 2010.

[12] N. Pujol-Moix, E. Muñiz-Diaz, M. Moreno-Torres et al., "platelet syndrome. Two new cases in a Spanish family," *Annals of Hematology*, vol. 62, no. 6, pp. 235–237, 1991.

[13] D. De Rocco, N. Pujol-Moix, A. Pecci et al., "Identification of the first duplication in *MYH9*-related disease: a hot spot for unequal crossing-over within exon 24 of the *MYH9* gene," *European Journal of Medical Genetics*, vol. 52, no. 4, pp. 191–194, 2009.

[14] K. Miyazaki, S. Kunishima, W. Fujii, and M. Higashihara, "Identification of three in-frame deletion mutations in *MYH9* disorders suggesting an important hot spot for small rearrangements in *MYH9* exon 24," *European Journal of Haematology*, vol. 83, no. 3, pp. 230–234, 2009.

[15] A. Pecci, E. Panza, D. De Rocco et al., "*MYH9* related disease: four novel mutations of the tail domain of myosin-9 correlating with a mild clinical phenotype," *European Journal of Haematology*, vol. 84, no. 4, pp. 291–297, 2010.

[16] K. H. Han, H. Lee, H. G. Kang et al., "Renal manifestations of patients with *MYH9*-related disorders," *Pediatric Nephrology*, vol. 26, no. 4, pp. 549–555, 2011.

[17] A. Pecci, C. Klersy, P. Gresele et al., "*MYH9*-related disease: a novel prognostic model to predict the clinical evolution of the disease based on genotype-phenotype correlations," *Human Mutation*, vol. 35, no. 2, pp. 236–247, 2014.

7

A Case Report on *Pasteurella multocida* Peritoneal Dialysis-Associated Peritonitis: When Cats Think Medical Equipment are Toys

Saeid Mirzai ,[1] Ahmad Oussama Rifai ,[2] Aron Tidrick,[1] Qitan Huang,[1] and Justin Hale[1]

[1]*Alabama College of Osteopathic Medicine, 445 Health Sciences Blvd, Dothan, AL 36303, USA*
[2]*The Virtual Nephrologist, INC., PO Box 1750, Lynn Haven, FL 32444, USA*

Correspondence should be addressed to Ahmad Oussama Rifai; aorifai@gmail.com

Academic Editor: Władysław Sułowicz

Pasteurella multocida is an aerobic gram-negative coccobacillus usually found in the oral cavities of most healthy cats and dogs as part of their natural oral flora. This zoonotic pathogen can cause a variety of infections in humans through bites, scratches, or licking. Infections range from less severe cases, such as infected animal bites and cellulitis, to more severe cases of pneumonia, septic arthritis, osteomyelitis, sepsis, and meningitis. However, the number of reported cases of peritoneal dialysis-associated peritonitis caused by *P. multocida* has been limited worldwide. Here, we report the case of a 59-year-old man undergoing continuous cycling peritoneal dialysis who developed *P. multocida* peritonitis, believed to be secondary to domestic cat exposure to dialysis equipment. Due to the increasing trend of pet ownership, patients maintained on peritoneal dialysis should be educated on the importance of strict hygiene and avoiding pet contact with the dialysis equipment, especially in bag exchange areas. Although the best means of preventing such infections is to avoid having pets at home, the positive psychological effects of pet ownership should also be considered. Thus, patients in such situations should be continuously educated and encouraged to be mindful of the importance of environmental hygiene.

1. Introduction

Aside from kidney transplantation, hemodialysis and peritoneal dialysis (PD) are two artificial renal replacement therapeutic methods used to treat patients with end-stage renal disease (ESRD). Both methods have their own limitations; thereby, one is not considered superior to the other. However, the application of PD is increasing, possibly owing to its lower cost and usage convenience since it can be performed at home and does not require travel to hospitals or satellite outpatient dialysis units [1].

Acute bacterial peritonitis in patients undergoing PD is a major cause of hospitalizations, transfer to hemodialysis, and catheter removal, presenting significant limitations to its utilization [2]. The major pathogens associated with peritoneal dialysis-associated peritonitis (PD-peritonitis) are the gram-positive cocci, *Staphylococcus aureus* and *S. epidermidis*, accounting for 42% of cases. These bacteria, originating from the skin, move through and along the dialysis catheter [3]. Gram-negative organisms are less commonly detected, accounting for 19% of cases [4]. A rare organism that has been shown to cause PD-peritonitis is *Pasteurella multocida*, with only 43 cases reported in the literature to date (Table 1).

P. multocida is an aerobic gram-negative coccobacillus found in the oral cavities of both domestic and wild animals [5]. It is part of their normal oropharyngeal flora, is spread through bites or scratches, and leads to various human diseases. Here, we report a case of PD-peritonitis caused by *P. multocida* in a patient with ESRD undergoing continuous cycling peritoneal dialysis (CCPD), believed to be caused by close contact with household cats.

2. Case Presentation

A 59-year-old Caucasian man with ESRD due to glomerulonephritis and failed kidney transplant who was undergoing CCPD for 7 months presented to the emergency department

TABLE 1: Previous case reports on peritoneal dialysis peritonitis caused by *Pasteurella multocida*.

Case	Citation	Year of publication	Age (years)/sex	Etiology of ESRD	Animal exposure	Treatment
1	11	1987	55/F	Hypertension	Cat	Vancomycin, gentamicin
2	12	1991	55/M	Polyarteritis nodosa	Cat	Vancomycin, gentamicin, ciprofloxacin
3	13	1991	54/M	Hypertension	Cat	Vancomycin, gentamicin, cefazolin
4	14	1991	25/M	Alport syndrome	Cat	Gentamicin, cephradine
5	15	1996	75/M	Hypertension	Cat	Vancomycin, cefamandole
6	16	1996	42/F	Hypertension	Cat	Vancomycin, gentamicin, penicillin
7	17	1997	12/F	Focal segmental glomerulosclerosis	Cat	Cephapirin, gentamicin
8	18	1997	73/M	Chronic glomerulonephritis	Cat	Vancomycin, ceftazidime
9	19	1998	55/M	Polyarteritis nodosa	Cat	Vancomycin, gentamicin, ampicillin-sulbactam
10	20	1998	47/F	Type 1 diabetes mellitus	Cat	Piperacillin, ciprofloxacin
11	21	1999	49/M	IgA nephropathy	Cat	Cefazolin, tobramycin
12	22	1999	18/M	Interstitial nephritis	Cat	Ticarcillin, clindamycin
13	23	2000	69/F	—	—	—
14	23	2000	46/F	—	—	—
15	23	2000	64/M	—	—	—
16	24	2000	22/F	Medullary cystic kidney disease	Cat	Vancomycin, amikacin, ciprofloxacin
17	25	2002	24/F	Chronic pyelonephritis	Cat	Ciprofloxacin
18	26	2004	48/F	—	Cat	Cefazolin, gentamicin, ampicillin
19	7	2004	73/F	Autosomal dominant polycystic kidney disease	Cat	Vancomycin, gentamicin, Ciprofloxacin
20	27	2005	52/M	IgA nephropathy	Cat	Amikacin, cefazolin
21	28	2005	21/F	Congenital small kidneys	Cat	Gentamicin, ceftazidime
22	28	2005	58/M	Cyclosporine nephrotoxicity	Cat	Gentamicin, vancomycin
23	29	2006	46/F	—	Cat	Ceftazidime
24	30	2007	48/F	—	Dog	Cefazolin, gentamicin
25	31	2008	29/F	—	Cat	Cefazolin, tobramycin
26	6	2010	38/M	ANCA-related vasculitis	Cat	Ampicillin, levofloxacin
27	10	2010	36/F	Systemic lupus erythematosus, diabetes mellitus, hypertension	Cat	Ciprofloxacin
28	32	2010	58/M	Type 2 diabetes mellitus	Cat	Cefazolin, ceftazidime
29	2	2012	45/M	IgA nephropathy	Cat	Vancomycin, ceftazidime, levofloxacin
30	33	2012	57/M	Autosomal dominant polycystic kidney disease	Cat, dog	Vancomycin, ceftazidime
31	34	2013	49/M	Diabetes mellitus	Cat, dog	Vancomycin, tobramycin, cefazolin, ceftazidime, amoxicillin/clavulanate
32	4	2013	7/F	CKD secondary to prior cardiac arrest	Cat	Ampicillin
33	3	2014	62/F	Hypertension	Cat	Ciprofloxacin, trimethoprim-sulfamethoxazole, cephalothin
34	5	2014	25/F	—	Cat	Cefazolin, gentamicin
35	35	2015	28/F	Hypertension, congenital solitary kidney	Cat	Cefazolin, tobramycin, ceftazidime

Table 1: Continued.

Case	Citation	Year of publication	Age (years)/sex	Etiology of ESRD	Animal exposure	Treatment
36	35	2015	37/M	Diabetes mellitus	Cat	Cefazolin, tobramycin
37	35	2015	41/M	Diabetes mellitus, hypertension	Cat	Cefazolin, tobramycin
38	35	2015	51/F	Hypertension	Cat	Cefazolin, tobramycin, Amoxicillin-clavulanic acid
39	35	2015	37/F	Chronic interstitial nephropathy	Cat	Ceftriaxone, amoxicillin
40	35	2015	59/F	Diabetes mellitus	Cat	Cefazolin, tobramycin, ceftazidime
41	35	2015	69/F	Diabetes mellitus	Cat	Cefazolin, tobramycin, ceftazidime, amoxicillin/clavulanic acid
42	36	2017	72/M	Diabetes mellitus	Cat	Vancomycin, ceftazidime
43	9	2018	3/F	Congenital nephrotic syndrome	Cat	Cefazolin, piperacillin, cefdinir
44	Our case	2019	59/M	Glomerulonephritis, failed kidney transplant	Cat	Vancomycin, ceftazidime

with periumbilical pain for several days. This was the first time the patient had experienced these symptoms since the initiation of CCPD. His medical history additionally included hypertension, valvular heart disease, degenerative arthritis, parathyroidectomy, and tobacco use. He had discontinued all of his immunosuppressive medications because his kidney transplant had been nonfunctional for several years.

Physical examination revealed a well-built, seemingly healthy man weighing 157 pounds with a blood pressure of 144/92 mmHg and a heart rate of 85 beats/min, without distress, and without jaundiced sclerae. He had clear lungs and systolic heart murmur. Abdominal examination revealed a soft abdomen with some fullness on the right lower quadrant proximal to his previous renal transplant, periumbilical tenderness, and intact exit site with no tunnel tenderness. He had active bowel sounds.

Laboratory testing revealed a white blood cell (WBC) count of $9.1 \times 10^3/\mu L$ with 70% neutrophils, hemoglobin level of 12.9 g/dL, hematocrit count of 38.5%, and platelet count of $263 \times 10^3/\mu L$. Serum chemistry analysis showed the following levels: sodium 139 mmol/L, potassium 3.4 mmol/L, chloride 95 mmol/L, total carbon dioxide 28 mmol/L, glucose 127 mg/dL, blood urea nitrogen 31 mg/dL, and creatinine 12.46 mg/dL. The peritoneal fluid was colorless and appeared hazy. Initial analysis showed a WBC count of 4,470 cells/μL with 85% polymorphonuclear cells and 15% mononuclear cells. Gram staining of the peritoneal fluid was negative for any organisms, only showing WBCs.

Based on the available information, the patient was diagnosed with PD-peritonitis, and empiric treatment with 1 g of vancomycin and 1 g of ceftazidime was administered intravenously and daily infusions initiated. The final diagnosis was made through peritoneal fluid culture that showed light growth of *P. multocida* after 3 days. The isolate was sensitive to ampicillin, ceftriaxone, ceftazidime, gentamicin, and ciprofloxacin. Therefore, antibiotics were adjusted according to the bacterial cultures, where intravenous ampicillin-sulbactam was started and then switched to oral amoxicillin-clavulanate for a total of 3 weeks. Patient had subsequent improvement in symptoms and laboratory results. He was able to continue PD successfully without any interruption or the need for catheter removal.

Upon taking further history, the patient reported having several cats at home, none of which were kittens. At night, he would begin his PD treatment and go into a different room to watch television. Therefore, the cats were assumed to play with the dialysis equipment or chew on the tubing, possibly leading to infection, although the patient did not recall noticing any fluid leakage from the tubing. Prior to discharge, the patient's dialysis technique was confirmed by direct observation, and aseptic technique was ensured. The patient additionally decided to place his cats outside the home at night before starting PD treatment. He did not have any more episodes of PD-peritonitis caused by *P. multocida* after changing his routine.

3. Discussion

P. multocida is an aerobic gram-negative coccobacillus found as one of the normal upper respiratory flora in various domestic animals, particularly cats and dogs. It was named after Louis Pasteur who first described the organism in 1880 [3]. The pathogen can lead to a wide variety of human conditions ranging from less severe cases such as infected animal bites and cellulitis to more severe cases of pneumonia, septic arthritis, osteomyelitis, sepsis, and meningitis. These severe conditions are more likely to occur in immunocompromised individuals due to the opportunistic nature of the organism [6]. PD-peritonitis secondary to *P. multocida* is very rare, with only 43 reported cases worldwide (Table 1).

The first case of PD-related peritonitis caused by *P. multocida* was reported by Paul and Rostand in Alabama in 1987 where the patient had acquired the infection from cat bites or scratches to the dialysis tubing [7]. Since then, the number of such cases reported in the literature is continuously increasing. This could be related to the growing population of ESRD patients, and the corresponding increase in PD as a home modality, indicating a correlation between home environment and medical therapy. According to the American Veterinary Medical Association, an increasing number of households are housing pets, with 30% of households owning two or more cats and 36% of households owning one or more dogs in 2012 [8]. This has led to an increasing risk of zoonotic transmitted infections over time.

The current literature on PD-peritonitis caused by *P. multocida* is summarized in Table 1, with the vast majority of cases acquired from cats and a small number from dogs. The prevalence of colonization with *P. multocida* has also been higher in cats (70–90%) than in dogs (50–66%), made worse by the sharper teeth found in cats [6]. Additionally, 20% of cats are found to have *Pasteurella* spp. on their claws [2]. The organism is spread through bites, scratches, and licking. The most common method which causes *P. multocida* PD-peritonitis is close contact of the cats with the dialysis equipment, including the tubing or bags; however, it can also spread through patients with pets who do not practice proper hygiene when preparing their treatment [4].

With regard to the types of PD, PD-peritonitis caused by *P. multocida* more commonly occurs in patients utilizing CCPD than in those using continuous ambulatory peritoneal dialysis (CAPD). This is possibly secondary to the length of tubing required or the prolonged amount of time the equipment is in contact with the environment as compared to CAPD. Cats may also enjoy the warmth of the heat plate and lay on the dialysis machine [9].

Although the majority of cases had direct contact with animals, there have been cases with no cat contact, or spontaneous cases in immunocompromised patients or those who have chronic diseases (such as malignancy, cirrhosis, diabetes, human immunodeficiency virus infection, chronic pulmonary disease, ESRD) [7]. Additionally, studies showing spontaneous oropharyngeal colonization in healthy livestock breeders indicated the possibility of colonization in patients who have housed pets for long periods of time [4]. Therefore, improper hygiene could lead to the spread of the organism from the patient's own saliva to their hands and dialysis equipment [5].

In terms of presentation, no specific clinical signs are typically present to differentiate *P. multocida* peritonitis from other etiologies [4]. Therefore, history taking is important in order to find out whether the patient has any pets and whether those pets have access to the dialysis equipment. Typical symptoms of peritonitis include low-to-moderate-grade fever, severe abdominal pain, and cloudy dialysate, in addition to occasional nausea and vomiting. Peripheral WBC count may be normal or show severe leukocytosis with increased polymorphonuclear leukocyte levels, and peritoneal dialysate WBC count is usually very high. Gram staining of the dialysate is usually negative, as it was in our patient [6]. Symptoms typically begin within 24 hours and improve within 48–96 hours after initiating the antibiotic therapy [5].

PD-peritonitis caused by *P. multocida* is usually susceptible to penicillin, which is considered the treatment of choice. Tetracyclines, cephalosporins (third- or later-generations), and fluoroquinolones are considered alternatives. Its susceptibility to aminoglycosides varies [7]. The typical duration of treatment is estimated to be 3 weeks according to the current literature, and the preferred route of administration is intraperitoneal [6]. PD-peritonitis prevention through proper hygiene and technique, or immediate treatment upon its occurrence, is critical due to the risk of possible peritoneal membrane failure because of severe and prolonged peritonitis. This is a major cause of PD termination and switching to hemodialysis [2]. Most cases of PD-peritonitis caused by *P. multocida* are resolved without catheter removal; however, the catheter should be removed if the patient continues to have cloudy effluent after an appropriate antibiotic treatment for 5 days, indicating refractory peritonitis [2].

P. multocida is a rare organism that causes PD-associated peritonitis in patients who keep pets, especially cats, in the environment where PD is performed. With the increasing trend of pet ownership, PD patients should be educated on the importance of strict hygiene and avoiding pet contact with dialysis equipment, especially in bag exchange areas [7]. The best method of preventing these infections is to avoid having pets at home by possibly relocating them with friends or family members while the patient is on dialysis. However, the positive psychological effects of pets on the patients' health should be considered [10]. Therefore, pet contact with dialysis equipment should be prevented and environmental hygiene maintained in patients who wish to have their pets at home. Additionally, patients should be continuously educated and encouraged to be cautious, especially during their switch from CAPD to CCPD [2].

References

[1] C. Goodlad and E. Brown, "The role of peritoneal dialysis in modern renal replacement therapy," *Postgraduate Medical Journal*, vol. 89, no. 1056, pp. 584–590, 2013.

[2] M. Nishina, H. Yanagi, M. Koizumi et al., "*Pasteurellamultocida* peritonitis associated with a cat in a peritoneal dialysis patient using an automated cycler device," *CEN Case Reports*, vol. 1, no. 2, pp. 73–76, 2012.

[3] H. F. Dresselaars, B. Zwart, A. M. Pettersson, M. C. Rijnsburger, and M. M. Ho-dac-Pannekeet, "Peritoneal dialysis-associated peritonitis of zoonotic origin, when minor gets major," *The Netherlands Journal of Medicine*, vol. 72, no. 10, pp. 551–553, 2014.

[4] P. M. Sol, N. C. van de Kar, and F. S. Michiel, "Cat induced *Pasteurellamultocida* peritonitis in peritoneal dialysis: a case report and review of the literature," *International Journal of Hygiene and Environmental Health*, vol. 216, pp. 211–213, 2013.

[5] I. Kim, Y. W. Kim, S. Chung, H. E. Yoon, and S. J. Shin, "Cat-induced *Pasteurellamultocida* peritonitis in continuous ambulatory peritoneal dialysis," *Kidney Research and Clinical Practice*, vol. 33, no. 1, pp. 65–67, 2014.

[6] H. Rondon-Berrios and G. J. Trevejo-Nunez, "Pets or pest: peritoneal dialysis-related peritonitis due to *Pasteurellamultocida*," *Journal of Microbiology, Immunology and Infection*, vol. 43, no. 2, pp. 155–158, 2010.

[7] F. J. Cooke, A. Kodjo, E. J. Clutterbuck, and K. B. Bamford,

"A case of *Pasteurellamultocida* peritoneal dialysis-associated peritonitis and review of the literature," *International Journal of Infectious Diseases*, vol. 8, no. 3, pp. 171–174, 2004.

[8] Association American Veterinary Medical, *US Pet Ownership & Demographic*, Illinois, AVMA, 2012.

[9] H. Tamura, S. Kuraoka, T. Nishi, Y. Hidaka, H. Nagata, and H. Nakazato, "*Pasteurellamultocida*peritonitis in a 3-year-old patient undergoing peritoneal dialysis: case report and review of the literature," *American Journal of Pediatrics*, vol. 4, pp. 52–55, 2018.

[10] S. M. Mugambi and M. E. Ullian, "Bacteremia, sepsis, and peritonitis with *Pasteurellamultocida* in a peritoneal dialysis patient," *Peritoneal Dialysis International*, vol. 30, no. 3, pp. 381–383, 2010.

[11] R. V. Paul and S. G. Rostand, "Cat-bite peritonitis: *Pasteurellamultocida* peritonitis following feline contamination of peritoneal dialysis tubing," *American Journal of Kidney Diseases*, vol. 10, no. 4, pp. 318–319, 1987.

[12] A. H. Frankel and M. J. Cassidy, "*Pasteurellamultocida* peritonitis in CAPD: beware of the cats," *Peritoneal Dialysis International*, vol. 11, no. 2, pp. 184–185, 1991.

[13] R. D. London and E. J. Bottone, "*Pasteurellamultocida*: zoonotic cause of peritonitis in a patient undergoing peritoneal dialysis," *The American Journal of Medicine*, vol. 91, no. 2, pp. 202–204, 1991.

[14] R. M. Elsey, R. W. Carson, and T. D. DuBose Jr., "*Pasteurellamultocida* peritonitis in an HIV-positive patient on continuous cycling peritoneal dialysis," *American Journal of Nephrology*, vol. 11, no. 1, pp. 61–63, 1991.

[15] A. R. Kitching, A. Macdonald, and P. J. Hatfield, "*Pasteurellamultocida* infection in continuous ambulatory peritoneal dialysis," *New Zealand Medical Journal*, vol. 109, p. 59, 1996.

[16] J. Uribarri, E. J. Bottone, and R. D. London, "*Pasteurellamultocida* peritonitis: are peritoneal dialysis patients on cyclers at increased risk?," *Peritoneal Dialysis International*, vol. 16, pp. 648–649, 1996.

[17] M. Loghman-Adham, "*Pasteurellamultocida* peritonitis in patients undergoing peritoneal dialysis," *Pediatric Nephrology*, vol. 11, no. 3, pp. 353–354, 1997.

[18] K. MacKay, L. Brown, and F. Hudson, "*Pasteurellamultocida* peritonitis in peritoneal dialysis patients: beware of the cat," *Peritoneal Dialysis International*, vol. 17, no. 6, pp. 608–610, 1997.

[19] J. Joh, R. Padmanabhan, and B. Bastani, "*Pasteurellamultocida* peritonitis following cat bite of peritoneal dialysis tubing. With a brief review of the literature," *American Journal of Nephrology*, vol. 18, no. 3, pp. 258–259, 1998.

[20] F. Musio and A. Tiu, "*Pasteurellamultocida* peritonitis in peritoneal dialysis," *Clinical Nephrology*, vol. 49, no. 4, pp. 258–261, 1998.

[21] K. Hamai, H. Imai, H. Ohtani et al., "Repeated cat-associated peritonitis in a patient on automated nocturnal intermittent peritoneal dialysis," *Clinical and Experimental Nephrology*, vol. 3, no. 1, pp. 59–61, 1999.

[22] Vimal Chadha and B. A. Warady, "*Capnocytophag acanimorsus* peritonitis in a pediatric peritoneal dialysis patient," *Pediatric Nephrology*, vol. 13, no. 8, pp. 646–648, 1999.

[23] M. J. R. Breton, L. M. Salavert, F. A. Viudes, B. C. Perez, and S. M. Gobernado, "Abdominal infection by *Pasteurella* spp. a report of 3 cases," *Revista Clínica Española*, vol. 200, pp. 139–142, 2000.

[24] G. Van Langenhove, R. Daelemans, P. Zachee, and R. L. Lins, "*Pasteurellamultocida* as a rare cause of peritonitis in peritoneal dialysis," *Nephron*, vol. 85, pp. 283–284, 2000.

[25] N. Kanaan, P. Gavage, M. Janssens, V. Avesani, J. Gigi, and E. Goffin, "*Pasteurella multocida* in peritoneal dialysis: a rare cause of peritonitis associated with exposure to domestic cats," *Acta Clinica Belgica*, vol. 57, pp. 254–256, 2002.

[26] J. Sillery, J. Hargreaves, P. Marin, E. Lerma, C. Kuznia, and C. Abbe, "*Pasteurellamultocida* peritonitis: another risk of animal-assisted therapy," *Infection Control & Hospital Epidemiology*, vol. 25, no. 1, pp. 5–6, 2004.

[27] O. Mat, F. Moenens, R. Beauwens et al., "Indolent *Pasteurellamultocida* peritonitis in a CCPD patient. 25 years of "cat-bite peritonitis": a review," *Peritoneal Dialysis International*, vol. 25, pp. 88–90, 2005.

[28] A. Malik, K. S. Mailey, and B. Bastani, "*Pasteurellamultocida* peritoneal dialysis-associated peritonitis: a report of two cases and review of the literature," *Journal of Nephrology*, vol. 18, pp. 791–793, 2005.

[29] T. Olea, C. Hevia, M. A. Bajo, and R. Selgas, "*Pasteurellamultocida* and *Candida albicans* peritonitis," *Nefrología*, vol. 26, pp. 136–138, 2006.

[30] S. J. Antony and K. A. Oglesby, "Peritonitis associated with *Pasteurella multocida* in peritoneal dialysis patients—case report and review of the literature," *Clinical Nephrology*, vol. 68, pp. 52–56, 2007.

[31] I. Kazuko, T. Yoshihiro, T. Tsutomu et al., "Two case reports of *Pasteurella peritonitis* in peritoneal dialysis," *Journal of the Japanese Society for Dialysis Therapy*, vol. 41, no. 3, pp. 213–218, 2008.

[32] A. Satomura, M. Yanai, T. Fujita et al., "Peritonitis associated with *Pasteurellamultocida*: molecular evidence of zoonotic etiology," *Therapeutic Apheresis and Dialysis*, vol. 14, no. 3, pp. 373–376, 2010.

[33] G. A. Weiss and M. Panesar, "*Pasteurellamultocida* peritonitis with bacteremia on initiation of peritoneal dialysis," *Peritoneal Dialysis International*, vol. 32, no. 3, pp. 363–364, 2012.

[34] Y. S. Al-Fifi, C. Sathianathan, B. L. Murray, and M. J. Alfa, "Pets are risky business for patients undergoing continuous ambulatory peritoneal dialysis," *Canadian Journal of Infectious Diseases and Medical Microbiology*, vol. 24, no. 3, pp. e96–e98, 2013.

[35] P. G. Poliquin, P. Lagacé-Wiens, M. Verrelli, D. W. Allen, and J. M. Embil, "*Pasteurella* species peritoneal dialysis-associated peritonitis: household pets as a risk factor," *Canadian Journal of Infectious Diseases and Medical Microbiology*, vol. 26, pp. 52–55, 2015.

[36] F. F. Girón, J. M. S. Martín, E. R. Gómez et al., "Simultaneous *Streptococcus canis* and *Pasteurellamultocida* peritonitis in a peritoneal dialysis patient," *Peritoneal Dialysis International*, vol. 37, pp. 483–484, 2017.

[37] J. A. Akoh, "Peritoneal dialysis associated infections: an update on diagnosis and management," *World Journal of Nephrology*, vol. 1, no. 4, pp. 106–122, 2012.

8

A Novel Homozygous Mutation in the *COL4A4* Gene (Gly1436del) Causing Alport Syndrome Exposed by Pregnancy: A Case Report and Review of the Literature

Ulrich Jehn,[1] Cornelie Müller-Hofstede,[2] Barbara Heitplatz,[3] Veerle Van Marck,[3] Stefan Reuter,[1] Hermann Pavenstädt,[1] and Britta George[1]

[1]*Department of Medicine D, Division of General Internal Medicine, Nephrology and Rheumatology, University Hospital of Münster, Münster 48149, Germany*
[2]*Institute of Human Genetics, University Hospital of Münster, Münster 48149, Germany*
[3]*Gerhard Domagk Institute of Pathology, University Hospital Münster, Münster 48149, Germany*

Correspondence should be addressed to Ulrich Jehn; ulrich.jehn@ukmuenster.de

Academic Editor: Hern n Trimarchi

Background. Alport syndrome results from a hereditary defect of collagen IV synthesis. This causes progressive glomerular disease, ocular abnormalities, and inner ear impairment. *Case Presentation.* Herein, we present a case of Alport syndrome in a 28-year-old woman caused by a novel mutation (Gly1436del) in the *COL4A4* gene that was not unveiled until her first pregnancy. Within the 29th pregnancy week, our patient presented with massive proteinuria and nephrotic syndrome. Light microscopic examination of a kidney biopsy showed typical histological features of segmental sclerosis, and electron microscopy revealed extensive podocyte alterations as well as thickness of glomerular basement membranes with splitting of the lamina densa. One and a half years after childbirth, renal function deteriorated to a preterminal stage, whereas nephrotic syndrome subsided quickly after delivery. *Conclusion.* This case report highlights the awareness of atypical AS courses and emphasizes the importance of genetic testing in such cases.

1. Background

Alport syndrome (AS) is a hereditary disease that impairs the synthesis of type IV collagen. It clinically presents with progressive glomerular disease, ocular abnormalities, and sensorineural hearing loss [1]. Atypical manifestations include leiomyomatosis and vascular alterations [2].

AS is inherited either X-linked (XLAS, ~ 80–85% of cases), autosomal dominant (ADAS, ~ 5%), or autosomal recessive (ARAS, ~ 10–15%). Mutations can affect the genes *COL4A3*, *COL4A4* (both located on chromosome 2, ADAS or ARAS), and *COL4A5* (located on the X-chromosome, XLAS), which encode $\alpha3$, $\alpha4$, and $\alpha5$ chains of type IV collagen, respectively. To date, at least 1422 mutations causing AS have been reported [3].

The renal genotype-phenotype correlation of AS is variable, differs to some extent between males and females, and is among others dependent on the mode of inheritance (see below). The main clinical findings are microscopic hematuria, proteinuria, and progressive loss of renal function culminating in end-stage renal disease (ESRD) [4]. Heterozygous mutations in *COL4A3* or *COL4A4* usually present as thin basement membrane nephropathy without impairment of renal function [5].

In women, the first clinical manifestation of AS may appear as nephrotic syndrome during pregnancy, as pregnancy-related hyperfiltration may acutely worsen renal function [6, 7]. However, due to the unspecific and variably graded clinical manifestations and the possible progression towards a renal phenotype with histological patterns of more common glomerular entities associated with proteinuria, AS remains a highly under- or misdiagnosed entity [4].

Therapeutic options to slow down the progression of renal failure and proteinuria in AS are limited. They include the administration of angiotensin-converting enzyme-inhibitors (ACE-I), in second-line angiotensin-receptor blockers (ARBs) or aldosterone inhibitors [4], and strict treatment of arterial hypertension. Other therapeutical options such as antisense oligonucleotides or stem-cell administration are at an experimental stage [8]. An anti-inflammatory approach using bardoxolone methyl, which inhibits NF-$\kappa\beta$, is currently being investigated in a phase-3 clinical trial [9].

In this manuscript, we present a case of AS caused by a novel *COL4A4* mutation in a 28-year-old woman, which was fulminantly exposed by pregnancy.

2. Case Presentation

A 28-year-old woman from Syria presented with nephrotic syndrome starting during the 29th week of her first pregnancy. Clinically, she showed anasarca with pleural effusions, ascites, and peripheral edema. At admission to our hospital, the patient showed normal blood pressure without antihypertensive medication. Initial laboratory findings included spot urine proteinuria of 17.2 g/g creatinine, hypoproteinemia of 3.8 g/dl [6.6–8.3 g/dl], serum albumin of 1.83 g/dl [3.9–5.0 g/dl], and serum creatinine of 1.4 mg/dl [<0.9 mg/dl] with an eGFR of 51 ml/min/1.73 m^2 (CKD-EPI formula).

For an overview of the patient's baseline characteristics, see Table 1.

There were no preexisting diseases in her medical history. Unfortunately, data on the renal function prior to her pregnancy are not available. Medical history revealed that her only sibling, an older sister, who still lives in Syria, was also diagnosed with nephrotic syndrome, which progressed to ESRD and was treated with a kidney transplantation. Interestingly, the cause of ESRD in the patient's sister has not yet been identified, but the onset of the sister's kidney disease also manifested during pregnancy. Both parents, who also live in Syria, do not knowingly suffer from any renal disease to the knowledge of our patient. Nevertheless, they have not been tested for asymptomatic microhematuria and/or microalbuminuria.

Extensive diagnostic workup was performed. Among others, phospholipase A2- (PLA2-) receptor- and thrombospondin type 1 domain-containing 7A (THSD7A) antibodies were negative, as well as ANA, ANCA, and anti-GBM antibodies. Preeclampsia was excluded by negative soluble fms-like tyrosine kinase-1/placental growth factor (sFlt/PlGF) ratio.

Given the clinical presentation, steroid therapy with prednisolone 1 mg/kg body weight was commenced.

At 37 + 0 weeks of gestation, our patient was admitted to the obstetrics department for pharmacological induction of labor. Because cardiotocography revealed fetal distress and profuse vaginal bleeding caused by premature placental detachment during the opening period, an emergency C-section was performed. After transfusion of six red blood cell concentrates, the further postpartum course was unremarkable both for our patient and the newborn from a gynaecological and pediatric point of view, respectively.

Two weeks after delivery, a kidney biopsy was performed. Light microscopic examination showed segmental sclerosis in 4 of 15 glomeruli (see Figure 1). Electron microscopy revealed extensive podocyte alterations with subtotal loss and effacement of the foot processes, as well as an irregular aspect of the glomerular basement membranes. Areas of remarkable thinning up to 130 nm alternated with areas with a multilamellar appearance with splitting of the lamina densa, the latter accounting for approximately 75% of the total basement membrane surface (see Figure 2).

Based on her medical history and actual findings suggestive of a hereditary AS, our patient underwent genetic evaluation.

Molecular genetic analysis proved an inframe deletion c.4307_4309del p.(Gly1436del) in the *Col4A4* gene causing loss of the amino-acid glycine. A wild-type allele was not detectable. Therefore, the mutation in our patient is probably present in a homozygous form. The patient believes that her parents are not consanguineous.

Treatment with ACE-I at the maximum dosage and good blood pressure control resulted in a significant decrease in proteinuria from 17.2 to 1 g/g creatinine three months postpartum, while eGFR further decreased to 37 ml/min/1.73 m^2. During the following eighteen months, renal function deteriorated to a preterminal stage (eGFR 15 ml/min/1.73 m^2), paralleled by a moderate increase in proteinuria to 2.4 g/g creatinine.

Of note, there is no clinical evidence of manifest ocular or inner ear involvement in our patient to date.

3. Discussion and Conclusions

Herein, we report the clinical manifestation of AS caused by the present inframe deletion c.4307_4309del p (Gly1436del) in the *Col4A4* gene, which is described here for the first time.

Based on the suggested homozygosity found in our patient and the fact that her parents were not noticeably affected, this constellation points towards an autosomal-recessive mode of inheritance.

At present, our patient's AS presents exclusively with significant renal involvement. Interestingly, in ARAS females, ocular and inner ear involvement is only present in a minority of patients [6, 10]. Basically, genotype-phenotype correlation in AS is variable. Most data addressing this question are available on the more common (85%) XLAS, whereas data on genotype-phenotype correlation in ARAS (15%) are sparse [11]. In XLAS, severe mutations as deletions, rearrangements, indels, and nonsense mutations are associated with earlier onset of ESRD compared to missense mutations (mean age 22.5 vs. 26.7 years) [11, 12]. Fitting to that, individuals with splice mutations or truncating mutations show a two-fold greater probability of developing ocular or hearing abnormalities [12].

In ARAS patients, mean age at ESRD onset was not found to be different for *COL4A3* or *COL4A4* mutations

Table 1: Initial patient's characteristics and laboratory results.

Baseline characteristics	
Age	28 years
Pregnancy week	29th
Symptoms	Nephrotic syndrome anasarca
Medical history	Empty
Family history	Sister with unknown nephrotic ESRD also unveiled by pregnancy
Initial laboratory results	
Serum creatinine	1.4 mg/dl [<0.9 mg/dl]
eGFR	51 ml/min/1.73 m^2
Protein/creatinine ratio	17.2 g/g creatinine
Total serum protein	3.8 g/dl [6.6–8.3 g/dl]
Serum albumin	1.8 g/dl [3.9–5.0 g/dl]
Initial blood pressure	130/70 mmHg

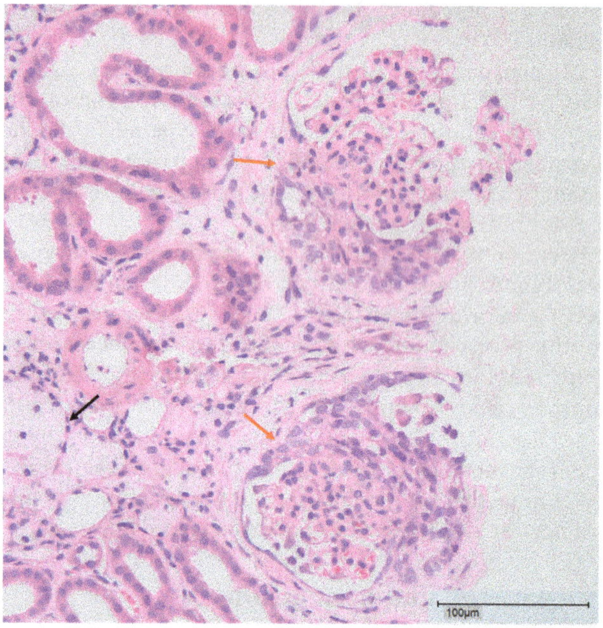

Figure 1: Photomicrography of the patient's kidney biopsy. It shows segmental sclerosis of 2 glomeruli (red arrows). The black arrow marks interstitial foamy macrophages, often seen in AS as well as in other types of chronic nephrosis. Bar: 100 μm.

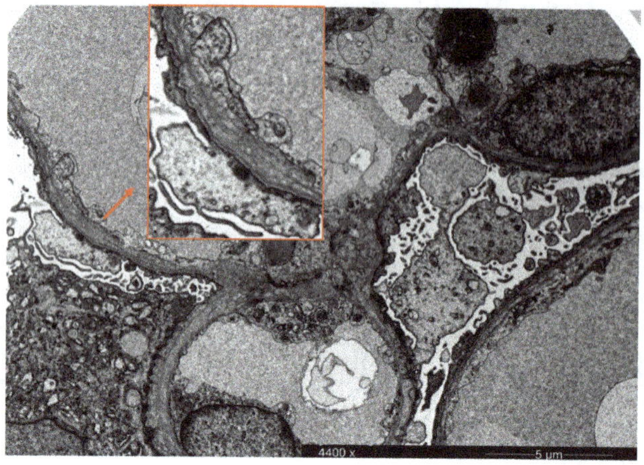

Figure 2: Electron micrography of the patient's kidney biopsy. It visualizes irregular thickness of glomerular basement membranes with splitting of the lamina densa (inset red box, 2-fold magnification) and severe podocyte foot process effacement. Bar: 5 μm.

compared to those individuals with X-linked *COL4A5* mutations. Furthermore, Savige et al. did not detect differences for age at ESRD onset between homozygous and compound heterozygous mutations [11]. Congruent to XLAS, homozygous or compound heterozygous deletions, rearrangements, indels, and nonsense mutations enhance the onset of ESRD compared to those cases with missense mutations [11].

The patient's sister, who still lives in Syria, also suffered from nephrotic syndrome with initial presentation during pregnancy and has since received a kidney transplant. Although the underlying cause of the kidney failure has not been evaluated, the constellation strongly suggests that the sister may also have inherited AS.

Even if the patient denies a kinship relationship between her parents, this seems to be the most likely mode of inheritance [13]. In Middle Eastern countries, consanguinity is still a common phenomenon with 30.3% of marriages in urban and 39.8% in rural areas [14].

It is known that heterozygous mutations in the *Col4A4* gene are associated with benign forms of familiar hematuria, which are usually neither progressive nor lead to renal failure. This explains the bland parental medical history regarding renal disease [8]. However, neither our patient's parents nor her sister have been genetically evaluated in Syria.

In our patient, nephrotic syndrome occurred during the 29th week of pregnancy with massive proteinuria and acute kidney failure. According to the literature, presentation of AS with these symptoms during the 29th–32nd pregnancy week is typical for pregnant women with AS [7, 15].

The age at the time of clinical manifestation in the presented case of AS, which is highly suggestive for ARAS, was 28 years. Referring to the literature, this tends to be a relatively late onset of ARAS [10, 11].

Histologically, AS presented as segmental sclerosis in this case. In another case report of ARAS caused by a *Col4A4* mutation with manifestation during pregnancy, Drury et al. described the histological presentation of their patient as global segmental glomerulosclerosis with collapsing features, which might be caused by the additive effect of hyperfiltration during pregnancy [6]. Generally, the literature review shows an association of collagen IV mutations with segmental sclerosis [5, 16], which may lead to misdiagnosis of collagen IV nephropathies as FSGS [6].

The present case report is intended to raise awareness of atypical courses of AS and emphasizes the importance of medical family history and genetic testing in such cases.

Abbreviations

ACE-I:	Angiotensin-converting enzyme-inhibitors
ADAS:	Autosomal dominant Alport syndrome
ANA:	Antinuclear antibodies
ANCA:	Antineutrophil cytoplasmic antibodies
ARAS:	Autosomal recessive Alport syndrome
ARB:	Angiotensin-receptor blockers
AS:	Alport syndrome
CKD-EPI:	Chronic kidney disease epidemiology collaboration
ESRD:	End-stage renal disease
FSGS:	Focal segmental glomerulosclerosis
eGFR:	Estimated glomerular filtration rate
GBM:	Glomerular basement membrane
Indel:	Insertion/deletion
NF-$\kappa\beta$:	Nuclear factor "kappa-light-chain-enhancer" of activated B-cells
PlGF:	Placental growth factor
PLA2:	Phospholipase A2
sFlt:	Soluble fms-like tyrosine kinase-1
THSD7A:	Thrombospondin type 1 domain-containing 7A
XLAS:	X-linked Alport syndrome.

Consent

Written informed consent was obtained from the patient prior to research participation and for publication of this case report and any accompanying images.

Disclosure

The research and publication of this case report was performed as part of the employment of all contributing authors at the University Hospital of Münster, Germany.

Authors' Contributions

UJ, CMH, and BG wrote the case report. SR and HP wrote the case report and supervised the work. VVM and BH performed histopathological analysis of biopsy specimens. All authors read and approved the manuscript.

Acknowledgments

The APC was funded by the Open Access Fund of the University of Münster.

References

[1] C. E. Kashtan, J. Ding, G. Garosi et al., "Alport syndrome: a unified classification of genetic disorders of collagen IV $\alpha345$: a position paper of the alport syndrome classification working group," *Kidney International*, vol. 93, no. 5, pp. 1045–1051, 2018.

[2] J. Kruegel, D. Rubel, and O. Gross, "Alport syndrome-insights from basic and clinical research," *Nature Reviews Nephrology*, vol. 9, no. 3, pp. 170–178, 2013.

[3] P. Vos, R. Zietse, M. van Geel, A. S. Brooks, and K. Cransberg, "Diagnosing alport syndrome: lessons from the pediatric ward," *Nephron*, vol. 140, no. 3, pp. 203–210, 2018.

[4] A. L. Pedrosa, L. Bitencourt, R. M. Paranhos, C. A. Leitáo, G. C. Ferreira, and R. M. Simões E Silva, "Alport syndrome: a comprehensive review on genetics, pathophysiology, histology, clinical, and therapeutic perspectives," *Current Medicinal Chemistry*, vol. 28, no. 27, pp. 5602–5624, 2021.

[5] K. Voskarides, A. Pierides, and C. Deltas, "COL4A3/COL4A4 mutations link familial hematuria and focal segmental glomerulosclerosis. glomerular epithelium destruction via basement membrane thinning?" *Connective Tissue Research*, vol. 49, no. 3, pp. 283–288, 2008.

[6] E. R. Drury, I. E. Stillman, M. R. Pollak, and B. M. Denker, "Autosomal recessive alport syndrome unveiled by pregnancy," *Nephron*, vol. 143, no. 4, pp. 288–292, 2019.

[7] F. Brunini, B. Zaina, D. Gianfreda et al., "Alport syndrome and pregnancy: a case series and literature review," *Archives of Gynecology and Obstetrics*, vol. 297, no. 6, pp. 1421–1431, 2018.

[8] K. Nozu, K. Nakanishi, Y. Abe et al., "A review of clinical characteristics and genetic backgrounds in alport syndrome," *Clinical and Experimental Nephrology*, vol. 23, no. 2, pp. 158–168, 2019.

[9] G. M. Chertow, G. B. Appel, S. Andreoli et al., "Study design and baseline characteristics of the CARDINAL trial: a phase 3 study of bardoxolone methyl in patients with alport syndrome," *American Journal of Nephrology*, vol. 52, no. 3, pp. 180–189, 2021.

[10] M. Oka, K. Nozu, H. Kaito et al., "Natural history of genetically proven autosomal recessive alport syndrome," *Pediatric Nephrology*, vol. 29, no. 9, pp. 1535–1544, 2014.

[11] J. Savige, H. Storey, H. Il Cheong et al., "X-linked and autosomal recessive alport syndrome: pathogenic variant features and further genotype-phenotype correlations," *PLoS One*, vol. 11, no. 9, Article ID e0161802, 2016.

[12] M. R. Bekheirnia, B. Reed, M. C. Gregory et al., "Genotype-phenotype correlation in X-linked alport syndrome," *Journal of the American Society of Nephrology*, vol. 21, no. 5, pp. 876–883, 2010.

[13] E. D. Avner, *Pediatric Nephrology*, Springer, Berlin, Germany, 2009.

[14] H. Othman and M. Saadat, "Prevalence of consanguineous marriages in Syria," *Journal of Biosocial Science*, vol. 41, no. 5, pp. 685–692, 2009.

[15] F. Pepe, F. Di Guardo, E. Zambrotta et al., "Renal impairment in alport syndrome pregnant woman: case report and review of the literature," *Clinical Case Reports*, vol. 8, no. 12, pp. 3003–3007, 2020.

[16] K. Voskarides, L. Damianou, V. Neocleous et al., "COL4A3/COL4A4Mutations producing focal segmental glomerulosclerosis and renal failure in thin basement membrane nephropathy," *Journal of the American Society of Nephrology*, vol. 18, no. 11, pp. 3004–3016, 2007.

9

A Case of De Novo Antiglomerular Basement Membrane Disease Presenting during Pregnancy

F. A. K. Lodhi,[1] T. Akcan,[1] J. N. Mojarrab,[1] S. Sajjad,[2] and R. Blonsky[3]

[1]*Department of Internal Medicine, Marshfield Clinic Health System, Marshfield, WI, USA*
[2]*Department of Pathology, Marshfield Clinic Health System, Marshfield, WI, USA*
[3]*Department of Nephrology, Marshfield Clinic Health System, Marshfield, WI, USA*

Correspondence should be addressed to F. A. K. Lodhi; lodhi.fahad@marshfieldclinic.org

Academic Editor: Rumeyza Kazancioglu

Background. Acute kidney injury (AKI) requiring dialysis during pregnancy is uncommon. We present a case of a young female diagnosed with antiglomerular basement membrane (anti-GBM) disease during pregnancy. *Case Presentation.* A 23-year-old woman approximately 15 weeks pregnant experienced weakness, nausea, vomiting, and anorexia for one week and anuria for 48 hours. No known drug allergies and no significant social or family history for kidney or genitourinary disease were reported. Laboratory analysis revealed anemia, life-threatening hyperkalemia, AKI, and elevated antiglomerular basement membrane (GBM) antibodies. Renal biopsy revealed 100% cellular crescents, confirming the diagnosis. The patient was treated using plasmapheresis and methylprednisolone followed by oral steroids, azathioprine, and tacrolimus. At 24 weeks and 4 days of gestation, the patient had hypoxic respiratory failure as well as preterm premature rupture of membranes. Due to the development of infection and lack of renal recovery, immunosuppression was discontinued. At 28 weeks and 0 days of gestation, the patient developed uncontrollable hypertension requiring emergent delivery. Postpartum, her hypertension improved without signs of preeclampsia though still requires dialysis. *Discussion.* Pregnancy presents a unique challenge for providers treating patients with anti-GBM disease. Fetal safety should be considered and risks thoroughly discussed with the patient when choosing an immunosuppressive regimen for this condition.

1. Introduction

Antiglomerular basement membrane (anti-GBM) disease is a rare, life-threatening, small vessel vasculitis usually presenting as rapidly progressive glomerulonephritis characterized by glomerular cellular crescents and linear deposits of IgG along the GBM [1]. Anti-GBM disease is reported to have an incidence of less than 1 per million population per year [2]. Standard therapy today consists of a combination of plasmapheresis, corticosteroids, and immunosuppressive drugs [3]. Levy et al. [4] reported that patients with anti-GBM disease who are dialysis-dependent on presentation showed only 8% renal survival at 1 year despite immunosuppression and plasma exchange. Given its rarity, there are only a handful of case reports documenting the occurrence of anti-GBM disease during pregnancy, treatments offered and long-term follow-up revealing the outcome of pregnancy, or the disease process itself, as a majority of pregnancies are terminated prior to term delivery to prevent worsening of conditions [5–8].

Here, we present a young woman diagnosed with anti-GBM disease early in her pregnancy and later giving birth prematurely with pre- and postpartum maternal, fetal, and neonatal course of events.

2. Case Presentation

A 23-year-old previously healthy woman at 15 weeks and 3 days gestation of her third pregnancy presented to the emergency department with complaints of persistent watery diarrhea, nausea, and vomiting for one week, bilateral lower extremity numbness, tingling, and weakness for five days, and anuria for 48 hours. Her past medical history was significant for obesity with a body mass index of 37.2 kg/m^2, vaginal delivery of a healthy female infant at 41 weeks of gestation 10 months prior to the current presentation, and a first-trimester miscarriage six months prior to presentation. Her medications included prenatal vitamins, folic acid, vitamin C, and ondansetron for nausea. She denied alcohol intake, tobacco use, or substance abuse. She had no known drug allergies. There was no previous history of renal or pulmonary disease. No family disease was known and she had no other relevant findings in her medical history.

The patient was afebrile on presentation with a blood pressure of 114/53 mmHg, a heart rate of 68 beats/minute, a respiratory rate of 31 breaths/minute, and an oxygen saturation of 98% on room air. The remainder of her systemic examination findings, including those for her chest, were within normal limits.

Initial laboratory workup included a complete blood count and comprehensive metabolic panel which showed anemia and electrolyte imbalance. Blood cell analysis revealed a normal total protein level, white blood cell count of 10.1×10^3 μL, mean corpuscular volume (MCV) of 72 fL, low serum albumin of 3.1 g/dL, hemoglobin level of 7.8 g/dL, and hematocrit of 24.1 % and elevated red cell distribution width (RDW). Electrolyte and metabolite analysis revealed low sodium level (129 mmol/L) and elevated potassium, creatinine, and blood urea nitrogen (BUN) levels of 7.1 mmol/L, 19.8 mg/dL, and 113 mg/dL, respectively, with a decreased estimated glomerular filtration rate (eGFR) of 2.2 mL/min compared to normal values from a metabolic profile checked six months prior and an elevated hemoglobin level of 12.3 g/dL one month prior to presentation. Transaminases were within normal limits. Urinalysis showed hematuria with >100 red blood cells per field and proteinuria with 100 mg/dL protein. Furthermore, the patient was found to have an elevated erythrocyte sedimentation rate (ESR) of 117 mm/hr and mildly elevated haptoglobin of 298 mg/dL. Hematological analysis and workup for evidence of disseminated intravascular coagulation revealed a normal (INR) of 1.0, activated partial thromboplastin time (APTT) of 36.0 seconds, and normal platelet response yet elevated levels of fibrinogen (798 mg/dL) and D-dimer (2,461 ng/mL). Iron panel detected a normal serum iron level of 46 μg/dL and low total iron-binding capacity (TIBC) of 225 μg/dL with a corresponding transferrin saturation percentage of 20%, reticulocyte count of 25.5×10^2 μL, and reticulocyte percentage of 0.78.

Further laboratory workup for autoimmune conditions, infectious disease, or history of drug use revealed elevated levels of serum anti-GBM antibodies at 7.6 units (U)/mL and no evidence for underlying microbial infection or drug-induced toxicity. Serum samples were negative for cryoglobulins, antiphospholipid, antinuclear, and cytoplasmic antibodies as well as extractable nuclear antigen and antibodies to red blood cells or ADAMS TS 13. Complement levels (C3 and C4) were within normal limits.

A renal ultrasound was performed and measured the right kidney at $14.6 \times 7.7 \times 7.8$ cm and $13.7 \times 7.2 \times 7.2$ cm for the left kidney and increased resistance pattern in the renal vasculature with no evidence of hydronephrosis, renal calculi, or focal lesions. The bladder appeared normal. No cause of acute renal failure was identified by diagnostic imaging. Obstetrical extended ultrasound revealed a single, living intrauterine gestation at 15 weeks and 3 days based on menstrual dates and fetal biometric measurements. Fetal growth was found to be appropriate for gestational age. Anatomic survey was limited due to early gestational age but overall appeared to be unremarkable. The fetus was found to be active in normal amniotic fluid volume. No CT chest was obtained on the initial presentation due to the absence of pulmonary symptoms and in an effort to avoid radiation exposure.

The patient received hemodialysis on day one via the right internal jugular temporary hemodialysis catheter placed emergently in ICU. The urgent need for pathological diagnosis and its associated risk to the mother and the fetus was thoroughly discussed with the patient and obstetrics/gynecology with the decision made to proceed with renal biopsy with continuous fetal monitoring and administration of desmopressin for bleeding risk associated with acute kidney injury and uremic platelets. Renal biopsy revealed findings consistent with rapidly progressing glomerulonephritis with 100% cellular crescents and immunofluorescence exhibiting diffuse linear staining along the glomerular basement membrane with IgG (3+), C3 (3+), kappa (3+), and lambda (2+) stains (Figures 1(a)–1(d)). Electron microscopy supported light microscopy findings of a diagnosis of anti-GBM disease. The patient underwent intermittent hemodialysis six days a week, four hours each (24 hours/week) to maintain electrolytes and laboratory numbers as close to normal as possible with pregnancy. Plasmapheresis was done for a total of seven treatments via the same right internal jugular access as used for hemodialysis. 1 plasma volume was exchanged, and for replacement, 5% albumin was used. However, for initial treatment, two units of fresh frozen plasma were used as it was the day following renal biopsy. Blood flow was 85 mL/min with a schedule of two days on with one day off to allow for clotting factors to reform. No anticoagulation was used for in-patient hemodialysis, and citrate with calcium infusion was used during plasmapheresis. She was treated with 1 g intravenous methylprednisolone every three days followed by oral prednisone daily with a slow taper, azathioprine 50 mg oral daily with tapering to a goal dose of 150 mg daily after a thiopurine methyltransferase (TPMT) enzyme assay tested negative, and 3 mg tacrolimus every 12 hours with a goal trough level of 3–7. Pneumocystis carinii pneumonia prophylaxis was also initiated with atovaquone. Other treatments included intravenous ferric gluconate for a total of five doses followed by darbepoetin alfa weekly. Renal function was monitored during the patient's hospital stay which showed mild improvement in creatinine, but unfortunately, she continued to be dialysis-dependent. A tunneled dialysis catheter was placed, and the patient was discharged in a stable condition after a 10-day hospital stay with the fetus at a gestational age of 16 weeks and 6 days. The patient followed up with her primary care physician, nephrologist, and obstetrician in the outpatient setting and remained stable on hemodialysis and immunosuppressive regimen until two months later when she was admitted again with

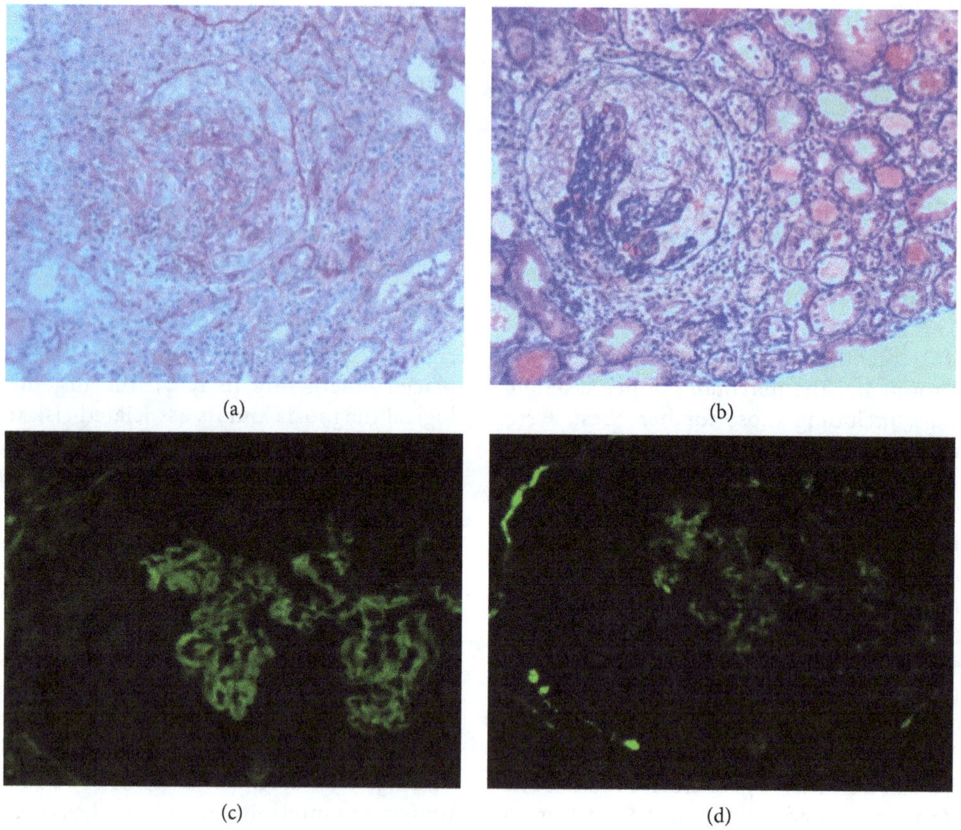

Figure 1: 27 glomeruli were seen on the renal biopsy specimen with the following histological findings. (a) Fibrocellular crescents in the glomeruli and lymphocyte infiltration around the tubule-interstitium near the glomerulus (periodic acid-Schiff (PAS) staining ×200). (b) Glomerulus with large crescent and collapsed tuft (Jones Silver staining ×200). (c, d) Immunofluorescence staining revealed linear staining along the glomerular capillary loops (IgG staining ×400).

preterm premature rupture of membranes at 24 weeks and 4 days of gestation. The patient had experienced shortness of breath and chest tightness for several weeks which were considered to be secondary to her pregnancy.

Given concerns for shortness of breath and chest tightness, a chest X-ray and chest computed tomography (CT) scan (Figure 2) were performed and were negative for pulmonary embolism though she developed bilateral patchy infiltrates of undetermined etiology while being on chronic immunosuppression for the last two months with tacrolimus, azathioprine, and prednisone. She was transferred to the critical care unit for airway monitoring. On admission, her systolic blood pressure was elevated at 130 mmHg, and her oxygen saturation rose to 96% on 6 L via oxygen mask. Medication history included tacrolimus, azathioprine, nifedipine, labetalol, prednisone, progesterone vaginal suppositories, and six times per week hemodialysis. Physical examination revealed 2+ pedal edema bilaterally, and fetal examination revealed baseline fetal heart tones of 150 s, moderate variability, no decelerations, and cephalic presentation. The serum microbial panel for hepatitis B surface antigen, rubella, syphilis, gonococcal, chlamydia, and HIV was negative. The respiratory viral panel was positive for parainfluenza virus. The patient was continued on antibiotics with symptomatic management for parainfluenza infection.

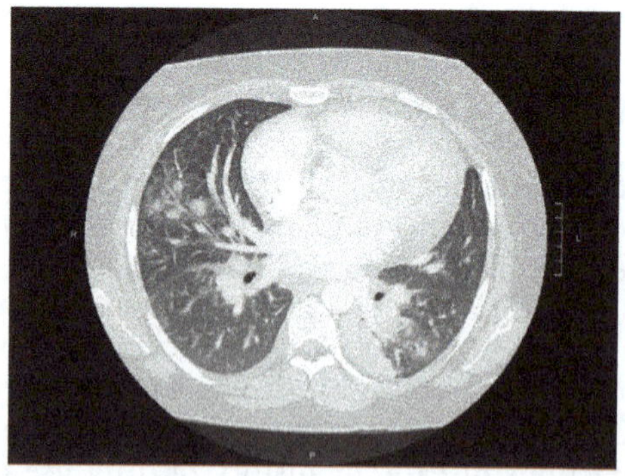

Figure 2: Computed tomography pulmonary angiogram showing no pulmonary embolism; multifocal pulmonary infiltrates; small right-sided pleural effusion; very small pericardial effusion; cardiomegaly.

Later, the patient developed severe hypertension which was not manageable with antihypertensive drugs, and the decision was made to deliver the fetus. Emergent cesarean section was performed at 28–0/7 weeks, and a male neonate, 1.1 kg with Apgar scores of 1/6/7, was delivered. The patient's postpartum course was relatively uncomplicated with no development of postpartum preeclampsia. The patient remained on hemodialysis until the end of her postpartum period, following which she transitioned to peritoneal dialysis and is currently awaiting a transplant.

3. Discussion

Anti-GBM antibody disease during pregnancy is a very rare occurrence. There are a few case reports in the literature with biopsy-proven anti-GBM disease and varied presentations. The outcomes of infants from mothers with anti-GBM disease during pregnancy are generally poor, often resulting in stillbirth and both natural and artificial abortion [5–8]. Moreover, to date, only five cases resulted in successful delivery which are summarized as follows.

Deubner et al. [9] described a case of a pregnant woman with rapidly progressive glomerulonephritis (RPGN) secondary to anti-GBM disease which flared postpartum with the development of precipitous renal failure. The patient experienced a full-term pregnancy and gave birth to a healthy infant. Deubner et al. postulated that the placenta may have served as an adsorptive surface for the autoantibody and may have ameliorated her symptoms. Yankowitz et al. [10] reported the case of a 28-year-old woman who was diagnosed with anti-GBM disease three months prior to her pregnancy and was treated with intensive hemodialysis and corticosteroids along with cyclophosphamide and who delivered an infant at 37 weeks of gestation. The patient's anti-GBM antibody levels became negative during pregnancy and were detected again after delivery. Al Harbi et al. [11] reported a case of a 30-year-old woman who presented with acute renal failure at 28 weeks of gestation and was treated with antibiotics, intensive hemodialysis, and corticosteroids and delivered an infant at 34 weeks of gestation. Sprenger-Maehr et al. [12] also described a case of a 30-year-old woman with anti-GBM disease who was treated with plasma exchange, corticosteroids, cyclophosphamide, and rituximab and delivered an infant at 38 weeks of gestation. Lastly, Vasiliou et al. [13] reported a 34-year-old woman who presented with RPGN and was diagnosed with anti-GBM disease during 18 weeks of gestation. She was treated with hemodialysis, intermittent plasmapheresis, and immunosuppressive therapy with tapering steroids and azathioprine. In all cases, reduction of anti-GBM antibodies via placental adsorption or combination immunosuppressive treatment and hemodialysis appears to improve pregnancy outcome.

The present case is unique in terms of diagnosis, flare-up, and treatment for anti-GBM disease during the course of pregnancy followed by a successful preterm delivery. In our case, the patient presented with anti-GBM disease during the early phase of her third pregnancy with no evidence of kidney dysfunction during her previous pregnancies. The anti-GBM antibody titers were very high at the time of diagnosis and unlike the cases reported by Deubner et al. [9] and Yankowitz et al. [10] did not become negative after treatment during pregnancy or 5 months postpartum. Our patient experienced a precipitous decline in renal function with only moderate improvement with immunosuppression along with intensive plasma exchange and hemodialysis. Treatment with immunosuppressive agents such as tacrolimus and azathioprine in addition to steroids allowed us to defer administration of cyclophosphamide use and resulted in a successful delivery. To our knowledge, this is the first report in the literature of a woman diagnosed with anti-GBM disease during early pregnancy who was treated with a combination of immunosuppressive drugs tacrolimus and azathioprine to result in a successful delivery.

Maternal, pregnancy, and fetal outcomes of anti-GBM disease in pregnancy are poor and are associated with uncontrolled vasculitis [5–8]. The treatment of choice in anti-GBM antibody disease is intensive plasmapheresis combined with immunosuppressive agents such as steroids, cyclophosphamide, and azathioprine [3, 4]. Plasmapheresis removes circulating anti-GBM antibodies and other mediators of inflammation while immunosuppressive agents minimize new antibody formation. Plasmapheresis is generally considered safe in pregnancy [14]. Systemic corticosteroids are generally considered low risk for teratogenicity although there are historical associations of this regimen to cleft palate [15]. Cyclophosphamide is the main immunosuppressive drug that has been used in anti-GBM disease for over 30 years. The challenge arises in pregnant patients where the literature does not support the use of cyclophosphamide, as there is a risk of teratogenicity, especially in the first trimester [16]. Growth retardation, suppression of fetal hematopoiesis, and impaired neurological development have been reported with use later in pregnancy in the second and third trimesters [17, 18]. Cyclophosphamide is excreted in breast milk and is also contraindicated during breastfeeding [19]. The use of rituximab for the treatment of anti-GBM disease has also been explored in the medical literature. However, limited data exist, but the use of this B-cell depleting agent may be considered as a viable option in anti-GBM disease that is refractory to standard treatment [20]. Pregnancy complicates its use, and after a detailed discussion regarding risks and benefits, the decision was made to not proceed with this agent due to maternal concerns of fetal B-cell depletion and other hematological abnormalities [21]. The use of tacrolimus and azathioprine is compatible in pregnancy and breastfeeding as per current literature [16, 22, 23]. Our patient presented in the second trimester during which time the use of cyclophosphamide is acceptable, but due to the lack of sufficient evidence regarding renal recovery with its use in anti-GBM disease, the decision was made to proceed with tacrolimus and azathioprine. The present case is an example that successful deliveries can be achieved in pregnant patients presenting with anti-GBM who are treated with immunosuppressive agents such as tacrolimus and azathioprine in addition to steroids; moreover, use of these agents may permit deferral of cyclophosphamide use until after pregnancy.

4. Conclusion

Anti-GBM disease should be considered in pregnant patients presenting with oligoanuric renal failure. Plasmapheresis and immunosuppression remain the treatments of choice. When choosing an immunosuppressive regimen in pregnancy, fetal safety should be considered and risks thoroughly discussed prior to treatment.

Acknowledgments

The authors acknowledge the Scientific Writing and Publications division of the Marshfield Clinic Research Institute for manuscript editing and submission.

References

[1] K. Gulati and S. P. McAdoo, "Anti-glomerular basement membrane disease," *Rheumatic Disease Clinics of North America*, vol. 44, no. 4, pp. 651–673, 2018.

[2] S. P. McAdoo and C. D. Pusey, "Anti-glomerular basement membrane disease," *Clinical Journal of the American Society of Nephrology*, vol. 12, no. 7, pp. 1162–1172, 2017.

[3] C. O. Savage, C. D. Pusey, C. Bowman, A. J. Rees, and C. M. Lockwood, "Antiglomerular basement membrane antibody mediated disease in the British Isles 1980-4," *Bmj*, vol. 292, no. 6516, pp. 301–304, 1986.

[4] J. B. Levy, A. N. Turner, A. J. Rees, and C. D. Pusey, "Long-term outcome of anti-glomerular basement membrane antibody disease treated with plasma exchange and immunosuppression," *Annals of Internal Medicine*, vol. 134, no. 11, pp. 1033–1042, 2001.

[5] S. Nair, J. George, S. Kumar, N. Gracious, and M. Das, "A case of Goodpasture's syndrome complicating pregnancy with dialysis requiring renal failure responding to plasmapheresis and termination of pregnancy," *Renal Failure*, vol. 35, no. 8, pp. 1173–1175, 2013.

[6] A. Shah, E. Bailey, and S. Hughes, "Goodpasture's syndrome, haemodialysis and pregnancy," *British Journal of Hospital Medicine*, vol. 68, no. 1, pp. 48-49, 2007.

[7] D. E. Nilssen, T. Talseht, and E. K. Brodwall, "The many faces of Goodpasture's syndrome," *Acta Medica Scandinavica*, vol. 220, no. 5, pp. 489–491, 1986.

[8] M. M. Adnan, J. Morton, S. Hashmi, S. Abdul Mujeeb, W. Kern, and B. D. Cowley Jr, "Anti-GBM disease in pregnancy," *Journal of Investigative Medicine High Impact Case Reports*, vol. 4, no. 1, 2016.

[9] H. Deubner, J. P. Wagnild, M. H. Wener, and C. E. Alpers, "Glomerulonephritis with anti-glomerular basement membrane antibody during pregnancy: potential role of the placenta in amelioration of disease," *American Journal of Kidney Diseases*, vol. 25, no. 2, pp. 330–335, 1995.

[10] J. Yankowitz, J. A. Kuller, and R. L. Thomas, "Pregnancy complicated by Goodpasture syndrome," *Obstetrics and Gynecology*, vol. 79, no. 5, pp. 806–808, 1992.

[11] A. Al-Harbi, G. H. Malik, S. A. Al-Mohaya, and M. Akhtar, "Anti-glomerular basement membrane antibody disease presenting as acute renal failure during pregnancy," *Saudi Journal of Kidney Diseases and Transplantation*, vol. 14, no. 4, pp. 516–521, 2003.

[12] H. Sprenger-Mähr, E. Zitt, A. Soleiman, and K. Lhotta, "Successful pregnancy in a patient with pulmonary renal syndrome double-positive for anti-GBM antibodies and p-ANCA," *Clinical Nephrology*, vol. 91, no. 2, pp. 101–106, 2019.

[13] D. M. Vasiliou, C. Maxwell, P. Shah, and M. Sermer, "Goodpasture syndrome in a pregnant woman," *Obstetrics & Gynecology*, vol. 106, no. 5, pp. 1196–1199, 2005.

[14] W. J. Watson, V. L. Katz, and W. A. Bowes Jr, "Plasmapheresis during pregnancy," *Obstetrics and Gynecology*, vol. 76, no. 3 Pt 1, pp. 451–457, 1990.

[15] B. Thomson, G. Joseph, W. F. Clark et al., "Maternal, pregnancy and fetal outcomes in de novo anti-glomerular basement membrane antibody disease in pregnancy: a systematic review," *Clinical Kidney Journal*, vol. 7, no. 5, pp. 450–456, 2014.

[16] M. Østensen, M. Khamashta, M. Lockshin et al., "Anti-inflammatory and immunosuppressive drugs and reproduction," *Arthritis Research & Therapy*, vol. 8, no. 3, p. 209, 2006.

[17] A. N. Baer, F. R. Witter, and M. Petri, "Lupus and pregnancy," *Obstetrical & Gynecological Survey*, vol. 66, no. 10, pp. 639–653, 2011.

[18] G. Lannes, F. R. Elias, B. Cunha et al., "Successful pregnancy after cyclophosphamide therapy for lupus nephritis," *Archives of Gynecology and Obstetrics*, vol. 283, no. S1, pp. 61–65, 2011.

[19] P. Wiernik and J. H. Duncan, "Cyclophosphamide in human milk," *The Lancet*, vol. 297, no. 7705, p. 912, 1971.

[20] R. Jain, H. Dgheim, and A. S. Bomback, "Rituximab for anti-glomerular basement membrane disease," *Kidney International Reports*, vol. 4, no. 4, pp. 614–618, 2019.

[21] E. F. Chakravarty, E. R. Murray, A. Kelman, and P. Farmer, "Pregnancy outcomes after maternal exposure to rituximab," *Blood*, vol. 117, no. 5, pp. 1499–1506, 2011.

[22] A. Jain, R. Venkataramanan, J. J. Fung et al., "Pregnancy after liver transplantation under Tacrolimus1," *Transplantation*, vol. 64, no. 4, pp. 559–565, 1997.

[23] A. B. Jain, R. Shapiro, V. P. Scantlebury et al., "Pregnancy after kidney and kidney-pancreas transplantation under tacrolimus: a single center's experience," *Transplantation*, vol. 77, no. 6, pp. 897–902, 2004.

10

Rifampicin-Associated Secondary Minimal Change Disease Presenting with Nephrotic Syndrome in a Pulmonary Tuberculosis Patient

Satyanand Sathi, Anil Kumar Garg, Manoj Kumar Singh, Virendra Singh Saini, and Devinder Vohra

Department of Medicine, S.M.M.H. Government Medical College, Saharanpur, Uttar Pradesh, India

Correspondence should be addressed to Satyanand Sathi; satyanandsathi@yahoo.com

Academic Editor: Phuong Chi Pham

Various extraglomerular disease processes have been associated with drug-induced secondary minimal change disease (MCD). In a majority of cases, preferably, a hypersensitivity reaction appears to be involved, and in some cases, there is direct toxic effect over glomerular capillaries. There are several reports to demonstrate that rifampicin has been associated with various nephrotoxic adverse effects, but rifampicin-induced secondary minimal change disease (MCD) is very rare. Here, we report the case of a young adult male who presented with nephrotic proteinuria with bland urine sediment after one month of initiation of rifampicin treatment for pulmonary tuberculosis. The patient had no proteinuria before the start of antituberculosis treatment. Renal biopsy showed nonproliferative glomerulopathy and immunofluorescence did not show significant glomerular immune deposits. Electron microscopy showed diffuse effacement of visceral epithelial cell foot processes and did not show any presence of glomerular immune complexes and thickening of glomerular basement membrane, promoting the diagnosis of minimal change nephrotic syndrome. The patient got complete remission after discontinuation of rifampicin.

1. Introduction

Primary minimal change disease (MCD) is characterized by a disorder of charge selective glomerular permselectivity and typical morphological changes in glomerular capillaries without well-defined extra-glomerular disease process [1]. In secondary MCD, the characteristic changes in glomerular permselectivity and morphology are elicited, directly or indirectly by extraglomerular disease process [1]. These extraglomerular disease processes may be neoplasm, toxic reactions to drugs, hypersensitivity, and idiosyncratic reaction [1]. Rifampicin is one of the commonly used standard antituberculosis drugs. However, it has been described to have some nephrotoxic adverse effects [2–6]. The most common type of rifampicin-induced nephrotoxicity is acute renal failure with acute tubular necrosis. Other types of nephrotoxicity are acute interstitial nephritis, light chain proteinuria, and rapidly progressive glomerulonephritis [3]. We herein report a case of rifampicin-associated secondary minimal change disease. Our case patient developed nephrotic syndrome after the start of rifampicin therapy for pulmonary tuberculosis, and there was no associated acute renal failure, acute interstitial nephritis, or acute tubular necrosis. After discontinuation of rifampicin, the patient had complete remission of nephrotic syndrome.

2. Case Presentation

A 26-year-old male was admitted to the hospital with a 2-week history of cough with expectoration and high-grade fever. He had a history of loss of appetite for ten days. On admission, his blood pressure was 116/76 mm Hg and his body temperature was 37.8°C. Rest of the physical examination was unremarkable, and urine analysis did not show any abnormal findings. The patient's laboratory profile was as follows: hemoglobin: 10.6 g/dL; total leukocyte count: 4,100/mm^3; platelet count: 2.6×10^5/mm^3; erythrocyte sedimentation rate (ESR): 58 mm/hr; serum creatinine: 0.86 mg/dL; sodium: 138 mEq/L; potassium: 3.7 mEq/L; and serum albumin: 4.2 g/dL. The chest X-ray showed dense homogenous opacity in right upper zone area of lung. PPD (purified protein derivative of tuberculin) skin test showed a positive reaction, and sputum smear for acid-fast bacilli was found to be positive. On the basis of clinical symptoms, high ESR, positive PPD skin test, positive sputum smear for acid-fast bacilli, and chest X-ray findings, the diagnosis of pulmonary tuberculosis was made. The antituberculosis treatment was started with rifampicin 450 mg/day, isoniazid 300 mg/day, ethambutol hydrochloride 800 mg/day, and pyrazinamide 1000 mg/day.

After one month of daily treatment, the patient became sputum smear negative for acid-fast bacilli, but he developed sudden onset swelling whole over the body. The patient's laboratory profile at that time was as follows: hemoglobin: 12.9 g/dL; total leukocyte count: 9,700/mm^3; platelet count: 2.6×10^5/mm^3; urinary protein: 3+; urinary sugar: 0; urine microscopy—white blood cell count: 2-3/high-power field; red blood cell count: 0-1/high-power field; urinary pH: 6.2; urinary albumin: 3+; serum albumin: 2.7 g/dL; serum sodium: 136.4 mEq/L; serum potassium: 4.4 mEq/L; blood urea: 36 mg/dL; serum creatinine: 0.82 mg/dL; serum cholesterol: 296 mg/dl; serum glutamic oxaloacetic transaminase (SGOT): 32 U/L; serum glutamic pyruvic transaminase (SGPT): 36 U/L; serum bilirubin total: 0.9 mg/dL; C3: 106.0 mg/dL (normal range: 90–180); C4: 18 mg/dL (normal range: 10–40); serum antinuclear antibody: negative; serum antistreptolysin O titer (ASO titer): <110 IU/mL; cytoplasmic antineutrophil cytoplasmic antibody: negative; perinuclear antineutrophil cytoplasmic antibody: negative; HIV I and II: negative; HBsAg: negative; and anti-HCV: negative. A 24-hour urinary protein value was 10.8 grams/day. Ultrasonography abdomen showed bilateral normal size kidneys with normal echogenicity. A renal biopsy showed nonproliferative glomerulopathy (22 glomeruli) (Figure 1). Tubular atrophy involved less than 10% of the sampled cortex. Tubules showed focally prominent cytoplasmic vacuolar changes, and the arteries sampled appeared unremarkable. Direct immunofluorescence did not show significant glomerular immune deposits. Renal electron microscopy showed diffuse effacement of visceral epithelial cell foot processes (Figure 2). Rifampicin-induced secondary minimal change disease was suspected, and the culprit drug rifampicin was stopped immediately. The other antitubercular drugs were continued with the addition of levofloxacin 500 mg/day. The proteinuria started to decline, and 24-hour urinary protein was 1.2 grams/day after two weeks of stopping of rifampicin. After 30 days of cessation of rifampicin, proteinuria was undetectable in 24-hour urinary samples, and serum albumin and serum cholesterol were found to be normal. The pulmonary tuberculosis was well managed by isoniazid, ethambutol hydrochloride, and levofloxacin, and there was no recurrence of proteinuria.

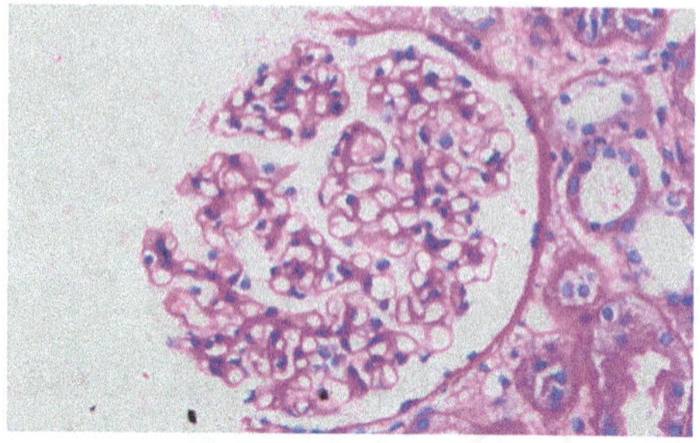

Figure 1: Kidney biopsy specimen on light microscopy showing normal appearing glomerulus without any proliferation or capillary wall thickening (PAS 40x).

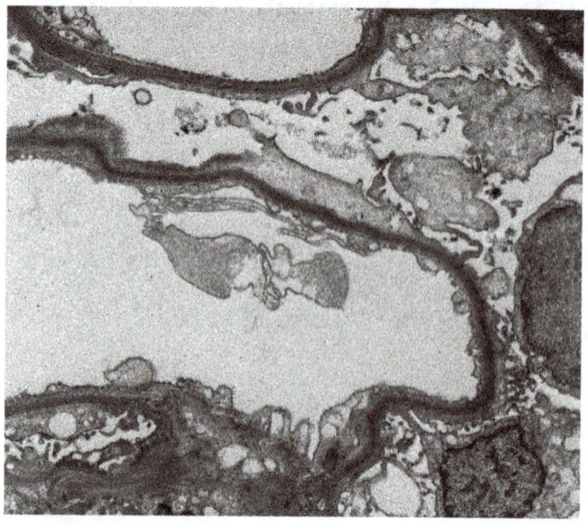

Figure 2: Kidney biopsy specimen with electron microscopy showing diffuse effacement of visceral epithelial cell foot processes (TEM 2000x).

3. Discussion

Various extraglomerular disease processes have been associated with drug-induced secondary minimal change disease (MCD). In the majority of cases, preferably a hypersensitivity reaction appears to be involved, and in some cases, there is a direct toxic effect (e.g., lithium, interferon, and daunomycin) over glomerular capillaries [1]. Nonsteroidal anti-inflammatory drugs (NSAIDs) can cause nephrotic proteinuria and may be associated with glomerular lesions similar to primary minimal change disease. In the majority of NSAID-induced MCD cases, there is an accompanying acute interstitial nephritis specified by the invasion of polyclonal T and B cells [1]. Clinically, NSAID-associated secondary MCD usually presents as acute renal failure. Our case patient developed sudden onset nephrotic proteinuria after one month of continuous use of rifampicin. The glomeruli did not show any immunoglobulins and complement deposition on immunofluorescence examination. Electron microscopy did not show any presence of glomerular immune complexes and thickening of the glomerular basement membrane, promoting the diagnosis of minimal change nephrotic syndrome.

According to De Vriese and coworkers, the most common clinical presentation of rifampicin-associated nephrotoxicity was acute renal failure, and it was due to acute tubular necrosis in the majority of cases, while acute interstitial nephritis was found in some cases [3]. They reported that rifampicin-induced acute renal failure occurred commonly in those patients who had intermittent or interrupted treatment. Our case patient was on continuous rifampicin treatment, and there was no concomitant acute renal failure and acute interstitial nephritis. Richard J. Glassock stated that there is a possibility of development of peculiar changes in permselectivity and morphology of glomerular capillaries in case of secondary MCD, and these changes are similar to primary MCD [1]. Re-exposure to the drug may cause recrudescence, and it is suggestive of a functioning cell-mediated hypersensitivity reaction [1]. Disappearance of proteinuria and full recovery are usually associated with withdrawal of the offending drug. The activated inflammatory or immune cells release permselectivity promoting factors, and this may be the reason for the association between MCD and drug exposure [1]. We thoroughly scrutinized his medical history including medication use. He had no other relevant medical history. We observed that he developed heavy proteinuria only after the start of antitubercular treatment. Favourably, his proteinuria improved after discontinuation of rifampicin. However, it is not yet proven, but there is a possibility that genetic susceptibility can play a role in the occurrence of MCD after drug exposure [1]. There was no such type of family history in our case patient. Yoshioka K and coworkers reported rapidly progressive glomerulonephritis due to rifampicin therapy [6]. Antirifampicin antibody was detected in a patient with crescentic glomerulonephritis by Ogata and coworkers, and they suggested a relationship between renal histology and antibody [3]. De Vriese and coworkers explained that antirifampicin antibody detection was restricted to only those patients who had acute renal failure after rifampicin therapy [3].

Neugarten and coworkers reported the first case of rifampicin-associated nephrotic syndrome with acute interstitial nephritis [7]. There was no immunoglobulin and complement deposition in the glomeruli. The electron microscopy showed dense deposits in the mesangial matrix, subendothelial, and paramesangial areas. They postulated the hypothesis that there was a development of humoral and cell-mediated immune responses to rifampicin treatment [7]. Tada and coworkers also reported rifampicin-associated secondary minimal change disease [3]. They hypothesized that rifampicin-induced endothelial injury was responsible for the development of nephrotic syndrome. Dong Hyuk Park and coworkers reported that rifampicin-induced minimal change disease was improved after cessation of rifampicin without the need of steroid therapy [8]. There were no immune complex or electron dense deposits in the glomeruli, and it was not suggestive of a humoral immune mechanism. They hypothesized that rifampicin-induced MCD was due to a direct toxic effect of the drug [8]. Jee-Seon Kim and coworkers reported rifampicin-induced minimal change disease with acute renal failure in a patient with latent tuberculosis [9]. This patient required temporary dialysis and recovered after discontinuation of rifampicin with steroid therapy [9]. However, our case patient did not demonstrate any renal failure, interstitial edema, or inflammatory cell infiltration or fibrosis, and the patient recovered without the need of steroid therapy.

4. Conclusion

From the clinical point of view, we should be aware that sometimes apparently looking primary MCD may be a representation of a secondary lesion due to an extra-glomerular disease process. Although secondary MCD is a rare side effect of rifampicin, it is advisable for monitoring of proteinuria during follow-up of patients who are on rifampicin therapy.

Consent

Guardians have given their written informed consent to publish this case, including publication of images.

Authors' Contributions

Satyanand Sathi and Anil Kumar Garg contributed to manuscript design, data interpretation, manuscript review, and drafting of the manuscript. Manoj Kumar Singh contributed to the manuscript review. Devinder Vohra and Virendra Singh Saini contributed to the final drafting and critical revision of the manuscript. All authors approved the final version of the manuscript.

Acknowledgments

The authors express their gratitude to the patient and his guardians for providing medical records to prepare the manuscript. The authors are also highly thankful to Dr. Alok Sharma, a senior renal biopsy pathologist at Lal Pathology, New Delhi, for reporting the renal biopsy specimens.

References

[1] R. J. Glassock, "Secondary minimal change disease," *Nephrology Dialysis Transplantation*, vol. 18, 2003.

[2] A. Covic, D. Goldsmith, L. Segall et al., "Rifampicin-induced acute renal failure: a series of 60 patients," *Nephrology Dialysis Transplantation*, vol. 13, no. 4, pp. 924–929, 1998.

[3] K. Kohno, Y. Mizuta, T. Yoshida et al., "Minimal change nephrotic syndrome associated with rifampicin treatment," *Nephrology Dialysis Transplantation*, vol. 15, no. 7, pp. 1056–1059, 2000.

[4] T. Muthukumar, M. Jayakumar, E. M. Fernando, and M. A. Muthusethupathi, "Acute renal failure due to rifampicin: a study of 25 patients," *American Journal of Kidney Diseases*, vol. 40, no. 4, pp. 690–696, 2002.

[5] V. V. Rekha, T. Santha, and M. S. Jawahar, "Rifampicin-induced renal toxicity during retreatment of patients with pulmonary tuberculosis," *The Journal of the Association of Physicians of India*, vol. 53, pp. 811–813, 2005.

[6] K. Yoshioka, N. Satake, Y. Kasamatsu, Y. Nakamura, and N. Shikata, "Rapidly progressive glomerulonephritis due to rifampicin therapy," *Nephron*, vol. 90, no. 1, pp. 116–118, 2002.

[7] J. Neugarten, G. R. Gallo, and D. S. Baldwin, "Rifampin-induced nephrotic syndrome and acute interstitial nephritis," *American Journal of Nephrology*, vol. 3, no. 1, pp. 38–42, 1983.

[8] H. Dong, S. A. Lee, S.-W. Kang, and H. Jung Oh, "Rifampicin-induced minimal Change disease is improved after cessation of rifampicin without steroid therapy," *Yonsei Medical Journal*, vol. 56, no. 2, pp. 582–585, 2015.

[9] J.-S. Kim, K.-J. Kim, and E.-Y. Choi, "Minimal change disease related to rifampicin presenting with acute renal failure during treatment for latent tuberculosis infection: a case report," *Medicine*, vol. 97, p. 22, Article ID e10556, 2018.

11

Targeting Cytokine Storm in COVID-19: A Role of Online Hemodiafiltration with Asymmetric Cellulose Triacetate in Maintenance Hemodialysis Patients—A Report of 10 Cases

José C. De La Flor,[1] **Francisco Valga**,[2] **Alexander Marschall**,[3] **Tania Monzon**,[4] **Cristina Albarracín**,[1] **Elisa Ruiz**,[1] **and Miguel Rodeles**[1]

[1]*Department of Nephrology, Central Defense Gomez Ulla Hospital, Madrid, Spain*
[2]*Department of Nephrology, Doctor Negrín University Hospital, Las Palmas de Gran Canaria, Spain*
[3]*Department of Cardiology, Central Defense Gomez Ulla Hospital, Madrid, Spain*
[4]*Department of Hemodialysis, Avericum S.L., Las Palmas de Gran Canaria, Spain*

Correspondence should be addressed to José C. De La Flor; josedelaflor81@yahoo.com

Academic Editor: Manel Vera

Early reports have suggested that maintenance hemodialysis (MHD) patients could be more susceptible to a severe course of COVID-19. Among the therapeutic approaches, the use of drugs that reduce the cytokine storm characteristic of this disease has been proposed. Some dialyzers, such as the new generation of asymmetric cellulose triacetate (ATA) membranes, could favor the effective elimination of medium-sized molecules and other inflammatory mediators. In this case series, we describe in depth the clinical, analytical, and radiological details, therapeutic aspects, and outcomes of the case series of 10 MHD patients of our dialysis unit, who tested positive for SARS-CoV-2 from 5 October to 30 November 2020. Furthermore, we evaluate the removal of hyperinflammatory parameters with the ATA membrane in postdilution online hemodiafiltration (OL-HDF) in these patients through a variety of biomarkers of systemic inflammation from the diagnosis until stripping. Biochemical blood analysis was carried out at baseline and at days 7 and 14 after diagnosis, respectively. 50% of the patients presented COVID-19 pneumonia and required hospital admission. Median hospitalization time was 21 days. A total of 4 patients developed severe pneumonia (3 of them died) and 1 patient developed moderate pneumonia. Patients who died ($n = 3$) were more likely to present bilateral pneumonia (100% vs 14.3%) at diagnosis and less reduction in interleukin 6 (IL-6) at day 14, as compared to those who survived. The use of the ATA membrane could be considered a therapeutic option, due to its immunomodulatory effect in MHD patients with SARS-CoV-2 infection, especially at the beginning of the disease, where the inflammatory component is predominant.

1. Introduction

In early December 2019, a respiratory disease caused by a novel coronavirus, named severe acute respiratory syndrome coronavirus 2 (SARS-CoV-2), emerged in Wuhan, China. This disease, which the World Health Organization (WHO) denominated coronavirus disease 2019 (COVID-19), spread rapidly throughout China and worldwide [1]. The WHO declared COVID-19 a pandemic in March 2020 [2]. At the beginning of June 2020, Spain was already recovering from the high infection rates, after it implemented one of the most draconian COVID-19 lockdowns in Europe. However, two months after lifting the restrictions, the virus spread faster than in any of Spain's neighboring countries. During the second wave of COVID-19, the therapeutic approach of targeting the virus replication and the hyperinflammation remains limited and its pathophysiologic basis is not yet not fully understood. Patients with end-stage kidney disease (ESKD), undergoing maintenance hemodialysis (MHD), may be more vulnerable to a SARS-CoV-2 infection, due to their suppressed immune system [3, 4]. Prompt identification of SARS-CoV-2 infection, isolation, and treatment according to the different manifestations of the disease are essential to reduce the spread of the disease. This is especially important in this population, given the logistical aspects of MHD that may increase the risk for disease transmission [5].

Among the therapeutic options for COVID-19, the use of drugs that reduce the hyperinflammation (cytokine storm) has been proposed [6–9]. The ERA/EDTA recommends in patients undergoing hemodialysis the use of the medium cut-off membranes (MCO) filter, with the aim of increasing the efficiency of removal of middle size molecules and, therefore, inflammation mediators implicated in the pathogenesis of SARS-CoV-2 infection, as established by the "Brescia Renal COVID-19 Task Force" [10]. However, their efficacy and safety are not been validated so far. After the first outbreak of SARS-CoV-2 in our dialysis unit [11], we established an action protocol for the management of patients in MHD with COVID-19. We used postdilution online hemodiafiltration (OL-HDF) with a dialyzer of asymmetric cellulose triacetate (ATA) membrane. This is a new generation of the cellulose triacetate membrane, with an increase in the coefficient of ultrafiltration (72 mL/h/mmHg) [12]; this could favor the elimination of medium-sized molecules and other inflammatory mediators. The aim of the present study was to describe in depth the clinical, analytical, and radiological details, therapeutic aspects, and outcomes of the case series of patients diagnosed with COVID-19 in our dialysis unit. In addition, we evaluate the removal of hyperinflammatory parameters with the ATA membrane in MHD patients with COVID-19, through a variety of biomarkers of systemic inflammation (neutrophil-to-lymphocyte (NLR), platelet-to-lymphocyte (PLR), monocyte-lymphocyte (MLR) lymphocyte-to-C-reactive protein (LCR) ratios, and interleukin 6 (IL-6)).

2. Case Reports

This is a case series of 10 adult MHD patients (13.2%) that tested positive for SARS-Cov-2 infection in the dialysis unit (with a total of 76 patients) of the Central Defense Gomez Ulla Hospital in Madrid, Spain. The patients were diagnosed from 5 October to 30 November 2020. The diagnosis was established according to the Spanish health system diagnostic criteria, which includes a positive result of the nasopharyngeal swab for SARS-CoV-2 nucleic acid, using reverse transcription-polymerase chain reaction (RT-PCR) [13]. If the RT-PCR resulted negative, however, the clinical suspicion remained strong, a second RT-PCR and/or a thoracic CT scan were performed. RT-PCR assay was performed according to the manufacture´s protocol by our center´s laboratory using Seegene's COVID-19 test kit. All SARS-Cov-2-infected patients received 3 HD sessions a week with the ATA membrane in postdilution OL-HDF and venous line administration of low-molecular-weight heparin (LMWH, Enoxaparin) at a dose of 40 to 60 mg at every HD session in nonhospitalized patients and a dose of 1 mg/kg/day (maximum dose of 80 mg) in hospitalized patients until stripping.

Initially, suspected or confirmed SARS-CoV-2 infected patients were dialyzed in a single isolation room. The patients were deisolated after two negative nasopharyngeal PCR tests taken 48 hours apart, obtained at days 14 and 15, or only one RT-PCT test if negative IgM and positive IgG results from the SARS-CoV-2 serological test. We collected demographic and epidemiological information, clinical features at diagnosis, and chest X-rays as well as technical parameters of dialysis and vascular access (Table 1). The treatments and outcomes are described in Table 2. For each patient, a blood test for systemic inflammation biomarkers was performed every 7 days from the diagnosis of infection Day 0 to Day 14. IL-6 analysis was performed at the time of diagnosis and 15 days after the start of the first session with the ATA membrane in OL-HDF.

The median age was 72 years (IQR: 69–80), and 50% were women. Fever and cough resulted to be the most prevalent symptoms (Table 1). According to the classification of the consensus document of the Spanish health system, half of the patients had COVID-19 pneumonia and required hospital admission. Four patients developed severe pneumonia (3 of them died) and 1 had moderate pneumonia. The median hospitalization time was 21 days. The 3 patients who died required a prolonged in-hospital stay of 24 days due to bacterial superinfection. Patients who died presented more often with fever than survivors (100% versus 43%, p value = 0.200), cough (100% vs 57.1%, p value = 0.475), diarrhea (66.7% vs 0%, p value = 0.067), and bilateral pneumonia (100% vs 14.3%, p value = 0.040) at diagnosis (Table 1).

Among the analytical parameters, we found no significant differences with regard to the laboratory data at 14 days and compared to baseline except for the white blood cell (WBC) count and NLR. See Table 3 for details. At diagnosis, the patients who died had higher mean C-reactive protein (CRP) levels (1.7 versus 0.8 mg/L) and higher IL-6 levels (41.4 versus 31.1 pg/mL), as compared to survivors, however, not reaching statistical significance. The median LCR at 7 (0.5 vs 0.9, p value = 0.017) and 14 days (0.4 vs 3.04, p value = 0.033) was lower in patients who died as compared to those who survived. We also found a higher reduction in IL-6 at 14 days in patients who survived (47% vs increases of 440%) as compared to those who died (Figure 1). The rest of the analytical parameters are presented in Table 4.

With regard to the treatment of the SARS-Cov-2 infection, high flow oxygen therapy >30 l.p.m. was prescribed in 4 patients, and dexamethasone was used in 6 (60%) cases. One of them received Anakinra for 5 days and none of them received Tocilizumab. The comparison of the treatment and outcome between patients who died and survivors is detailed in Table 2.

3. Discussion

Recent studies have described the incidence, clinical and radiologic features, laboratory characteristics, and hyperinflammatory parameters, therapeutic strategies, recovery, evolution, outcome, and screening of COVID-19 in MHD patients [10, 11, 14–18, 23]. However, there are few studies on the technique and the dialyzer used in patients with COVID-19 undergoing hemodialysis [10, 19, 20], as well as

Table 1: Patients characteristics, dialysis parameters, and clinical findings at COVID-19 diagnosis.

Characteristics	All patients ($n = 10$)	Death patients ($n = 3$)	Survivors ($n = 7$)	p value*
Demographics				
Age (years)	71.5 [69.0–80.0]	69 [58–82]	72 [70–80]	0.45
Male, n (%)	5 (50)	2 (67)	3 (43)	0.50
Diabetes mellitus, n (%)	4 (40)	1 (33.3)	3 (42.9)	0.8
Hypertension, n (%)	10 (100)	3 (100)	7 (100)	1
Initial nephropathy, n (%)				0.35
Diabetic nephropathy	2 (20)	1 (33.3)	1 (14.3)	—
Hypertension	3 (30)	—	3 (42.9)	—
Chronic interstitial nephritis	3 (30)	1 (33.3)	2 (28.6)	—
Vasculitis	1 (10)	1 (33.3)	—	—
Amyloidosis	1 (10)	—	1 (14.3)	—
Dialysis details				
Vascular access, n (%)				
Tunneled CVCs	6 (60)	2 (66.7)	4 (57.1)	0.79
AVF native	3 (30)	1 (33.3)	2 (28.6)	—
Prosthetic fistula	1 (10)	—	1 (14.3)	—
ESA (UI/week)	12000 [9000–18000]	15000 [9000–15000]	9000 [6000–30000]	0.91
Dialysis time (h)	3.75 [3.5–4.0]	4.0 [3.5–4.0]	3.75 [3.5–4.0]	0.46
Dry weight (kg)	67.3 [0.54–73.5]	68.5 [49–70]	66.0 [54.0–76.0]	0.73
Ultrafiltration volume (ml)	1867 (1587–2145)	1494 [1422–1587]	1984 [1819–2235]	0.02
Blood flow rate (ml/min)	343.9 [322.5–350.3]	344.1 [322.5–346.6]	343.6 [321.6–350.4]	0.91
Dialysis vintage (month)	49.4 [30.7–62.7]	30.7 [12.3–56.2]	56.2 [37.1–91.9]	0.29
Signs and symptoms, n (%)				
Fever	6 (60)	3 (100)	3 (42.9)	0.09
Cough	7 (70)	3 (100)	4 (57.1)	0.18
Diarrhea	2 (20)	2 (66.7)	0	0.02
Bilateral pneumonia	4 (40)	3 (100)	1 (14.3)	0.04

Data are shown as median [interquartile range] or percentage (%). AVF: arteriovenous fistula; CVC: central venous catheter; ESA: erythropoiesis-stimulating agents. *Mann–Whitney U or Chi-square.

Table 2: Patients' treatment and outcome.

	All patients ($n = 10$)	Death patients ($n = 3$)	Survivors ($n = 7$)	p value*
Antibiotic therapy, n (%)	6 (60)	3 (100)	3 (43)	0.2
Cephalosporin (third generation)	3 (30)	2 (50)	1 (14.3)	0.2
Macrolidc	1 (10)	—	1 (14.3)	1
Carbapenems	4 (40)	3 (100)	1 (14.3)	0.03
Others	3 (30)	2 (66.7)	1 (14.3)	0.2
Steroids, n (%)	6 (60)	3 (100)	3 (43)	0.2
Anakinra, n (%)	1 (10)	1 (33.3)	0	0.3
Tocilizumab, n (%)	0	0	0	
High flow oxygen therapy >30 lpm, n (%)	4 (40)	3 (100)	1 (14.3)	0.03
Anticoagulation, n (%)	5 (50)	3 (100)	2 (28.6)	0.2

Data are shown as number and percentage. *Chi-square/Fisher's exact test.

Table 3: Inflammatory parameters at baseline, 7 days, and 14 days after diagnosis.

	At baseline	At 7 days	At 14 days	p value*
CRP (mg/dL)	1.54 [0.52–4.31]	1.63 [0.49–12.89]	3.23 [0.35–8.49]	0.28
PCT (mg/dL)	0.54 [0.37–0.75]	0.88 [0.21–1.17]	0.42 [0.20–0.84]	0.54
Ferritin (ng/mL)	1020 [601–1952]	1639 [702–2958]	1706 [603.5–3286]	0.28
WBC count ($10^3/\mu L$)	4.8 [4.5–6.9]	7.4 [4.3–11.1]	8.7 [6.6–12.4]	0.007
NLR	3.1 [2.6–7.5]	5.8 [2.5–22]	13.3 [3.2–22.6]	0.04
LCR	1.7 [0.4–1.9]	0.65 [0.08–1.01]	0.9 [0.01–4.9]	0.88
MLR	2.3 [1.7–3.5]	2.5 [1.7–4.0]	2.7 [1.7–3.3]	0.33
Fibrinogen (mgl/dL)	529.5 [328–610]	530 [411–718]	491.5 [468–517]	0.58
IL-6 (pg/mL)	36.0 [28.4–70.3]		80.6 [11.3–220.4]	0.721

*Wilcoxon matched-pairs signed-ranks test (14 days vs baseline). CRP: C-reactive protein; PCT: procalcitonin; WBC: white blood cell; NLR: neutrophil-to-lymphocyte ratio; LCR: lymphocyte-to-C-reactive protein ratio; MLR: monocyte-lymphocyte ratio; IL-6: interleukin 6.

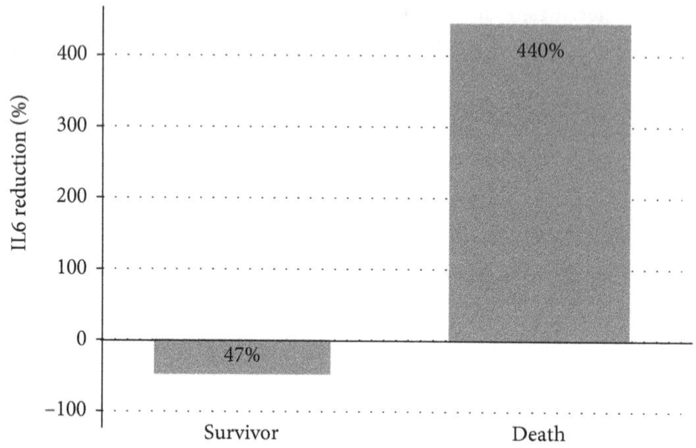

Figure 1: Interleukin-6 level reduction at 14 days according to vital status.

Table 4: Laboratory data at diagnosis according to vital status.

	All patients ($n = 10$)	Death patients ($n = 3$)	Survivors ($n = 7$)	p value*
Hemoglobin (g/dL)	10.7 [10.5–11.9]	10.6 [8.3–11.9]	10.8 [10.5–13.8]	0.49
ALT (UI/L)	12.5 [10.0–15.0]	13.0 [10.0–170]	12.0 [10.0–15.0]	0.56
AST (UI/L)	18 [14–22]	16 [14–17, 23]	28 [23–2064]	0.02
NT-proBNP (pg/dL)	3926 [3200–9145]	9145 [2500–10023]	3900 [3200–4760]	0.57
Troponin (g/l)	60 [48.7–80.9]	80.9 [56.1–81.0]]	60.0 [44–60.7]	0.3
GGT (UI/L)	23.0 [15.0–38.0]	30.0 [17.0–38.0]	18.0 [14.0–38.0]	0.49
D-dimer (ng/dL)	1489 [780–2476]	1753 [426–1982]	1225 [780–3302]	0.73
CPK (UI/L)	59 [31–81]	81.0 [23.0–780]	58 [31–80]	0.43
Fibrinogen (mgl/dl)	529 [328–610]	531 [275–651]	528 [328–610]	0.91
IL-6 (pg/ml)	36.0 [28.4–70.3]	41.4 [31.8–95.4]	31.1 [21.3–70.3]	0.31
WBC ($10^3/\mu$L)	4.8 [4.5–6.9]	5.4 [4.5–9.5]	4.8 [4.3–6.9]	0.31
MLR	2.3 [1.7–3.5]	2.5 [1.4–55.3]	2.0 [1.7–3.5]	0.91
NLR	3.1 [2.6–7.5]	2.7 [2.6–6.5]	3.3 [2.5–9.4]	0.57
LCR	1.7 [0.4–1.9]	0.4 [0.3–0.6]	1.8 [1.6–2.1]	0.09
Ferritin (ng/mL)	1020 [601–1952]	1062 [978–19083]	915 [336–1952]	0.31
PCT (mg/dL)	0.54 [0.37–0.75]	0.54 [0.33–100]	0.53 [0.37–0.75]	0.91
CRP (mg/dL)	1.5 [0.5–4.3]	1.7 [1.7–7.9]	0.8 [0.3–4.3]	0.21

*Mann–Whitney *U*. ALT: alanine aminotransferase; AST: aspartate aminotransferase; NT-proBNP: NT-proB-type natriuretic peptide; GGT: gamma-glutamyl transferase; CPK: creatine phosphokinase; IL-6: interleukin 6; WBC: white blood cell; NLR: neutrophil-to-lymphocyte ratio; LCR: lymphocyte-to-C-reactive protein ratio; MLR: monocyte-lymphocyte ratio; PCT: procalcitonin; CRP: C-reactive protein.

on the response of this infection on the removal of the inflammatory parameters. We present a single-center experience of the use of the ATA membrane dialyzer in postdilution OL-HDF in 10 MHD patients with COVID-19. We used this dialyzer since it may reduce the concentration of inflammatory cytokines. In addition, it minimizes the loss of albumin, thus not altering the coagulation patterns. Furthermore, it may avoid adverse hypersensitivity reactions, reduce additional inflammation, and achieve a good clearance of uremic toxins. ATA membranes are characterized by presence of low electrical charge, allowing a low adsorption capacity [19], which influences the properties of antithrombotic agents described for these membranes [20].

The incidence of COVID-19 in our HD unit during the second pandemic wave was 13.2%, which is very similar compared to other cohorts [10, 14, 21, 23]. Mortality and complication rates are high in MHD patients. This is probably due to a very high number of comorbid conditions. We observed that 4 of the 10 patients presented a severe form of COVID-19. In our cohort, we found a 30% death rate in COVID-19-infected MHD patients, which is in line with other reports in Europe (29% in Italy and 28–31% in Spain), although higher than 16% reported in China [10, 14, 21, 22].

MHD patients with COVID-19 could be detected early because they are admitted to the centers of HD three times a week. This has allowed various biomarkers of inflammation to be proposed to predict severe forms of COVID-19 and mortality [24]. Elevation of common parameters associated with inflammation, such as CRP, procalcitonin (PCT), and cytokines, is very frequently found in COVID-19 [25, 26]. However, the NLR, PLR, MLR, and LCR are biomarkers of systemic inflammation, available in almost all laboratories, and are rarely used in this infection. The first of them has been the most thoroughly studied and has shown prognostic ability in multiple clinical settings, such as acute kidney injury [27], kidney disease [28], cardiovascular disease [29], ANCA-associated vasculitis [30], cancer patients [31], renal transplantation [32], and recently COVID-19 as a short-term predictor marker associated with severe forms of COVID-19 in HD patients [15, 18, 33]. In our study, the CRP levels at diagnosis were almost double in patients who died, as compared to survivors. Luo et al.[34] found in a study of 298 patients that CRP performed better than other parameters (age, neutrophil count, and platelet count) in predicting adverse outcomes. Admission serum CRP levels were identified as a moderate discriminator of disease severity. However, PCT levels in our patients at diagnosis were higher in survivors, as compared to deceased.

Several reports of non-MHD patients with COVID-19 have described elevated levels of neutrophils and CRP with lymphopenia [13, 23, 26], but very few reports have considered the cost-effective markers NLR, PLR, MLR, and LCR to aid complication predictions and response to the therapeutic measures performed. We observed that the blood test based on the combination of these biomarkers performed on Days 7 and 14, rather than at diagnosis (Day 0), better discriminates patients who will develop severe forms of COVID-19 and died, from those with the nonsevere forms and survivors. Out of all these ratios, in our study, NLR and LCR were associated with the severe form and mortality. Very similar observer data by Qin et al. [26] showed that an NLR >5.2 was associated with the most severe form of COVID-19 within a cohort of 452 patients, while Mutinelli-Szymanski et al. [15], in a prospective, observational, and multicentric study of 62 adult HD patients, observed that an NLR >3.7 at day 7 was associated with the severe form and with poor survival. Therefore, we believe that NLR and LCR could be helpful for clinicians to identify patients who may develop a severe form of the disease at an early stage.

Severe forms of COVID-19 induce an inflammatory reaction triggered by a cytokine storm, causing direct tissue damage and organ failure [25, 35]. Some studies have suggested that the dynamic change of IL-6 and IL-1 levels and other cytokines can be used as a marker in disease monitoring in patients with severe COVID-19 [36]. Del Valle et al.[37] investigated, in a study of 1814 non-hemodialysis patients of the Mount Sinai Health System in New York, several cytokines upon admission. The authors propose that serum IL-6 and tumor necrosis factor-alpha (TNF-α) levels should be considered in the management and treatment of patients with COVID-19 to stratify prospective clinical trials, guide resource allocation, and inform therapeutic options. In a recent Spanish observational, single-center, prospective study, Quiroga et al.[38] evaluated the impact of reducing IL-6 using a cytokine adsorbent filter in 16 COVID-19 hemodialysis patients. IL-6 levels were obtained before and after the first admission hemodialysis session and at 1 week. The authors concluded that a positive IL-6 balance during the admission hemodialysis session was associated with higher mortality. We observed in our study that at admission, predialysis IL-6 levels were very similar in patients who died, as compared to those who survived. However, on day 14, IL-6 levels were higher in patients who died. Despite having been prescribed an ATA dialyzer, patients who died did not show a decrease in IL-6 levels during the first 2 weeks after the diagnosis of COVID-19 compared to those who survived. However, we observed a 68.6% reduction in IL-6 levels in the surviving patients.

COVID-19 is associated with a syndrome of hypercoagulability with implications in the coagulation of extracorporeal hemodialysis circuits [39]. Nephrologists should consider using dialyzer membranes with poor platelet and coagulation activity in order to minimize the use of LMWH during the dialysis session and to maximize its efficacy with systemic anticoagulation for the management of the hypercoagulation state of this infection. Several studies have described the benefits of the use of LMWH in patients with COVID-19 for the prevention of activation of the coagulation cascade, induced by inflammation [40]. In addition, Perna et al.[41] recommend the use of LMWH in each hemodialysis session and propose to monitor these patients with Anti-Factor Xa activity assay and D-dimer levels to possibly increase the LMWH dosage. In our study, we monitor patients only with D-dimer levels. Patients during their follow-up presented a bad clinical respiratory course, associated with a progressive increase in these levels. In these patients, the dose of LMWH was increased. This underscores the need for a dialyzer membrane that requires little anticoagulation such as the ATA membrane, therefore maximizing the effectiveness of the LMWH.

Several studies have evaluated the coagulation parameter D-dimer in the progression of COVID-19. Bilaloglu et al.[42] observed, in 3334 consecutive patients admitted to 4 hospitals in New York City, that a thrombotic event occurred in 16.0%. Higher D-dimer levels at presentation were independently associated with thrombotic events, consistent with early coagulopathy. In our study, during COVID-19 infection, our MHD patients at diagnosis presented an increase in D-dimer of >1400 ng/mL. However, this increase did not correlate with mortality. Furthermore, in MHD hemodialysis patients infected with COVID-19, the D-dimer levels, even though they may not be higher than those of the non-COVID hemodialysis population, should be evaluated with caution due to the wide dispersion of values.

So far, only glucocorticoids have shown a beneficial effect in severe COVID-19 situations in controlled clinical trials [43, 44]. The usefulness of Tocilizumab in COVID-19 is being controversial, since its use in most retrospective studies has been associated with improved survival, but the result of different clinical trials does not seem favorable [45–47]. On the other hand, the use of inhibitory molecules of other interleukins is currently being studied, with Anakinra as the most commonly investigated anti-interleukin molecule studied after Tocilizumab for the treatment of COVID-19 [48]. In our case series, only one patient received treatment with Tocilizumab and, given the poor evolution, Anakinra was added. Despite having received both immunomodulatory treatments, the patient was one of the 3 patients who died. However, it is worth mentioning that the 3 patients who did not survive were patients with high comorbidity due to tumor history, autoimmune, and cardiovascular disease.

The main limitations of our study were the small sample size, the observational retrospective design, a possible selection bias, and the difficulty to assess the response in the decrease in inflammatory parameters with the use of ATA dialyzer, since at the moment there is no standard treatment regimen for this type of patients. Secondly, we collected IL-6 levels at the time of diagnosis and after 2 weeks. Therefore, we were only able to assess the removal of IL-6 in those patients who did not present a severe form of the disease. However, one of the strengths of our study is the measurement of the markers NLR, PLR, MLR, and LCR, which were carried out systematically every 7 days in all patients.

In conclusion, our understanding of treatment in COVID-19 has changed substantially in the past months, in both the nonrenal and renal population in HD. Some dialyzers, such as ATA membranes, may be helpful in the modulation of an immune dysregulated response in COVID-19 infection in MHD patients. Further observations and studies will be needed to fully understand the removal of inflammatory parameters with the use of these dialysis membranes in patients with COVID-19.

Consent

Each patient signed an informed consent to collect anonymous data and to publish cases (including publication of images).

References

[1] W.-j. Guan, Z.-y. Ni, Y. Hu et al., "Clinical characteristics of coronavirus disease 2019 in China," *New England Journal of Medicine*, vol. 382, no. 18, pp. 1708–1720, 2020.

[2] Coronavirus Disease (COVID-19), https://www.who.int/emergencies/diseases/novel-coronavirus-2019?gclid=EAIaIQobChMIv9ygwaq87gIV0N_tCh2TDQT4EAAYASAAEgK54fD_BwE.

[3] S. Kato, M. Chmielewski, H. Honda et al., "Aspects of immune dysfunction in end-stage renal disease," *Clinical Journal of the American Society of Nephrology*, vol. 3, no. 5, pp. 1526–1533, 2008.

[4] C. J. Kelly, "T cell function in chronic renal failure and dialysis," *Blood Purification*, vol. 12, no. 1, pp. 36–41, 1994.

[5] D. E. Weiner and S. G. Watnick, "Hemodialysis and COVID-19: an achilles' heel in the pandemic health care response in the United States," *Kidney Medicine*, vol. 2, no. 3, pp. 227–230, 2020.

[6] J. B. Moore and C. H. June, "Cytokine release syndrome in severe COVID-19," *Science*, vol. 368, no. 6490, pp. 473-474, 2020.

[7] G. Monteleone, P. C. Sarzi-Puttini, and S. Ardizzone, "Preventing COVID-19-induced pneumonia with anticytokine therapy," *The Lancet Rheumatology*, vol. 2, no. 5, pp. e255–e256, 2020.

[8] M. Z. Tay, C. M. Poh, L. Rénia, and P. A. MacAry, "The trinity of COVID-19: immunity, inflammation and intervention," *Nature Reviews Immunology*, vol. 20, no. 6, pp. 363–374, 2020.

[9] J. Zhong, J. Tang, C. Ye, and L. Dong, "The immunology of COVID-19: is immune modulation an option for treatment?" *The Lancet Rheumatology*, vol. 2, no. 7, pp. e428–e436, 2020.

[10] F. Alberici, E. Delbarba, C. Manenti et al., "Management of patients on dialysis and with kidney transplantation during the SARS-CoV-2 (COVID-19) pandemic in brescia, Italy," *Kidney International Reports*, vol. 5, no. 5, pp. 580–585, 2020.

[11] J. C. d. l. F. Merino, F. V. Amado, A. Marschall et al., "COVID-19 in chronic hemodialysis patients: a report of 9 cases in Madrid, Spain," *Clinical Nephrology*, vol. 95, no. 1, pp. 45–53, 2021.

[12] F. Maduell, R. Ojeda, M. Arias-Guillén et al., "Una nueva generación de triacetato de celulosa adecuado para hemodiafiltración on-line," *Nefrologia*, vol. 38, pp. 220-221, 2018.

[13] C. Huang, Y. Wang, X. Li et al., "Clinical features of patients infected with 2019 novel coronavirus in Wuhan, China," *The Lancet*, vol. 395, no. 10223, pp. 497–506, 2020.

[14] M. Goicoechea, L. A. Sánchez Cámara, N. Macías et al., "COVID-19: clinical course and outcomes of 36 hemodialysis patients in Spain," *Kidney International*, vol. 98, no. 1, pp. 27–34, 2020.

[15] P. Mutinelli-Szymanski, I. Hude, E. Merle et al., "Neutrophil: lymphocyte ratio predicts short-term outcome of COVID-19 in haemodialysis patients," *Clinical Kidney Journal*, vol. 14, no. 1, p. 124, 2021.

[16] C. Creput, C. Fumeron, D. Toledano, M. Diaconita, and H. Izzedine, "COVID-19 in patients undergoing hemodialysis: prevalence and asymptomatic screening during a period of high community prevalence in a large Paris center," *Kidney Medicine*, vol. 2, no. 6, pp. 716–723, 2020.

[17] C. Ronco, T. Reis, and M. Cozzolino, "Rationale for medium cutoff membranes in COVID-19 patients requiring renal replacement therapy," *Nephron*, vol. 144, no. 11, pp. 550–554, 2020.

[18] F. Valga, N. Vega-Díaz, T. Monzón et al., "Papel de la hemodiálisis extendida en COVID-19: a propósito de un caso," *Nefrología*, vol. 40, no. 4, pp. 487–490, 2020.

[19] F. Maduell, L. Rodas, J. J. Broseta et al., "Medium cut-off dialyzer versus eight hemodiafiltration dialyzers: comparison using a global removal score," *Blood Purification*, vol. 48, no. 2, pp. 167–174, 2019.

[20] M. Belmouaz, J. Diolez, M. Bauwens et al., "Comparison of hemodialysis with medium cut-off dialyzer and on-line hemodiafiltration on the removal of small and middle-sized molecules," *Journal of Clinical Nephrology*, vol. 89, pp. 50–56, 2018.

[21] Y. Ma, B. Diao, X. Lv et al., *Novel Coronavirus Disease in Hemodialysis (HD) Patients: Report from One HD Center in Wuhan*, Wuhan, China, 2019.

[22] H. Trujillo, F. Caravaca-Fontán, Á. Sevillano et al., "SARS-CoV-2 infection in hospitalized patients with kidney disease," *Kidney International Reports*, vol. 5, no. 6, p. 905, 2020.

[23] D. Wang, B. Hu, C. Hu et al., "Clinical characteristics of 138 hospitalized patients with 2019 novel coronavirus-infected pneumonia in Wuhan, China," *Jama*, vol. 323, no. 11, pp. 1061–1069, 2020.

[24] C. Danwang, F. T. Endomba, J. R. Nkeck, D. L. A. Wouna, A. Robert, and J. J. Noubiap, "A meta-analysis of potential biomarkers associated with severity of coronavirus disease 2019 (COVID-19)," *Biomarker Research*, vol. 8, no. 1, 2020.

[25] G. Chen, D. Wu, W. Guo et al., "Clinical and immunological features of severe and moderate coronavirus disease 2019," *Journal of Clinical Investigation*, vol. 130, no. 5, pp. 2620–2629, 2020.

[26] C. Qin, L. Zhou, Z. Hu et al., "Dysregulation of immune response in patients with coronavirus 2019 (COVID-19) in Wuhan, China," *Clinical Infectious Diseases*, vol. 71, no. 15, pp. 762–768, 2020.

[27] M. Abu Alfeilat, I. Slotki, and L. Shavit, "Single emergency room measurement of neutrophil/lymphocyte ratio for early

detection of acute kidney injury (AKI)," *Internal and Emergency Medicine*, vol. 13, no. 5, pp. 717–725, 2018.

[28] I. Kocyigit, E. Eroglu, A. Unal et al., "Role of neutrophil/lymphocyte ratio in prediction of disease progression in patients with stage-4 chronic kidney disease," *Journal of Nephrology*, vol. 26, no. 2, pp. 358–365, 2013.

[29] D. Martínez-Urbistondo, A. Beltrán, O. Beloqui, and A. Huerta, "The neutrophil-lymphocyte ratio as a marker of systemic endothelial dysfunction in asymptomatic subjects," *Nefrología (English Edition)*, vol. 36, no. 4, pp. 397–403, 2016.

[30] J. A. Fonseca, J. Gameiro, I. Duarte, S. Jorge, and J. A. Lopes, "The neutrophil-to-lymphocyte ratio as a marker of vasculitis activity, severe infection and mortality in anca-associated vasculitis: a retrospective study," *Nefrología*, 2020.

[31] R.-M. Wen, Y.-J. Zhang, S. Ma et al., "Preoperative neutrophil to lymphocyte ratio as a prognostic factor in patients with non-metastatic renal cell carcinoma," *Asian Pacific Journal of Cancer Prevention*, vol. 16, no. 9, pp. 3703–3708, 2015.

[32] M. Naranjo, A. Agrawal, A. Goyal, and J. Rangaswami, "Neutrophil-to-lymphocyte ratio and platelet-to-lymphocyte ratio predict acute cellular rejection in the kidney allograft," *Annals of Transplantation*, vol. 23, pp. 467–474, 2018.

[33] D. M. Simadibrata, J. Calvin, A. D. Wijaya, and N. A. A. Ibrahim, "Neutrophil-to-lymphocyte ratio on admission to predict the severity and mortality of COVID-19 patients: a meta-analysis," *The American Journal of Emergency Medicine*, vol. 42, pp. 60–69, 2021.

[34] X. Luo, W. Zhou, X. Yan et al., "Prognostic value of C-reactive protein in patients with coronavirus 2019," *Clinical Infectious Diseases*, vol. 71, no. 16, pp. 2174–2179, 2020.

[35] P. Mehta, D. F. McAuley, M. Brown, E. Sanchez, R. S. Tattersall, and J. J. Manson, "COVID-19: consider cytokine storm syndromes and immunosuppression," *The Lancet*, vol. 395, no. 10229, pp. 1033-1034, 2020.

[36] C. Zhang, Z. Wu, J.-W. Li, H. Zhao, and G.-Q. Wang, "Cytokine release syndrome in severe COVID-19: interleukin-6 receptor antagonist tocilizumab may be the key to reduce mortality," *International Journal of Antimicrobial Agents*, vol. 55, no. 5, Article ID 105954, 2020.

[37] D. M. Del Valle, S. Kim-Schulze, H.-H. Huang et al., "An inflammatory cytokine signature predicts COVID-19 severity and survival," *Nature Medicine*, vol. 26, no. 10, pp. 1636–1643, 2020.

[38] B. Quiroga, P. Muñoz Ramos, M. Giorgi et al., "Dynamic assessment of interleukin-6 during hemodialysis and mortality in COVID 19," *Ther Apher Dial*, pp. 1–9, 2021.

[39] I. Portales-Castillo and A. S. Allegretti, "Dialysis filter life in COVID-19: early lessons from the pandemic," *Kidney360*, vol. 1, no. 12, pp. 1334–1336, 2020.

[40] L. Lin, L. Lu, W. Cao, and T. Li, "Hypothesis for potential pathogenesis of SARS-CoV-2 infection-a review of immune changes in patients with viral pneumonia," *Emerging Microbes & Infections*, vol. 9, no. 1, pp. 727–732, 2020.

[41] A. F. Perna, G. Capolongo, F. Trepiccione, M. Simeoni, M. Zacchia, and D. Ingrosso, "COVID-19, low-molecular-weight heparin, and hemodialysis," *Kidney and Blood Pressure Research*, vol. 45, no. 3, pp. 357–362, 2020.

[42] S. Bilaloglu, Y. Aphinyanaphongs, S. Jones, E. Iturrate, J. Hochman, and J. S. Berger, "Thrombosis in hospitalized patients with COVID-19 in a New York city health system," *Jama*, vol. 324, no. 8, pp. 799–801, 2020.

[43] R. Fadel, A. R. Morrison, A. Vahia et al., "Early short-course corticosteroids in hospitalized patients with COVID-19," *Clinical Infectious Diseases*, vol. 71, no. 16, pp. 2114–2120, 2020.

[44] J. A. C. Sterne, S. Murthy, J. V. Diaz et al., "Association between administration of systemic corticosteroids and mortality among critically ill patients with COVID-19: a meta-analysis," *The Journal of the American Medical Association*, vol. 324, pp. 1330–1341, 2020.

[45] P. Toniati, S. Piva, M. Cattalini et al., "Tocilizumab for the treatment of severe COVID-19 pneumonia with hyperinflammatory syndrome and acute respiratory failure: a single center study of 100 patients in Brescia, Italy," *Autoimmunity Reviews*, vol. 19, no. 7, Article ID 102568, 2020.

[46] F. Menzella, M. Fontana, C. Salvarani et al., "Efficacy of tocilizumab in patients with COVID-19 ARDS undergoing noninvasive ventilation," *Critical Care*, vol. 24, no. 1, 2020.

[47] O. Moreno-Pérez, M. Andres, J.-M. Leon-Ramirez et al., "Experience with tocilizumab in severe COVID-19 pneumonia after 80 days of follow-up: a retrospective cohort study," *Journal of Autoimmunity*, vol. 114, Article ID 102523, 2020.

[48] G. Cavalli, G. De Luca, C. Campochiaro et al., "Interleukin-1 blockade with high-dose anakinra in patients with COVID-19, acute respiratory distress syndrome, and hyperinflammation: a retrospective cohort study," *The Lancet Rheumatology*, vol. 2, no. 6, pp. e325–e331, 2020.

12

A Patient with SIADH, Urinary Retention, Constipation and Bell's Palsy following a Tick Bite

Mariana Leone, Anwar Iqbal, J. R. Hugo Bonatti, Samina Anwar, and Catherine Feaga

Meritus Health, Hagerstown, MD, USA

Correspondence should be addressed to J. R. Hugo Bonatti; hugo.bonatti@dr.com

Academic Editor: David Mudge

Introduction. Lyme disease is the most common vector borne disease in the USA caused by the bacterium *Borrelia burgdorferi*. If untreated, Lyme disease can cause a variety of secondary symptoms often difficult to interpret. Some of the rare manifestations of Lyme disease include SIADH-like syndrome, enteroparesis, and urinary retention. *Case Report*. A 69-year-old male presented with anorexia and constipation and was found to have hyponatremia. Several days after admission, Bell's palsy developed and he experienced urinary retention requiring catheterization. Lyme disease was confirmed on serology, and he recalled a rash on his elbow four weeks prior. Ceftriaxone was started and the patient improved; he had multiple bowel movements after receiving laxatives and the Foley catheter was removed; serum sodium normalized with fluid restriction. He was discharged home and was well with symptoms completely resolved at three-month follow-up. *Discussion*. There should be a high alert of atypical presentation of this common tick bite associated infection. Review of the literature revealed ten similar cases, but only three of these patients were reported to have a combination of SIADH, urinary retention, and enteroparesis.

1. Introduction

Lyme disease is the most common vector borne disease and is caused by bacterium *Borrelia burgdorferi* (and rarely *Borrelia mayonii*) [1]. Approximately 30000 cases are annually reported to the Centers of Disease Control (CDC); it is estimated that up to almost 500000 individuals acquire the infection every year, with Maryland and Southern Pennsylvania being hotspots [1]. Lyme disease may progress through three stages, characterized as early localized stage, early disseminated stage, and late disseminated stage. Untreated Lyme disease may be complicated by chronic manifestations such as Lyme arthritis, Lyme neuroborreliosis, or other neurological manifestations [1–3]. Peripheral neuropathy is one of the common long-term complications, but involvement of the autonomic nerve system has been rarely reported. Single symptom manifestations may be more common, but subsets of patients may present with an obscure mix of symptoms delaying the diagnosis. Enteroparesis causing constipation and ileus and urinary retention are extremely rare conditions associated with Lyme disease; only a few cases of SIADH have been reported [4–9]. We herein present a patient who developed an unusual combination of symptoms, which resolved after treatment of his Lyme disease was initiated. In addition, a review of the English literature with regard to enteroparesis, urinary retention, and SIADH associated with Lyme disease was completed.

2. Case Report

A 69-year-old male with a medical history of hypertension and hyperlipidemia was initially admitted for abdominal pain and hyponatremia. He had developed decreased appetite, anorexia, and abdominal "fullness" four weeks earlier. At the same time, he experienced chills, headache, fatigue, and myalgias and noted an erythematous and edematous rash on his left elbow, which spontaneously resolved within one week. He complained of acute onset of significant constipation with no issues with moving his bowels previously and laxatives did not help. In the ER, he complained of significant abdominal discomfort. On examination, his

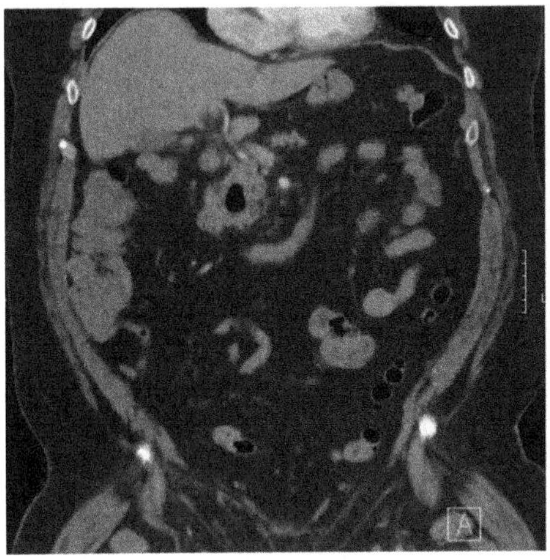

(a)

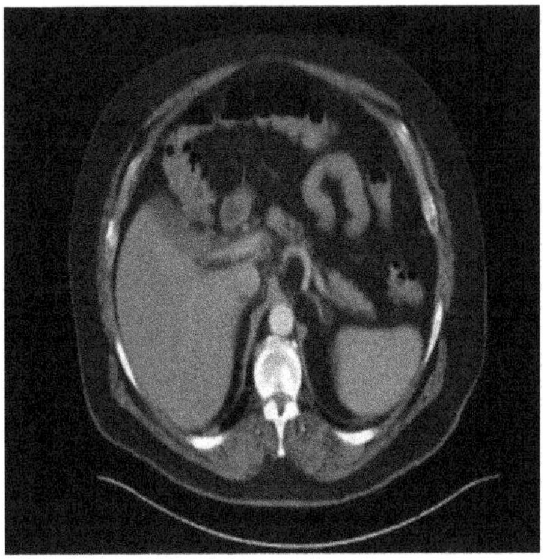

(b)

FIGURE 1: (a), (b) CT scan at initial presentation: moderate stool burden, no other findings.

abdomen was distended and moderately tender. WBC and CRP were normal, but sedimentation rate was elevated. He was hyponatremic with a serum sodium of 125.6 mmol/dL and potassium was 2.7 mmol/dL. Abdominal CT scan revealed no acute process but noted a moderate stool burden (Figures 1(a) and 1(b)). The patient was admitted for electrolyte correction and pain control and was started on a bowel regimen, and further work up of the obscure condition was initiated. He tested negative for SARS-COVID-19 on PCR.

Four days after his admission, the patient developed left lid ptosis and right lip numbness. He tested negative for CMV and HSV, but Lyme serology was found to be positive (total IgM and IgG antibodies). A lumbar puncture was performed. CSF was cloudy and revealed mild leukocytosis (WBC 53/microL, 45 mononucelar cells) with elevation in protein (278 mg/dl) and low glucose of 38 mg/dl (blood glucose of 95 mg/dl). Antibiotic therapy with intravenous ceftriaxone (2 g daily) was started on day 5 of his hospitalization. Late afternoon on day 7th of his hospitalization (corresponding to day 2 of antibiotic initiation), the patient was found to be tachycardic, weak, diaphoretic, and febrile. Serial troponins were elevated from 3.60 ng/ml to 4.70 ng/ml, and an EKG was performed which revealed no ST segment changes, no heart block, or arrythmia, and an echocardiogram showed no acute dysfunction, no valvular pathology, and an ejection fraction of 50%. These results suggested that Lyme carditis and NSTEMI were unlikely, and that these symptoms could be a Jarisch–Herxheimer reaction. Ceftriaxone was stopped and he was switched to IV doxycycline at a dose of 100 mg bid—a bacteriostatic agent seemed the better choice over a bactericidal antibiotic. The patient's acute symptoms improved within 24 hours. Serum sodium increased to >130 mmol/dL within 5 days but then dropped again to 122 mmol/dL.

On day 13th of hospitalization, the patient also began experiencing urinary retention; a Foley catheter was placed and Flomax (tamsulosin) was administered. The catheter remained in place for 72 hours and was then removed per hospital protocol, but voiding trials were unsuccessful. The Foley catheter was reinserted on day 16th of hospitalization. The hyponatremia also persisted, with sodium levels ranging from 122 mmol/L to 135 mmol/L. Diagnosis of SIADH secondary to Lyme disease was supported by serum osmolality of 261 mosmol/kg, TSH of 3.96 microIU/ml, and urine studies (osmolality 650 mosmol/kg, urine sodium 101 mmol/L). With fluid restriction, hyponatremia stepwise resolved. On day 17th of hospitalization, the patient was transitioned to oral doxycycline and was subsequently discharged to inpatient rehabilitation services where he remained for another 17 days with resolved urinary retention, nerve palsy and constipation, and normalized serum sodium and potassium. He was well and symptom free at the three month follow-up visit.

3. Discussion

Our case emphasizes that Lyme disease is capable of causing a mix of symptoms, which may be difficult to interpret, leading to a delay in diagnosis. Of note, these various symptoms may develop consecutively further obscuring the clinical picture. However, once the correct diagnosis was established and appropriate treatment was initiated, all symptoms resolved and the patient completely recovered.

The clinical manifestations of Lyme disease vary dependent on the stage of disease progression. Erythema migrans develops in approximately 50–80% of adults, and it is not uncommon that patients present with fever, malaise, fatigue, generalized pain, headaches, and other "flu-like" symptoms, during spirochete dissemination [1, 10].

Lyme disease may involve the central and less commonly the peripheral nervous system [10] with cranial neuritis most commonly involving the facial nerve, presenting with acute facial paralysis. Radiculoneuritis involving one or several dermatomes is another painful complication, and this may be accompanied by muscle weakness [10]. On rare occasions, Lyme disease may cause chronic epigastric pain [6] as well as

Table 1: Demographic and clinical data from review of the literature and our case.

Author	Year	Origin	Age	M/F	SIADH	Enteroparesis	Urinary retention	*n* symptoms	Other neurologic symptoms	Antibiotic treatment	Additional treatment	Outcome
Olivares	1995	France	54	M	No	No	Yes	1	None	Ceftriaxone to doxycycline	Alpha blocker, intermittent catheterization	Complete recovery
Chatila	1998	USA	61	M	No	Yes	No	1	Bells play	Doxycycline	Prednisone taper	Complete recovery
Shamim	2005	USA	64	M	Yes	Yes	Yes	3	Weakness, fatigue, hallucinations	Ceftriaxone	Fluid restriction	Complete recovery
Shamim	2005	USA	84	M	Yes	Yes	Yes	3	Weakness	Ceftriaxone	Fluid restriction, laxatives, physical therapy	Complete recovery
Perkins	2006	USA	73	F	Yes	No	No	1	Unsteady gait, falls, decreased mental activity, daytime somnolence	Ceftriaxone	Fluid restriction	Complete recovery
Schefte	2015	Denmark	66	F	No	Yes	Yes	2	Lower back pain	Ceftriaxone	Laxatives	Complete recovery
Siddiqui	2017	USA	83	F	Yes	No	No	1	Bilateral arm weakness	Ceftriaxone	Fluid restriction, salt tablets	Complete recovery
Dumic	2018	USA	25	M	No	No	Yes	1	Frequent falls, bilateral lower-extremity weakness and numbness	Ceftriaxone	Steroid taper, acyclovir, intermittent catheterization	Slow recovery
Saalami	2018	USA	62	F	Yes	Yes	Yes	3	Lower back pain, weakness	Ceftriaxone	Hypertonic saline, fluid restriction	Complete recovery
Da Porto	2019	Italy	62	M	Yes	No	No	1	Weakness, dizziness, confusion, backpain	Ceftriaxone	NS infusion, fluid restriction	Slow recovery
Leone	2020	USA	69	M	Yes	Yes	Yes	3	Bell's palsy, anorexia	Ceftriaxone to doxycycline	Fluid restriction, foley catheter, alpha blocker	Complete recovery

chronic diarrhea and ulcerative colitis [11] possibly accompanied by anxiety [6, 11].

In our patient, an extremely rare mix of symptoms including SIADH, urinary retention, and constipation together with facial neuritis was observed. In our review of the literature of ten similar cases, only three patients with such a symptom complex were found, but none had facial palsy. Table 1 provides the results of the literature review and our case. Eight reports were from the USA and three from Europe (France, Denmark, Italy). There were six men and five women with a median age of 64 (range 25–84) years. Seven patients had SIADH, six had enteroparesis, and seven had urinary retention, and all except one had additional neurologic symptoms with weakness being the most common presentation.

Most patients were treated with fluid restriction, and once the antibiotic treatment of Lyme disease was initiated, SIADH and the associated profound hyponatremia resolved [5, 7, 9, 12, 13]. SIADH may be an underreported manifestation of neuroinvasive Lyme disease.

Urinary retention was in most cases treated with catheterization, and several patients were given an alpha-adrenergic receptor antagonist. Olivares et al. were the first to report in 1995 a case of acute transverse myelitis related to Lyme neuroborreliosis leading to isolated acute urinary retention without lower-extremity impairment [14]. In our patient, transverse myelitis was suspected too, but MRI excluded this condition. Dumic et al. in 2019 reported a healthy 25-year-old man presenting with secondary erythema migrans, aseptic meningitis, and transverse myelitis causing bilateral lower-extremity motor and sensory deficits associated with urinary retention and constipation [15]. An additional four cases of enteroparesis causing constipation have been documented. Two of them were summarized by Shamin in 2005, both associated with other symptoms including hyponatremia, acute idiopathic polyneuritis with sensory deficits, constipation, and urinary retention, and patients also reported visual hallucinations [13]. Various gastrointestinal symptoms have been reported in Lyme disease, but enteroparesis is a rare symptom [13, 16]. The spectrum includes slow gastric emptying, constipation, and even acute and chronic intestinal pseudoobstruction [4, 8, 13, 17].

Our case highlights the importance of including neurological Lyme disease as a possible diagnosis in individuals who present with symptoms of autonomic dysregulation such as hyponatremia due to an SIADH-like syndrome, urinary retention, anorexia, constipation, and facial palsy.

References

[1] CDC, "Lyme disease. centers for disease control and prevention (CDC)," 2019, https://www.cdc.gov/lyme/index.html.

[2] J. Scieszka, J. Dabek, and P. Cieslik, "Post-lyme disease syndrome," *Reumatologia*, vol. 53, no. 1, pp. 46–48, 2015.

[3] J. A. Cardenas-De La Garza, E. De La Cruz-Valadez, J. Ocampo-Candiani, and O. Welsh, "Clinical spectrum of lyme disease," *European Journal of Clinical Microbiology and Infectious Diseases*, vol. 38, no. 2, pp. 201–208, 2019.

[4] R. Chatila and C. R. Kapadia, "Intestinal pseudoobstruction in acute lyme disease: a case report," *American Journal of Gastroenterology*, vol. 93, no. 7, pp. 1179-1180, 1998.

[5] A. Da Porto, M. Battellino, G. Colussi, V. Di Piazza, and L. Sechi, "Hiccups and inappropriate ADH secretion syndrome as presentations of tick-borne disease," *European Journal of Case Reports in Internal Medicine*, vol. 6, no. 8, Article ID 001188, 2019.

[6] B.-A. Hansen, T. Finjord, and O. Bruserud, "Autonomous dysfunction in lyme neuroborreliosis. a case report," *Clinical Case Reports*, vol. 6, no. 5, pp. 901–903, 2018.

[7] O. Salaami and D. M. Manning, "Woman with lower back pain, SIADH and a twist of lyme," *BMJ Case Reports*, vol. 7, 2018.

[8] D. F. Schefte and T. Nordentoft, "Intestinal pseudoobstruction caused by chronic lyme neuroborreliosis. a case report," *Journal of Neurogastroenterology and Motility*, vol. 21, no. 3, pp. 440–442, 2015.

[9] N. Siddiqui, D. M. St Peter, and S. Marur, "Ticks and salt: an atypical case of neuroborreliosis," *Journal of Community Hospital Internal Medicine Perspectives*, vol. 7, no. 6, pp. 358–362, 2017.

[10] J. J. Halperin, "Nervous system lyme disease," *Infectious Disease Clinics of North America*, vol. 29, no. 2, pp. 241–253, 2015.

[11] V. Sherr, "Bell's palsy of the gut and other GI manifestations of lyme and associated diseases," *Practical Gastroenterology*, vol. 30, no. 4, p. 74, 2006.

[12] M. P. Perkins, N. Shumway, and W. L. Jackson, "Lyme neuroborreliosis presenting as the syndrome of inappropriate antidiuretic hormone secretion," *MedGenMed: Medscape General Medicine*, vol. 8, no. 3, p. 71, 2006.

[13] E. A. Shamim, S. A. Shamim, G. Liss, E. Nylen, J. H. Pincus, and M. Yepes, "Constipation heralding neuroborreliosis," *Archives of Neurology*, vol. 62, no. 4, pp. 671–673, 2005.

[14] J.-P. Olivares, F. Pellas, M. Ceccaldi et al., "Lyme disease presenting as isolated acute urinary retention caused by transverse myelitis: an electrophysiological and urodynamical study," *Archives of Physical Medicine and Rehabilitation*, vol. 76, no. 12, pp. 1171-1172, 1995.

[15] I. Dumic, D. Vitorovic, S. Spritzer, E. Sviggum, J. Patel, and P. Ramanan, "Acute transverse myelitis—a rare clinical manifestation of lyme neuroborreliosis," *IDCases*, vol. 15, Article ID e00479, 2019.

[16] S. A. Zaidi and C. Singer, "Gastrointestinal and hepatic manifestations of tickborne diseases in the United States," *Clinical Infectious Diseases*, vol. 34, no. 9, pp. 1206–1212, 2002.

[17] R. Autschbach, A. Zaremba, and B. Ulrich, "Pseudo-obstruction of the colon following tick bite injury," *Chirurg*, vol. 60, no. 5, pp. 365–367, 1989.

13

Candida auris Invasive Infection after Kidney Transplantation

Javier Reque ,[1] Rosa Arlandis,[1] Nayara Panizo,[2] Maria José Pascual,[1] and Alejandro Perez-Alba[1]

[1]*Nephrology Department, Hospital General Universitario de Castellón, Castellón de la Plana, Spain*
[2]*Nephrology Department, Hospital Clínico Universitario Valencia, Valencia, Spain*

Correspondence should be addressed to Javier Reque; javier.reque@hotmail.com

Academic Editor: Sophia Lionaki

Introduction. C. auris has been associated not only with a variety of invasive fungal infections, including candidemia, sometimes related to central venous catheter, but also with pericarditis and respiratory tract and urinary tract infections. *Materials and Methods.* We describe the case of a patient with persistent fever despite antibiotics, who presented with *Candida* isolation in blood cultures, typified as *Candida auris* species. *Results.* A 57-year-old male receiving peritoneal dialysis underwent kidney transplantation which was complicated by primary nonfunction due to arterial thrombosis necessitating graft nephrectomy. During the postoperative period, he presented with *Pseudomonas aeruginosa* pneumonia that was treated with levofloxacin and catheter-related *Enterococcus faecalis* bacteremia treated with linezolid. After hospital discharge, he then presented with herpes zoster infection treated with valacyclovir. Ten days later, he developed peritonitis and exit site infection with multidrug-resistant *Pseudomonas aeruginosa* treated with intraperitoneal aztreonam and peritoneal dialysis catheter removal. Despite broad-spectrum antibiotic therapy, the patient remained febrile. All microbiology laboratory tests were negative, so it was decided to stop antibiotic therapy for 48 hours and repeat cultures in order to avoid possible false negatives. In new blood cultures performed after suspension of antibiotic therapy, candidemia was observed, later typified as *Candida auris* species. After completing antifungal treatment (three weeks with intravenous amphotericin B 100 mg qd and two weeks of intravenous anidulafungin 100 mg qd), microbiological cultures remained negative and the patient made uneventful recovery. *Conclusion. Candida auris* invasive infection has been mainly described in patients with severe underlying comorbidities and immunocompromise. Multidrug-resistant clusters of *Candida auris* are increasingly emerging.

1. Introduction

Combination treatment with micafungin and voriconazole has demonstrated efficacy for these multidrug-resistant isolates, but in case of urinary tract or central nervous system infection, amphotericin B added to 5 flucytosine is preferred, always guided by sensitivity tests.

2. Case Report

A 57-year-old man with kidney failure secondary to autosomal dominant polycystic kidney disease (ADPKD) receiving peritoneal dialysis (PD) therapy was admitted to the reference transplantation hospital to undergo kidney transplantation. The patient's medication prior to transplantation included valsartan as an antihypertensive drug and intravenous iron. He received basiliximab, tacrolimus, and mycophenolate as immunosuppressive induction therapy. Twenty-four hours after the procedure, he complained of severe abdominal pain. The Doppler ultrasound confirmed arterial thrombosis, so urgent kidney transplantectomy was indicated and PD restarted. All immunosuppressive medications were immediately discontinued. During this admission, he developed *Pseudomonas aeruginosa* pneumonia that was treated with levofloxacin for 12 days and catheter-related *Enterococcus faecalis* bacteremia treated with linezolid for 21 days. After hospital discharge, he presented with herpes zoster at the lumbar dermatomes infection treated with valacyclovir for 7 days. Ten days later, he developed PD peritonitis and exit site infection with multidrug-resistant *Pseudomonas aeruginosa* (only susceptible to colistin and aztreonam). Since the patient remained asymptomatic, treatment was started on an outpatient basis with intraperitoneal aztreonam. However, poor clinical course was observed, with increasing acute phase reactants and persistent fever. Hospital admission was decided to complete the study and treatment.

On admission, antifungal treatment with fluconazole was started and stopped after 10 days due to liver toxicity. Colistin was also commenced due to the history of multidrug-resistant *Pseudomonas aeruginosa* peritonitis. In addition, empirical coverage with intravenous vancomycin and metronidazole was initiated, and a microbiological screen was requested including blood, urine, and peritoneal fluid culture.

Given the persistence of elevated acute phase reactants and fever, we decided to remove the PD catheter 7 days after starting antibiotic treatment, and the patient was transferred to hemodialysis through a right temporary femoral catheter.

Despite broad-spectrum antibiotic therapy, the patient remained febrile. All microbiology laboratory tests were negative. At this time, it was decided to stop antibiotic therapy for 48 hours and repeat cultures in order to mitigate possible false negatives. In new blood cultures performed after suspension of antibiotic therapy, candidemia was observed, later typified as *Candida auris* species. Given these results, right femoral catheter removal was decided, antifungal treatment combined with caspofungin and amphotericin B was initiated, and contact isolation of the patient was established. Subsequently, insertion of the right internal jugular temporary catheter was made to continue hemodialysis sessions. Caspofungin was suspended two days after initiation due to liver toxicity, replacing it with anidulafungin.

After initiation of antifungal therapy, progressive clinical improvement was observed, with persistent decrease in acute phase reactants and fever. Serum blood cultures were performed every 72 hours after the first week of treatment and remained negative in all determinations. Given these results, after one month of antifungal treatment, insertion of a right internal jugular permanent tunnelled hemodialysis catheter was performed.

After completing antifungal treatment (three weeks with intravenous amphotericin B 100 mg qd and two weeks of intravenous anidulafungin 100 mg qd) with negative microbiological cultures and given the clinical stability of the patient, he was discharged with subsequent outpatient follow-up.

3. Discussion

This is one of the few cases reported in patients on peritoneal dialysis and the first in our region. The newest *Candida* species called *Candida auris* was first reported in Japan in 2009 and named so as it was first described and isolated from the ear canal of a Japanese patient. It has been subsequently isolated from several body sites of patients in multiple countries on five continents [1]. It has been associated with nosocomial outbreaks in intensive care settings, and its transmission despite the implementation of enhanced infection prevention and control (IPC) measures is a particular concern.

The *Candida auris* genome is approximately 12.5 Mb [2]. Genome analysis suggests that there are between 6,500 and 8,500 protein-coding sequences, with a number of these genes coding for proteins characterized as virulence factors in other *Candida* species, such as biofilm formation [3]. In addition, multiple transporter genes and protein kinases, which may facilitate the acquisition of drug resistance, have been identified [2]. Colonization with *C. auris* has been detected at multiple body sites, including the nares, groin, axilla, and rectum [4,5], suggesting the need for systemic swabs/cultures and patient isolation after treatment and upon readmission to healthcare facilities.

C. auris has not only been associated with a variety of invasive fungal infections, including candidemia, sometimes related to central venous catheters, but also presents as pericarditis and respiratory tract and urinary tract infections [4,5]. Most of the cases have been described in intensive care facilities, usually in patients with severe underlying comorbidities including hematological malignancies and other immunocompromised states [6]. *Candida auris* infection treatment is a major concern due to the increasing emergence of multidrug-resistant clusters. Reduced susceptibility to triazole antifungals has been demonstrated in different regions, and there is also variable susceptibility of isolates to amphotericin B [7]. Consequently, echinocandins were initially recommended as empirical treatment. However, because of the widespread use of echinocandins, *C. auris* isolates with reduced susceptibility are appearing [8]. Combination treatment with micafungin and voriconazole has demonstrated efficacy for these multidrug-resistant isolates in vitro [9].

Mortality rates have varied significantly across geographic regions. As such, the overall attributable mortality rate is unclear. In the United Kingdom, no deaths were considered directly attributable to *C. auris* for 22 patients who received targeted antifungal treatment [6]. The number of deaths attributable to candidemia, as opposed to an underlying medical condition, may be difficult to quantify.

In conclusion, invasive *Candida auris* infection is rare, and one of the main determinants of prognosis is early treatment.

References

[1] A. Jeffery-Smith, S. K. Taori, and S. Schelenz, "Candida auris: a review of the literature," *Clinical Microbiology Reviews*, p. 31, 2018.

[2] C. Sharma, N. Kumar, J. F. Meis, R. Pandey, and A. Chowdhary, "Draft genome sequence of a fluconazole-resistant candida auris strain from a candidemia patient in india," *Genome Announcements*, vol. 3, 2015.

[3] S. Chatterjee, S. V. Alampalli, R. K. Nageshan, S. T. Chettiar, S. Joshi, and U. S. Tatu, "Draft genome of a commonly misdiagnosed multidrug resistant pathogen Candida auris," *BMC Genomics*, vol. 16, no. 1, p. 686, 2015.

[4] S. Vallabhaneni, A. Kallen, and S. Tsay, “Investigation of the first seven reported cases of Candida auris, a globally emerging invasive, multidrug-resistant fungus-United States,” *American Journal of Transplantation: Official Journal of the American Society of Transplantation and the American Society of Transplant Surgeons*, vol. 17, pp. 296–299, 2017.

[5] S. Schelenz, F. Hagen, J. L. Rhodes et al., “First hospital outbreak of the globally emerging Candida auris in a European hospital,” *Antimicrobial Resistance and Infection Control*, vol. 5, no. 1, p. 35, 2016.

[6] B. Calvo, A. S. A. Melo, A. Perozo-Mena et al., “First report of Candida auris in America: clinical and microbiological aspects of 18 episodes of candidemia,” *Journal of Infection*, vol. 73, no. 4, pp. 369–374, 2016.

[7] S. R. Lockhart, K. A. Etienne, S. Vallabhaneni et al., “Simultaneous emergence of multidrug-ResistantCandida aurison 3 continents confirmed by whole-genome sequencing and epidemiological analyses,” *Clinical Infectious Diseases*, vol. 64, no. 2, pp. 134–140.

[8] C. Sharma, N. Kumar, R. Pandey, J. F. Meis, and A. Chowdhary, “Whole genome sequencing of emerging multidrug resistant Candida auris isolates in India demonstrates low genetic variation,” *New microbes and new infections*, vol. 13, pp. 77–82, 2016.

[9] H. Fakhim, A. Chowdhary, and A. Prakash, “In vitro interactions of echinocandins with triazoles against multidrug-resistant candida auris,” *Antimicrobial Agents and Chemotherapy*, p. 61, 2017.

14

Highest Recorded Serum Creatinine

Christine Persaud,[1] Uttsav Sandesara,[2] Victor Hoang,[1] Joshua Tate,[1] Wayne Latack,[1] and David Dado[1]

[1]Department of Medicine, Keesler Medical Center, Biloxi 39534, MS, USA
[2]Department of Medicine, University of Mississippi Medical Center, Jackson 39216, MS, USA

Correspondence should be addressed to Christine Persaud; christine.k.persaud@mail.mil

Academic Editor: Anja Haase-Fielitz

Serum creatinine is a commonly used laboratory marker to assess kidney function; however, there has not been an established level of serum creatinine to predict mortality. After extensive literature review, we present a case of the highest recorded serum creatinine of 73.8 mg/dL in a 23-year-old male with the history of pediatric deceased donor kidney transplant (DDKT). He initially presented with uremia and signs of acute renal allograft failure after two months of immunosuppressive medication non-adherence, ultimately requiring emergent hemodialysis, which was complicated by new onset seizures. This was the patient's fourth episode of late acute rejection and emphasizes the need for education of immunosuppressant adherence and periodic monitoring of renal function in high-risk patients. Though there is no known creatinine level incompatible with life, this patient appears to have the highest known serum creatinine in a uremic patient on record.

1. Introduction

Serum creatinine is a commonly used laboratory measurement to gauge renal function in clinical practice. Creatinine is a byproduct of the metabolism of creatine in skeletal muscle and dietary meat intake [1]. It is freely filtered across the glomerulus, and there is additional creatinine secretion in the proximal tubule of the nephron via organic cation secretory pathways [2]. Therefore, serum creatinine is a reflection of glomerular filtration rate, creatinine secretion in the renal tubule, creatine intake, and baseline skeletal muscle mass. Creatinine is also known to vary by gender and race, with average values of 1.14 mg/dL in men and 0.93 mg/dL in women in the United States [3]. The previously highest serum creatinine reported was 53 mg/dL [4]. In current clinical practice, there remains uncertainty regarding the role of serum creatinine and mortality, specifically in the context of the degree of creatinine elevation. We present a case of acute renal allograft rejection with the highest serum creatinine reported in previous literature.

2. Case Presentation

We report a 23-year-old African American male with a medical history of pediatric DDRT secondary to left-sided dysplastic kidney and right-sided obstructive uropathy. He presented to the emergency department with a one-week history of decreasing urine output, increased shortness of breath, generalized weakness, and nausea. He initially received his DDKT in 2010, which has been complicated by multiple episodes of both acute T cell-mediated and acute antibody-mediated rejection. The patient admitted to a two-month history of immunosuppressive medication non-adherence with tacrolimus, mycophenolate, and prednisone.

Physical examination revealed a young male, in no distress, weighing 142 pounds. He had a blood pressure of 153/102 mmHg and a heart rate of 77 beats/min. Exam findings are as follows: pale conjunctiva, lungs clear to auscultation, regular heart rate and rhythm, active bowel sounds, no abdominal tenderness, and no focal neurological deficit. Admission labs included a serum creatinine of

64.6 mg/dL (0.67–1.17 mg/dL) with a blood urea nitrogen (BUN) of 212 mg/dL (6–20 mg/dL), which increased to a serum creatinine of 73.8 mg/dL and BUN of 244 mg/dL prior to initiation of emergent dialysis. Serum chemistry included sodium 137 mmol/L (136–145 mmol/L), potassium 6.0 mmol/L (3.5–5.1 mmol/L), chloride 98 mmol/L (98–107 mmol/L), total carbon dioxide 7 mmol/L (22–29 mmol/L), glucose 68 mg/dL (74–106 mg/dL), and phosphorus 14.7 mg/dL (2.7–4.5 mg/dL).

The patient was initiated on emergent dialysis via a temporary dialysis catheter. Dialysis was complicated by new onset of seizures, initially thought to be secondary to dialysis disequilibrium syndrome. An electroencephalogram (EEG) was performed showing right temporal spikes epileptiform discharges with intermittent slow waves lateralized to the right hemisphere. Patient was thought to have epilepsy with initial seizure exacerbation secondary to severe metabolic derangements in setting of acute renal failure and severe azotemia. He was initiated on daily levetiracetam with resolution of seizures.

Patient received continuous renal replacement therapy (CRRT) while in the intensive care unit. After stabilization of his acute medical issues, a tunneled dialysis catheter was placed in his right internal jugular vein prior to discharge. Ultimately, the patient was diagnosed with renal allograft failure secondary to medication nonadherence and was discharged home on intermittent hemodialysis with improvement in serum creatinine to 23.8 mg/dL and BUN of 76 mg/dL at time of discharge, after completion of four hemodialysis sessions.

3. Discussion

This case demonstrated a record high serum creatinine of 73.8 mg/dL based on our review of previous literature [4–7]. Currently, there is not a known effect of creatinine levels on human physiology or survivability [5]. Even with its inherent limitations, previous studies have explored the relationship between increased serum creatinine and mortality. In a prospective population-based study of people >65 years old, 11.2% of the population had an elevated serum creatinine (>1.5 mg/dL in men and >1.3 mg/dL in women) which was associated with a higher overall mortality (76.7 vs. 29.5/1000 years) [8]. In a retrospective study of hospitalized patients, very low serum creatinine admission value of <0.4 mg/dL was significantly associated with increased mortality, exceeding the risk related to a creatinine value of >1.5 mg/dL [9].

This patient had elevated creatinine secondary to acute renal allograft rejection. Acute allograft rejection is a functional deterioration of the allograft caused by specific pathologic changes due to recipient's immune system recognizing nonself-antigens from the allograft [10]. Typically, such rejection leads to subsequent rise in serum creatinine indicating substantial histological damages without significant symptom manifestation [11]. The long-term function of a renal allograft is associated significantly with acute rejection episodes, especially late acute rejections [12]. Late acute rejections occur greater than 3 months after transplant, and this case represented the patient's fourth episode of such. In a previous historical cohort study, the late acute rejection group was shown to have the highest amount of graft loss when compared to the no rejection and early acute rejection groups [12]. This patient was ultimately diagnosed with renal allograft failure and remained dialysis dependent after discharge.

Our patient showed minimal symptoms initially, likely related more to azotemia and metabolic derangements rather than the elevated serum creatinine level. Chronic kidney disease (CKD) symptoms typically do not manifest until KDIGO CKD stages IV and V [13]. Chronic kidney disease is commonly detected by routine urine testing and labs, as it initially can present asymptomatically [13]. This case demonstrates the importance of periodic lab evaluation to assess kidney function in high-risk renal patients and the need for counseling on the importance of medication adherence. There is no known creatinine incompatible with life, and this patient appears to have the highest survivable serum creatinine recorded in the medical literature.

Disclosure

The views expressed in this material are those of the authors and do not reflect the official policy or position of the U.S. Government, the Department of Defense or the Department of the Air Force.

References

[1] A. S. Levey, R. D. Perrone, and N. E. Madias, "Serum creatinine and renal function," *Annual Review of Medicine*, vol. 39, no. 1, pp. 465–490, 1988.

[2] O. Shemesh, H. Golbetz, J. P. Kriss, and B. D. Myers, "Limitations of creatinine as a filtration marker in glomerulopathic patients," *Kidney International*, vol. 28, no. 5, pp. 830–838, 1985.

[3] C. Jones, G. McQuillan, J. Kusek et al., "Serum creatinine levels in the US population: third national health and nutrition examination survey," *American Journal of Kidney Diseases*, vol. 32, no. 6, pp. 992–999, 1998.

[4] A. A. Asif, H. Hussain, and T. Chatterjee, "Extraordinary creatinine level: a case report," *Cureus*, vol. 12, 2020.

[5] A. C. Storm, N. L. Htike, D. A. Cohen, and R. L. Benz, "A surviving patient with record high creatinine," *Open Journal of Nephrology*, vol. 3, no. 4, pp. 217–219, 2013.

[6] V. Master Sankar Raj, J. Garcia, and R. Gordillo, "17 year-old boy with renal failure and the highest reported creatinine in pediatric literature," *Case Reports in Pediatrics*, vol. 2015, Article ID 703960, 4 pages, 2015.

[7] S. D. Abuhasna, "Highest serum creatinine ever reported," *Hemodialysis International*, vol. 17, no. 1, pp. 137-138, 2012.

[8] L. F. Fried, M. G. Shlipak, C. Crump et al., "Renal insufficiency as a predictor of cardiovascular outcomes and mortality in elderly individuals," *Journal of the American College of Cardiology*, vol. 41, no. 8, pp. 1364–1372, 2003.

[9] C. Thongprayoon, W. Cheungpasitporn, W. Kittanamongkolchai, A. M. Harrison, and K. Kashani, "Prognostic importance of low admission serum creatinine concentration for mortality in hospitalized patients," *The American Journal of Medicine*, vol. 130, no. 5, pp. 545–554, 2017.

[10] R. Naik, *Renal Transplantation Rejection*, StatPearls Publishing, Treasure Island, FL, USA, 2020, https://www.statpearls.com/articlelibrary/viewarticle/17170/.

[11] H. Reisner, J. C. Jennette, and A. M. Hussein Gasim, "Chapter 13: pathology of medical renal disease," in *Pathology: A Modern Case Study*, McGraw-Hill, Chapel Hill, NC, USA, 2nd edition, 2015.

[12] M. Jalalzadeh, N. Mousavinasab, S. Peyrovi, and M. H. Ghadiani, "The impact of acute rejection in kidney transplantation on long-term allograft and patient outcome," *Nephro-Urology Monthly*, vol. 7, no. 1, Article ID e24439, 2015.

[13] S. Vaidya, *Chronic Renal Failure*, StatPearls Publishing, Treasure Island, FL, USA, 2020, https://www.statpearls.com/articlelibrary/viewarticle/28357/.

15

Langerhans Cell Histiocytosis Manifests with Acute Severe Hypernatremia during Hospitalization

Kullaya Takkavatakarn,[1] **Hansamon Poparn**,[2,3] **and Pisut Katavetin**[1]

[1]*Division of Nephrology, Department of Medicine, King Chulalongkorn Memorial Hospital, Faculty of Medicine, Chulalongkorn University, Bangkok, Thailand*
[2]*Department of Pediatric Hematology and Oncology, Department of Pediatrics, Faculty of Medicine, Chulalongkorn University, Bangkok, Thailand*
[3]*Integrative and Innovative Hematology/Oncology Research Unit, Faculty of Medicine, Chulalongkorn University, Bangkok, Thailand*

Correspondence should be addressed to Kullaya Takkavatakarn; koykullaya@hotmail.com

Academic Editor: Anja Haase-Fielitz

Central diabetes insipidus (DI) is characterized by a deficiency in arginine vasopressin (AVP), an antidiuretic hormone leading to excessive free water loss in the urine and hypernatremia. Central DI can be the first presentation of several occult diseases. However, patients with central DI who have functioning thirst mechanisms and access to water may initially exhibit normal sodium levels. We report a 57-year-old woman who was admitted to the hospital due to cholangitis. Her initial serum sodium was normal and she rapidly developed severe hypernatremia after fluid restriction. The results of the laboratory workup indicated DI, which dramatically responded to desmopressin. MRI showed an ill-defined faint hyper signal intensity in T1, T2/FLAIR lesions involving the bilateral hypothalamus. The histopathological findings confirmed the diagnosis of Langerhans cell histiocytosis (LCH) with multiorgan involvement. Serum sodium returned to normal after receiving desmopressin and water replacement therapy.

1. Introduction

Hypernatremia, defined as a serum sodium concentration greater than 145 mEq/L, is a common electrolyte disorder in hospitalized patients and is significantly associated with in-hospital mortality. The primary cause of hyponatremia is water deficit resulting from a deficiency in water intake or excessive water loss. Central diabetes insipidus (DI) is characterized by a lack of arginine vasopressin (AVP), an antidiuretic hormone (ADH), due to several disorders that arise from either the pituitary or the hypothalamus. The deficiency of AVP leads to hypotonic polyuria. Central DI patients who have intact thirst mechanisms increase their water intake to maintain water balance and sodium levels. In the setting of impaired or limited access to free water, hypernatremia might rapidly develop. Delay in diagnosis and treatment of central DI could result in severe hypernatremia and serious neurological complications. Central DI should be considered in patients who develop acute hypernatremia after hospitalization, especially in patients with polyuria, regardless of the history of hypothalamic-pituitary disease.

2. Case Report

A 57-year-old woman was admitted to the medical ward due to an acute fever for 2 days. She had palpable neck mass and progressive jaundice for 2 months. She developed nocturia and polydipsia with a daily fluid intake of 4–6 L per day for 2 weeks. On physical examination, her blood pressure was 82/50 mmHg, pulse rate 92 beats per minute, and body temperature 38°C. Her body weight was 58 kg. She had moderate icteric sclera and thyroid enlargement with a firm consistency. Her liver span was 14 cm. Her abdomen was soft with mild tenderness at the right upper quadrant. The computed tomography of the neck and abdomen revealed diffusely enlarged thyroid glands that caused tracheal effacement and marked hepatomegaly with many enlarged intra-abdominal lymph nodes that constricted the common bile duct. She was diagnosed with acute cholangitis with septic shock. Her vital signs were stable after receiving antibiotics and resuscitation with 2 L of normal saline. She was ordered to be NPO to monitor her abdominal signs. Her serum sodium was 138 mEq/L. Eighteen hours after admission, her serum sodium level increased to 169 mEq/L without overt neurological abnormalities. Total fluid intake was 3,800 ml (normal saline) and her urine output was 5,850 mL in 18 hours. Her body weight was 56.4 kg.

Routine laboratory values are shown in Table 1. Urine specific gravity and osmolality were 1.004 and 152 mOsm/Kg, respectively. Urine sodium was less than 20 mEq/L and urine potassium was 6.8 mEq/L. After two micrograms of desmopressin was prescribed, her urine output was substantially reduced to 20 mL per hour and urine osmolality was increased to 628 mOsm/Kg (313%), indicating complete central DI. The hormonal assay revealed normal serum morning cortisol and thyroid hormone. Magnetic resonance imaging (MRI) of the sellar and suprasellar regions was performed to determine the underlying pathology responsible for central DI. The pituitary gland and pituitary stalk were both normal in size. There was an ill-defined faint hyper signal intensity in T1, T2/FLAIR lesion involving the bilateral hypothalamus with modest perilesional edema (Figure 1). The pathology of the thyroid and lymph node biopsies revealed aggregation of histiocyte-like cells, some of which had nuclear grooves. The immunohistochemistry was positive for CD1a and S100, which was compatible with Langerhans cell histiocytosis (LCH) (Figure 2). She had no family history of LCH. Her bone and skin were unremarkable.

The final diagnosis was complete central DI due to LCH with the hypothalamus, thyroid, and lymph node involvement. To correct hypernatremia, 5% dextrose water was administered to replace the water deficit. In addition, daily intranasal desmopressin 2.5 mcg was prescribed. Her serum sodium level had returned to normal after three days. Figure 3 demonstrates the time course of the serum sodium concentration.

After treatment with intravenous antibiotics, acute cholangitis was significantly improved and the patient could be discharged from the hospital. Dexamethasone was started for treatment of LCH and chemotherapy was scheduled to begin. Two weeks later, the patient was still stable, with a normal serum sodium level.

Table 1: Laboratory data.

Parameter	Result	Reference
Serum		
Sodium, mEq/L	138	135–145
Potassium, mEq/L	3.4	3.5–5.0
Chloride, mEq/L	102	98–107
Bicarbonate, mEq/L	31	22–29
Urea nitrogen, mg/dL	9	7–20
Creatinine, mg/dL	0.78	0.5–1.0
Glucose, mg/dL	98	70–100
Calcium, mg/dL	7.7	8.8–10.2
Phosphorus, mg/dL	2.8	2.5–4.5
Albumin, g/dL	1.8	3.5–5.0
Total bilirubin, mg/dL	11.26	0.2–1.2
Direct bilirubin, mg/dL	8.65	0–0.5
SGOT, μ/l	121	5–35
SGPT, μ/l	21	0–40
Alkaline phosphatase, μ/L	900	40–120
Urine		
Specific gravity	1.004	1.003–1.030
Osmolality, mOsm/Kg	152	100–850
Sodium, mEq/L	<20	
Potassium, mEq/L	6.8	

SGOT-serum glutamic-oxaloacetic transaminase; SGPT-serum glutamic pyruvate transaminase.

3. Discussion

Hypernatremia is a common electrolyte disorder caused by either excessive sodium intake or net water loss. Only a few instances, such as administration of hypertonic sodium bicarbonate during resuscitation or hypertonic saline to correct hyponatremia, cause sodium retention. Therefore, the cause of hypernatremia in the vast majority of patients is water deficit due to decreased water intake or increased water loss. Thirst and ADH secretion are the two defense mechanisms against hypernatremia. Although stimulation of thirst occurs at a slightly higher serum osmolality than ADH secretion, thirst is the primary defense mechanism against hypernatremia. Thus, patients with normal thirst mechanisms and who can access water rarely have hypernatremia. In addition, ADH plays an essential role in preventing further electrolyte-free water loss by maximizing urine concentration [1]. Three primary conditions are necessary to concentrate urine: (1) a concentrated renal medullary interstitium, (2) ADH to insert aquaporin-2 channels into the apical membranes of the collecting duct, and (3) the ability of collecting duct cells to respond to ADH [2]. Patients with defective thirst mechanisms or limited access to water, such as neonates, the elderly, and patients with neurological disabilities, may develop hypernatremia due to insufficient water intake. DI and osmotic diuresis result in excess urinary water loss. While diarrhea, vomiting, and conditions that enhance insensible loss cause nonrenal water loss.

Hypernatremia is always accompanied by hyperosmolarity. As a result, patients with hypernatremia should have maximally concentrated urine. If defense mechanisms are intact and the renal concentrating mechanism is normal, patients would have urine osmolality greater than 600–800 mOsm/Kg and would not have polyuria [3]. A normal response is observed in patients with hypodipsia and nonrenal water loss. In contrast, patients with lower urine osmolality or polyuria usually have hypernatremia from diabetes insipidus or osmotic diuresis. In our patient, her

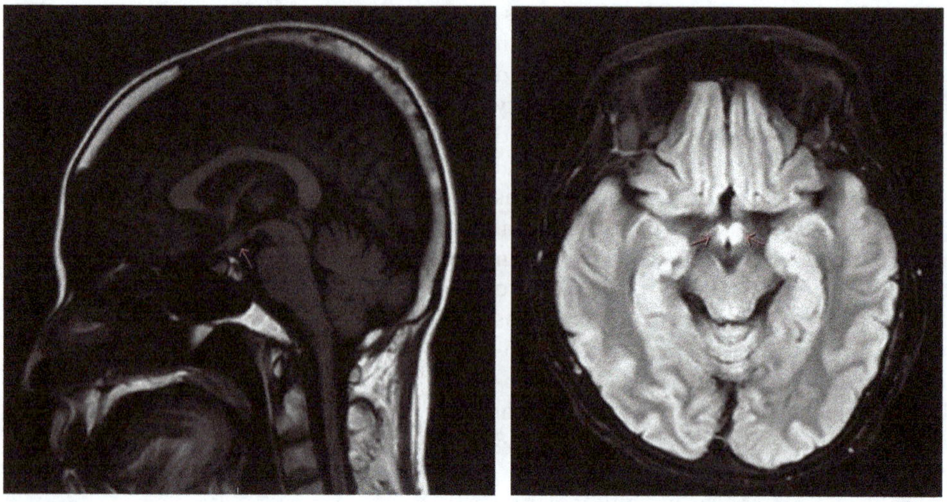

FIGURE 1: T1 and T2 FLAIR sections of magnetic resonance imaging show hyper signal intensity involving the bilateral hypothalamus.

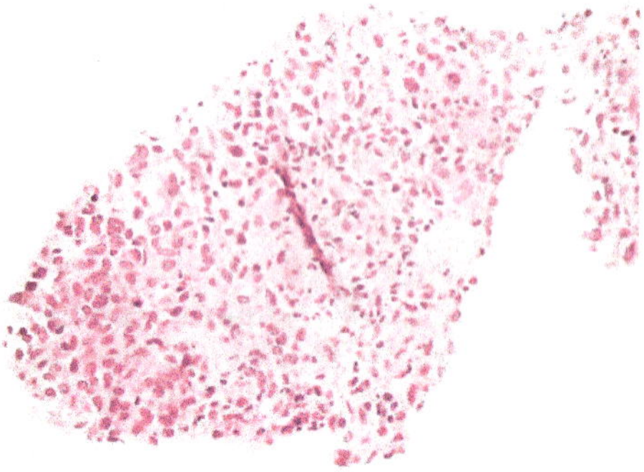

FIGURE 2: The core biopsy shows the aggregation of histiocyte-like cells, some of which show nuclear grooves. Mitosis and necrosis are not observed.

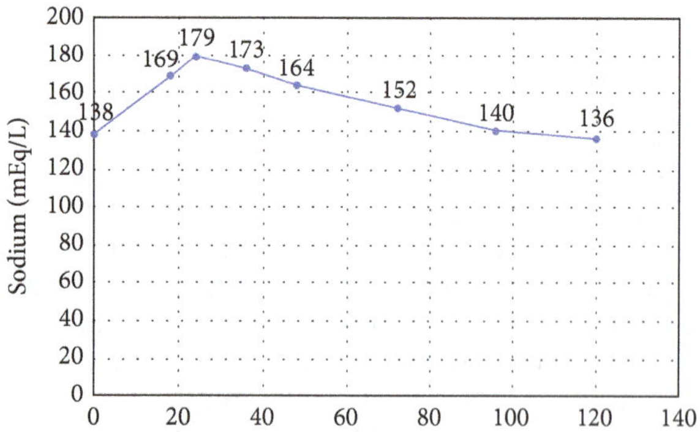

FIGURE 3: Time course of sodium levels.

serum sodium levels increased significantly (31 mEq/L in 18 hours) after being admitted to the hospital with oral fluid restriction. The patient did not have a history of hypertonic fluid administration and gastrointestinal loss. Moreover, the patient had low urine osmolality and polyuria (>3 L in 24 hours), suggesting renal water loss from diabetes insipidus (Figure 4).

The next step diagnostic process was to determine whether the DI is central or nephrogenic. Administration of desmopressin, a synthetic analog of ADH, after water deprivation, could help distinguish the various forms of DI. Patients with central DI are able to concentrate the urine after the deficiency of ADH is replaced with desmopressin, whereas patients with nephrogenic DI do not have a substantial response to desmopressin due to renal resistance to ADH activity. An increase of at least more than 50 percent in urine osmolality after desmopressin administration suggests complete central DI which is caused by several disorders that arise from either the pituitary or the hypothalamus [4]. A thorough clinical history and physical examination should be obtained to evaluate for the signs and symptoms of hormonal deficiency. Also, an MRI of the sellar and suprasellar regions is required to evaluate any pituitary or hypothalamic abnormalities.

LCH is a rare disorder characterized by clonal proliferation of CD1a+/CD207+ myeloid dendritic cells. The pathogenesis of LCH remains unclear, but recent studies support that activation of the mitogen-activated protein kinase (MAPK) pathway plays a major role in the development of LCH, with somatic mutation in $BRAF^{V600E}$ (50–65%) and MAP2K1 (25%) being the most common mutations resulting in the overactive MAPK pathway [5, 6]. LCH is primarily considered a pediatric disease with a case rate of approximately 5 per million; however, it can occur at any age. The incidence of LCH in an adult is very low (1–2 cases per million) [7]. Consequently, the diagnosis of LCH might be delayed due to the lack of suspicion.

The clinical manifestations of LCH depend on sites of accumulation or infiltration of abnormal proliferative cells, ranging from focal self-limited single organ involvement to aggressive multiorgan involvement. Bone and skin are the most common sites, followed by the central nervous system (CNS), liver, spleen, lungs, lymph nodes, and hematopoietic system [8]. Adult-onset LCH is typically multisystem involvement. The most common presenting symptom of CNS-LCH is central DI due to hypothalamic-pituitary involvement [9]. The prevalence of central DI in patients with LCH ranges from 10–30% and increases to 40% in patients with multisystem involvement [10, 11]. A previous case of adipsic

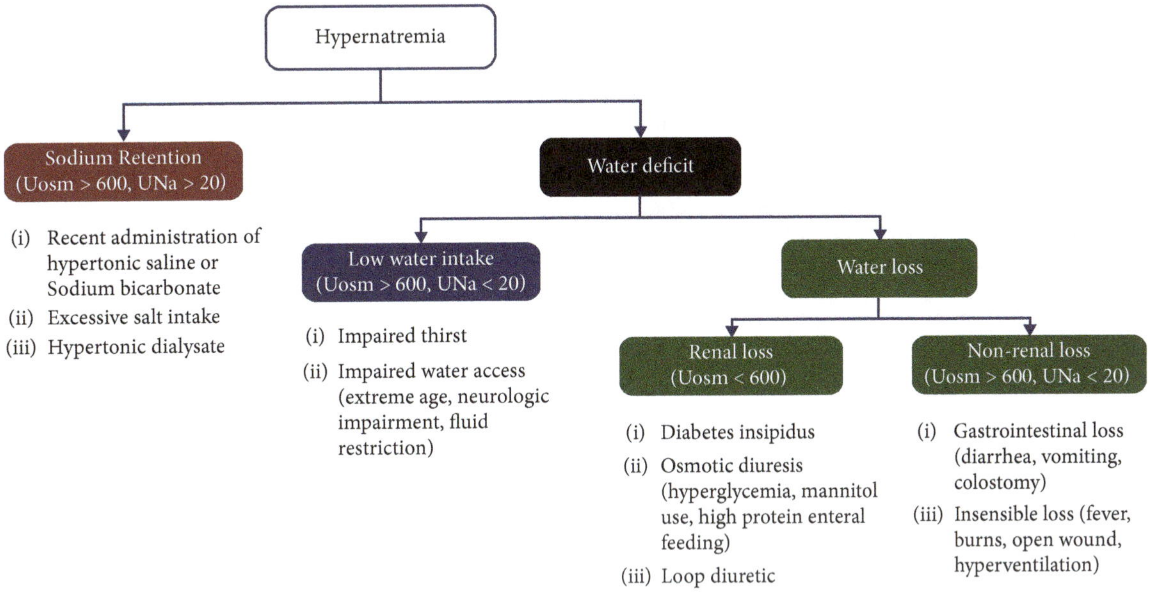

FIGURE 4: Diagnostic approach to hypernatremia.

DI caused by LCH has been previously reported. The infiltration of the thirst center in the hypothalamus could be the possible mechanism underlying adipsic DI [12]. In addition, CDI can be the first manifestation, even before LCH is diagnosed. Therefore, LCH should be considered in patients with central DI. MRI brain may show abnormal T2 hyper-intensity at hypothalamic or sella-suprasellar regions. The definitive diagnosis of LCH must be confirmed by a pathological study of affected tissue that should be positive for CD1a, CD207, and S100 in immunohistochemical studies [13].

4. Learning Points

(i) Central DI patients with intact thirst mechanisms and water accessibility can present with normal sodium levels. A detailed history of polyuria and polydipsia should be obtained in suspicious cases.

(ii) Central DI should be considered in acute severe hypernatremia patients with polyuria regardless of the history of hypothalamic-pituitary disease.

(iii) Langerhans cell histiocytosis, an uncommon illness that affects multiple organs, is one of the causes of central DI. Therefore, a biopsy of the affected tissue should be performed to confirm the diagnosis when the clinical picture is suspicious of this disease.

Acknowledgments

The authors thank Dr. Pinya Chanjaruvong for reviewing the MRI and Dr. Narittee Sukswai for preparation of the microscopic pictures of the pathology.

References

[1] S. N. Thornton, "Thirst and hydration: physiology and consequences of dysfunction," *Physiology & Behavior*, vol. 100, no. 1, pp. 15–21, 2010.

[2] J. M. Sands and H. E. Layton, "The physiology of urinary concentration: an update," *Seminars in Nephrology*, vol. 29, no. 3, pp. 178–195, 2009.

[3] M. M. Braun, C. H. Barstow, and N. J. Pyzocha, "Diagnosis and management of sodium disorders: hyponatremia and hypernatremia," *American Family Physician*, vol. 91, no. 5, pp. 299–307, 2015.

[4] S. Gubbi, F. Hannah-Shmouni, C. A. Koch, and J. G. Verbalis, "Diagnostic testing for diabetes insipidus," in *Endotext [Internet]*, K. R. Feingold, B. Anawalt, A. Boyce, G. Chrousos, W. W. de Herder, and K. Dhatariya, Eds., MDText.com, Inc, South Dartmouth, USA, 2000.

[5] G. Badalian-Very, J. A. Vergilio, M. Fleming, and B. J. Rollins, "Pathogenesis of langerhans cell histiocytosis," *Annual Review of Pathology: Mechanisms of Disease*, vol. 8, no. 1, pp. 1–20, 2013.

[6] J. Signorelli, S. Ravulapati, J. L. Patel, M. W. Deininger, and S. K. Tantravahi, "Disease characteristics and treatment of adult langerhans cell histiocytosis: a single center experience," *Blood*, vol. 132, no. Supplement 1, p. 4315, 2018.

[7] C. Lian, Y. Lu, and S. Shen, "Langerhans cell histiocytosis in adults: a case report and review of the literature," *Oncotarget*, vol. 7, no. 14, Article ID 18678, 2016.

[8] J. K. Suh, S. Kang, H. Kim, H. J. Im, and K. N. Koh, "Recent advances in the understanding of the molecular pathogenesis and targeted therapy options in langerhans cell histiocytosis," *Blood Research*, vol. 56, no. S1, pp. S65–S69, 2021.

[9] W. R. Duarte-Celada, S. Thakolwiboon, L. Brandi, C. Duarte-Celada, and M. Avila, "Adult langerhans cell histiocytosis of the central nervous system," *Baylor University Medical Center Proceedings*, vol. 33, no. 4, pp. 603–605, 2020.

[10] M. Aricò, M. Girschikofsky, T. Généreau et al., "Langerhans cell histiocytosis in adults: report from the international registry of the histiocyte society," *European Journal of Cancer*, vol. 39, no. 16, pp. 2341–2348, 2003.

[11] R. Al-Hader, A. Suneja, M. Ab, and A. B. Memon, "Adult-onset neurological langerhans cell histiocytosis and response

to treatment," *Austin Journal of Clinical Neurology*, vol. 8, no. 1, p. 1146, 2021.

[12] S. Kumar, P. Rohl, and T. Diamond, "A rare case of adipsic diabetes insipidus associated with Langerhans cell histiocytosis," *AACE Clinical Case Reports*, vol. 4, no. 5, pp. e388–e393, 2018.

[13] S. K. Lau, P. G. Chu, and L. M. Weiss, "Immunohistochemical expression of langerin in langerhans cell histiocytosis and non-langerhans cell histiocytic disorders," *The American Journal of Surgical Pathology*, vol. 32, no. 4, pp. 615–619, 2008.

16

Ten Cases of Biopsy-Proven Acute Tubulointerstitial Nephritis: Report from a Single Center in a Rural Area from 2008 to 2021

Kei Nagai[1,2] **Tsuyoshi Tsukada,**[1] **Akiko Sakata,**[3] **and Atsushi Ueda**[1]

[1]*Department of Nephrology, Hitachi General Hospital, 2-1-1 Jonan-Cho, Hitachi, Ibaraki 317-0077, Japan*
[2]*Department of Nephrology, Faculty of Medicine, University of Tsukuba, 1-1-1 Tennodai, Tsukuba, Ibaraki 305-8575, Japan*
[3]*Department of Pathology, Hitachi General Hospital, 2-1-1 Jonan-Cho, Hitachi, Ibaraki 317-0077, Japan*

Correspondence should be addressed to Kei Nagai; knagai@md.tsukuba.ac.jp

Academic Editor: Kouichi Hirayama

Acute tubulointerstitial nephritis (ATIN) can be caused by any number of factors, and it accounts for several percent of renal biopsy cases. In Japan, case reports exist, but there are few single-center series of ATIN cases. *Case 1.* A teenage male patient developed fever and cough on day X-61 and was found to have normal renal function and positive C-reactive protein (CRP) by his primary care physician. On day X-20, he presented with cough and nasal discharge in addition to low-grade fever, and his doctor noted renal dysfunction with serum creatinine of 2.12 mg/dL, negative urine occult blood, and positive urine glucose. Renal biopsy results showed diffuse interstitial nephritis with scarce glomerular involvement. There was no concurrent uveitis. Renal function normalized after 4 months of treatment with moderate-dose prednisolone. *Cases 2–10.* Of the 422 cases for which renal biopsies were performed at our institution from 2008 to 2021, acute tubulointerstitial nephritis was confirmed clinically and pathologically in 9 cases in addition to case 1, accounting for 2.4% of all biopsy cases. In the analysis of the 10 patients, the median age was 40 years old, eGFR at diagnosis was 19.4 (3.2–49.1) mL/min/1.73 m^2, and 2 of them underwent hemodialysis, but both were weaned from dialysis, and the eGFR after treatment was 53.6 (20.8–110.0) mL/min/1.73 m^2; all patients showed improvement ($P < 0.001$). Treatment consisted of steroids in 8 patients and no steroids in 2 patients, the latter being treated by discontinuation of the suspect drugs and treatment of infection; 7 of the 10 patients were examined for ocular uveitis, and uveitis was diagnosed in 5 patients. The causes and clinical course of ATIN are diverse, but it is treated according to individual judgment in addition to standard treatment, and it generally has a good renal prognosis.

1. Introduction

Acute tubulointerstitial nephritis (ATIN) accounts for approximately 1–3% of all renal biopsies and 6–27% of renal biopsies during the clinical course of acute kidney injury, depending on the patient population [1–4]. Classically, ATIN has been reported to be secondary to bacterial and viral infections and tuberculosis, but in recent years, antibiotics and anti-inflammatory drugs (non-steroidal anti-inflammatory drugs, NSAIDs), as well as proton pump inhibitors (PPIs), have been implicated. Sarcoidosis, IgG4-related disease, and tubulointerstitial nephritis and uveitis (TINU) syndrome have also been reported as immunological causes [1, 5–7]. Differences in causes are reflected in differences in the clinical course, which vary greatly depending on the subject under investigation, and there are fewer reported cases of ATIN than those of glomerular disease. Therefore, reports from specific spatiotemporal areas are important for an accurate understanding of the clinical epidemiology of ATIN. In this report, a representative case and a series of ATIN cases in a single center in a rural area, which have not been reported extensively in Japan to date, are presented.

2. Case Presentation

2.1. Case 1. A teenage male patient developed fever and cough on X-61 and was found to have normal renal function and positive C-reactive protein (CRP) of 4.76 mg/dL by his primary care physician. On day X-20, he presented with cough and nasal discharge in addition to a low-grade fever, and he was found to have serum CRP of 5.37 mg/dL, serum creatinine of 2.12 mg/dL, negative urine occult blood, and positive urine protein (1+) and urine sugar (1+). At the same time, he was on multiple medications, including antitussive expectorants and anti-allergic medications. At the subsequent visit on day X-6, positive CRP and renal impairment continued, and he was referred to our hospital for further investigation. On day X-4, the laboratory data indicated severe tubulointerstitial nephritis with positive urine protein (1+) and urine sugar (1+), along with urine β2-microglobulin of 56.73 mg/L and N-acetyl-β-D-glucosaminidase (NAG) of 14.5 IU/L, with eosinophilia (11% of white blood cells, 7100/μL) (Figure 1). He was hospitalized for a renal biopsy in our department, and laboratory test findings on admission are shown in Table 1. Anti-nuclear antibody was negative, and specific antibodies (anti-dsDNA-antibody, anti-SS-A, and anti-SS-B antibody) were negative on serum immunology. The renal specimen contained 8 glomeruli and was found to show no global sclerosis and no proliferative lesions or membranous alterations in the glomeruli (Figures 2(a) and 2(b)). The cortical interstitium was moderately diffusely expanded, with inflammatory cell infiltration consisting mainly of lymphocytes with plasma cells, histiocytes, and neutrophils. Diffuse areas of tubulitis were observed, with necrosis and desquamation of tubular epithelial cells (Figure 2(c)). These changes were also seen in the medullary interstitium as tubulitis (not shown). Immunoglobulins and complement were not specifically stained in the glomeruli (Figure 2(d)). Collectively, this was diagnosed as diffuse tubulointerstitial nephritis without glomerular involvement. There was no concurrent uveitis, and other serological findings did not indicate secondary interstitial nephritis such as due to Sjogren's syndrome. Since his renal injury and general symptoms (fever and fatigue) did not remit spontaneously, it was decided to treat him with corticosteroid for his nephritis possibly due to the prior common airway infection and/or a drug-induced mechanism. A low dose of oral prednisolone, 25 mg/day (approximately 0.45 mg/kg/day), was administered on an outpatient basis, and the dose was decreased each month; renal function normalized after 4 months of treatment with the gradually tapered prednisolone. The treatment of case 1 was based on the empirical methods commonly used in our hospital, but with a smaller steroid dose and a longer duration compared to description in textbooks based on case series from other countries [8].

2.2. Cases 2–10. Of the 422 cases for which renal biopsies with any reason for examination were performed at our center from 2008 to 2021, ATIN was confirmed clinically and pathologically in 9 cases in addition to case 1, accounting for 2.4% of all biopsy cases (Table 2). In the analysis of 10 patients, the median age was 40 years, eGFR at diagnosis was 19.4 (3.2–49.1) mL/min/1.73 m^2, and 2 of them underwent hemodialysis, but both patients were withdrawn from dialysis. The median eGFR after treatment was 53.6 (20.8–110.0) mL/min/1.73 m^2, and all patients showed improvement ($P < 0.001$). Treatment consisted of corticosteroids (15 to 50 mg) in 8 patients; the 2 patients who did not receive corticosteroids were treated by discontinuation of the suspected drugs and treatment of infection. Seven of the 10 patients were evaluated for ocular uveitis, and uveitis was found in 5 of them. Although cases 2 and 6 were elderly patients and the steroid dosage was relatively high compared to the other cases, they relapsed during the outpatient course and required re-treatment.

3. Discussion

TIN is a histopathologic disease concept and is a general term for renal lesions that are primarily inflammatory in the tubulointerstitial region. It is classified as ATIN, which mainly consists of acute lesions such as edema and cellular infiltration, and chronic TIN, which consists of chronic changes, such as interstitial fibrosis and tubular atrophy. As in case 1, ATIN can be properly diagnosed by examination of both the clinical and pathological aspects of the case. Causes of ATIN include infections, drug-related, immune abnormalities, urinary tract abnormalities, heavy metal and other poisonings, ischemia, and metabolic disorders [1–4, 8]. Systematic survey reports from western countries have estimated that 71% are antimicrobial and other drug-related, 15% are infectious, 8% are idiopathic, 5% are TINU syndrome, and 1% is sarcoidosis [9]. In Japan, ATIN, which has a wide variety of causes, has no definitive treatment protocols. Corticosteroid therapy has been reported to be effective in ATIN, but there are no controlled trials, and it is difficult to establish the optimal treatment, including its dosage [9]. Steroids are empirically administered at a dose of about 1 mg/kg/day of prednisolone orally for 2 or 3 weeks, followed by a gradually tapering dose over 3 to 4 weeks [10, 11], but small doses or steroid pulse therapy may be administered on a case by case basis.

Case 1 was diagnosed as ATIN due to prior common airway infection and/or drug-induced. In the setting of infection-related interstitial nephritis, eradication of the infection is often associated with renal function recovery. Treatment of drug-induced ATIN is more complicated and controversial. The most important intervention is early recognition of the disease and drug discontinuation. A drug-free trial should be undertaken to determine if renal function recovers without further intervention [8]. If no improvement is noted after a period of observation (several days) or if renal function decreases rapidly, a trial of corticosteroid is reasonable [8]. Despite early intervention including culprit drug discontinuation, a substantial proportion of patients (up to 35%) may develop CKD [8]. In our experience, 5 of 10 cases continued to have decreased renal function, with eGFR less than 60 mL/min/1.73 m^2 (Table 2). Nevertheless, at our hospital, we do not necessarily use high doses of steroids, but often use 0.4 to 0.6 mg/kg, to induce remission of ATIN and substantial recovery of renal function. Our practical view is to try to eliminate the cause of the disease by taking a detailed history, not to introduce treatment for a week until renal biopsy results are available if renal injury is not severe, and

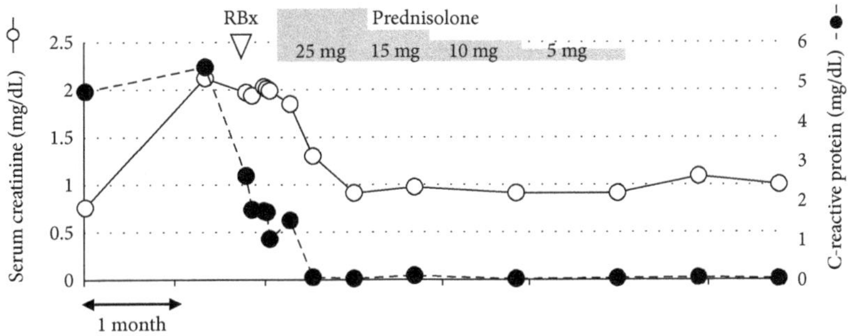

Urinary Glucose	2+	2+	2+	3+	1+	1+	1+	+/-	(-)	
Urinary Protein	1+	1+	2+	1+	+/-	+/-	(-)	(-)	(-)	
Urinary RBC	NA	1>	1>	1>	1>	1-4	1>		1>	(/HPF)
Urinary β2-MG		56.73	36.07	25.09	10.38	15.04	3.71	2.91	2.70	(mg/L)
Urinary NAG		14.5	21.1	9.4	6.5	6.3	6.6	4.9	5.3	(IU/dL)

FIGURE 1: Clinical features and course of case 1. Renal biopsy of case 1 was performed approximately 2 months after disease onset. Disease activity and effectiveness of treatment for acute tubulointerstitial nephritis were monitored by renal function (serum creatinine), inflammation (C-reactive protein), and tubular functional defects (urinary glucose, protein, β2-microglobulin, and N-acetylglucosaminidase). Abbreviations: RBx, renal biopsy; RBCs, red blood cells; NA, not available; HPF, high-power field; NAG, N-acetylglucosaminidase.

TABLE 1: Laboratory findings of case 1.

Urinalysis		Blood chemistry tests (cont.)	
Gravity	1.016	Sodium	138 mmol/L
Protein	2+	Chloride	102 mmol/L
Sugar	2+	Potassium	3.4 mmol/L
Blood	Negative	Corrected calcium	10.0 mg/dL
Sediment		Phosphate	4.0 mg/dL
Red blood cells	<1/HPF	Total bilirubin	0.4 mg/dL
White blood cells	5–9/HPF	Aspartate aminotransferase	15 U/L
Urinary biochemical tests		Alanine aminotransferase	13 U/L
Daily urinary protein	0.9 g/24 hr	Lactate dehydrogenase	192 U/L
N-Acetylglucosaminidase	21.1 IU/L	Alkaline phosphatase	136 U/L
β2-Microglobulin	36.07 mg/L	Creatin kinase	31 U/L
Complete blood count		Total cholesterol	224 mg/dL
White blood cells	7100/mL	LDL cholesterol	162 mg/dL
Neutrophils	65%	Triglyceride	110 mg/dL
Eosinophils	11%	Glucose	97 mg/dL
Basophils	0%	Hemoglobin A1c	6.0%
Lymphocytes	7%	Serology	
Monocytes	17%	C-reactive protein	1.71 mg/dL
Hemoglobin	11.2 g/dL	HBs antigen	Negative
Platelets	32.4 × 104/mL	Anti-HCV antibody	Negative
Coagulation tests		Immunoglobulin G	1723 mg/dL
PT-INR	1.06	Immunoglobulin A	194 mg/dL
APTT	30.4 sec	Immunoglobulin M	74 mg/dL
APTT, ctrl	32.5 sec	Immunoglobulin E	333 IU/mL
D dimer	1.4 μg/mL	Anti-streptolysin O	21 IU/mL
Blood chemistry tests		Complement 3	139 mg/dL
Total protein	8.0 g/dL	Complement 4	52 mg/dL
Albumin	4.2 g/dL	CH50	64.0 U/mL
Urea acid	4.1 mg/dL	Rheumatoid factor	33 IU/mL
Urea nitrogen	23.9 mg/dL	Anti-nuclear antibody	×40>
Creatinine	2.01 mg/dL	Anti-dsDNA-Ab	<10 U/cmL

PT-INR, prothrombin time-international normalized ratio; APTT, activated partial thromboplastin time; LDL, low-density lipoprotein; HBs, hepatitis B surface; HCV, hepatitis C virus; CH50, 50% hemolytic unit of complement; DNA, deoxyribonucleic acid.

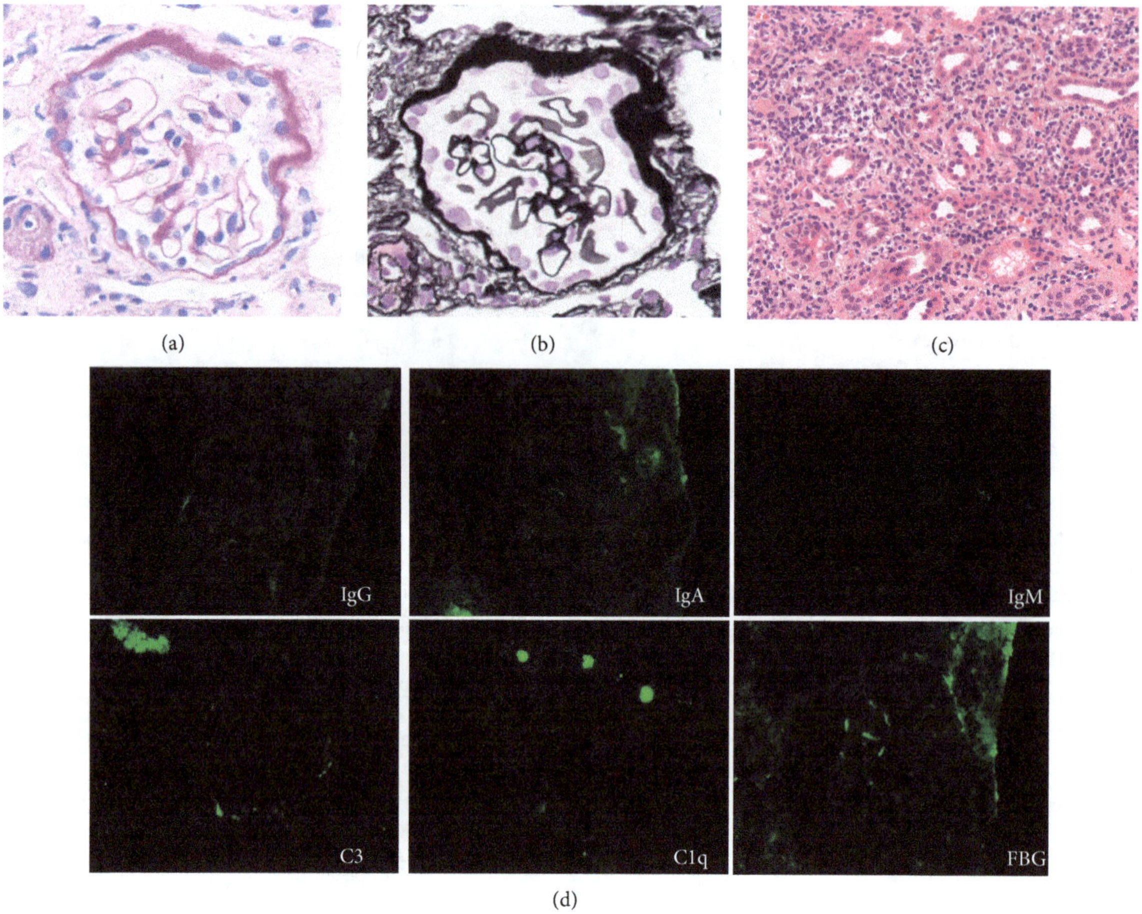

FIGURE 2: Renal pathological findings of case 1. Light microscopy findings show minor glomerular changes in case 1. Periodic acid-Schiff staining (a, c) and periodic acid methenamine silver staining (b). Immunofluorescence studies show no specific staining for immunoglobulin, complement, and fibrinogen (d).

TABLE 2: Ten cases of biopsy proven acute tubulointerstitial nephritis from a single center in a rural area from 2008 to 2021.

Case #	Age	Sex	eGFR at diagnosis	Renal pathology	Uveitis	Initial treatment	Outcome
1	Teens	M	38.5	ATIN	No	Prednisolone 25 mg	eGFR 97.1 mL/min/1.73 m^2
2	60 s	M	27.7	ATIN	Yes	Prednisolone 30 mg	Relapse+, eGFR 41.6 mL/min/1.73 m^2
3	30 s	F	9.4	ATIN	Yes	Prednisolone 30 mg	eGFR 60.9 mL/min/1.73 m^2
4	60 s	M	5.1	ATIN	Not examined	No steroid usage	eGFR 35.1 mL/min/1.73 m^2
5	20 s	M	49.1	ATIN	Yes	Prednisolone 30 mg	eGFR 110.0 mL/min/1.73 m^2
6	70 s	F	3.2	ATIN, Fibrosis	Not examined	Prednisolone 50 mg, HD	Relapse+, eGFR 23.1 mL/min/1.73 m^2
7	20 s	M	31.9	ATIN	Yes	Prednisolone 20 mg	eGFR 68.1 mL/min/1.73 m^2
8	Teens	F	43.7	ATIN, IgA deposition	Yes	Prednisolone 15 mg	eGFR 93.9 mL/min/1.73 m^2
9	50 s	M	7.4	ATIN	Not examined	No steroid usage, HD	eGFR 46.3 mL/min/1.73 m^2
10	40 s	F	11.1	ATIN	No	Prednisolone 30 mg	eGFR 20.8 mL/min/1.73 m^2

ATIN, acute tubulointerstitial nephritis; HD, hemodialysis.

to use outpatient steroid therapy if the exacerbation trend continues.

In addition to renal function as an indicator of treatment, disease-specific clinical findings of ATIN are used to determine the efficacy of interventions. Laboratory findings in ATIN feature eosinophilia, eosinouria on cytopathology, abnormal urinary sediment (hematuria, leukocyturia, and leukocyte casts), and mild proteinuria (less than 1 g/24 h). Tubular functional defects are represented by glycosuria, phosphaturia, hyperkalemia, acidosis, diabetes insipidus, and increased NAG and β2-microglobulin levels [8]. In case 1, a proximal tubular defect was observed as glycosuria and elevated NAG and β2-microglobulin levels. These abnormalities remitted gradually with corticosteroid therapy, suggesting that there is no guarantee that the amount of steroids is sufficient, but at least the required amount is reached.

A feature of this case series is that the patients were observed at our hospital, the only facility performing renal biopsies in a rural medical area of approximately 250,000 people, and thus they are less subject to bias due to indications for performing renal biopsies and inconsistent referral criteria to nephrologists than in a multicenter study. In the context of ATIN, we do not have any specific criteria for referral to nephrologist so far. However, our medical area (Hitachi, Japan) has recently developed collaboration between generalist and nephrologist to aim for improving prognosis of chronic kidney disease [12]. We believe that this collaboration will be effective in the early detection, diagnosis, and treatment of ATIN as well. The rate of TINU syndrome was much higher than expected based on previous reports from outside Japan (50% vs. 5% [9], 3% [1], and 2% [13], respectively). No papers have reported accurate international comparisons or ethnic differences in TINU, and it is difficult to generalize when differences in indications for renal biopsy and ophthalmological examination are taken into account, but there is no doubt that TINU is often diagnosed, at least in our region. However, familial occurrence or genetic background, that may involve in development of TINU syndrome [14], was not examined in this case series. We were unable to discuss exactly why our cases were older and male-dominant than the other evidence (young and female-dominant) [15]. Convincing clinical evidence for a role for steroid therapy, however, comes from studies of the idiopathic form of ATIN, particularly TINU syndrome. These manifestations of the cause of renal disease suggest the reason for the effectiveness of low-dose steroids in the present case series for improvement of renal function.

In conclusion, the causes and clinical course of ATIN are diverse, but it is treated according to individual judgment in addition to standard treatment and generally has a good renal prognosis. This report presents the results of treatment at a single institution in Japan, and treatment with a small dose of steroids results in recovery of renal function.

Disclosure

The corresponding author is employed by the University of Tsukuba.

References

[1] M. Prendecki, A. Tanna, A. D. Salama et al., "Long-term outcome in biopsy-proven acute interstitial nephritis treated with steroids," *Clinical Kidney Journal*, vol. 10, no. 2, pp. 233–239, 2017.

[2] J. S. Cameron, "Allergic interstitial nephritis: clinical features and pathogenesis," *Quarterly Journal of Medicine*, vol. 66, no. 250, pp. 97–115, 1988.

[3] K. Farrington, D. A. Levison, R. N. Greenwood, W. R. Cattell, and L. R. Baker, "Renal biopsy in patients with unexplained renal impairment and normal kidney size," *Quarterly Journal of Medicine*, vol. 70, no. 263, pp. 221–233, 1989.

[4] J. Rossert, "Drug-induced acute interstitial nephritis," *Kidney International*, vol. 60, no. 2, pp. 804–817, 2001.

[5] A. R. Berliner, M. Haas, and M. J. Choi, "Sarcoidosis: the nephrologist's perspective," *American Journal of Kidney Diseases*, vol. 48, no. 5, pp. 856–870, 2006.

[6] M. R. Clarkson, L. Giblin, F. P. O'Connell et al., "Acute interstitial nephritis: clinical features and response to corticosteroid therapy," *Nephrology Dialysis Transplantation*, vol. 19, no. 11, pp. 2778–2783, 2004.

[7] Y. Raissian, S. H. Nasr, C. P. Larsen et al., "Diagnosis of IgG4-related tubulointerstitial nephritis," *Journal of the American Society of Nephrology*, vol. 22, no. 7, pp. 1343–1352, 2011.

[8] U. C. Brewster and A. Rastegar, "35-acute interstitial nephritis," in *National Kidney Foundation Primer on Kidney Diseases*, S. J. Gilbert and D. E. Weiner, Eds., pp. 312–317, W. B. Saunders, Pennsylvania, USA, 6th edition, 2014.

[9] R. J. Baker and C. D. Pusey, "The changing profile of acute tubulointerstitial nephritis," *Nephrology Dialysis Transplantation*, vol. 19, no. 1, pp. 8–11, 2004.

[10] C. D. Pusey, D. Saltissi, L. Bloodworth, D. J. Rainford, and J. L. Christie, "Drug associated acute interstitial nephritis: clinical and pathological features and the response to high dose steroid therapy," *Quarterly Journal of Medicine*, vol. 52, no. 206, pp. 194–211, 1983.

[11] G. Eknjoyan, "Acute hypersensitivity interstitial nephritis," in *Current Therapy in Nephrology and Hypertension*, R. J. Glassock, Ed., pp. 99–101, Mosby, St. Louis, 4th edition, 1998.

[12] K. Nagai and A. Ueda, "Impact of collaboration between general practitioners and nephrologists on renal function: an experience in the Hitachi area," *Clinical and Experimental Nephrology*, 2022.

[13] A. K. Muriithi, N. Leung, A. M. Valeri et al., "Biopsy-proven acute interstitial nephritis, 1993–2011: a case series," *American Journal of Kidney Diseases*, vol. 64, no. 4, pp. 558–566, 2014.

[14] M. Morino, K. Inami, T. Kobayashi, K. Yanagisawa, and K. Maeda, "Acute tubulointerstitial nephritis in two siblings and concomitant uveitis in one," *Pediatrics International*, vol. 33, no. 1, pp. 93–98, 1991.

[15] J. T. Mandeville, R. D. Levinson, and G. N. Holland, "The tubulointerstitial nephritis and uveitis syndrome," *Survey of Ophthalmology*, vol. 46, no. 3, pp. 195–208, 2001.

17

A Case of Oxalate Nephropathy in a Known Diabetic Patient following Acute Alcoholic Pancreatitis

John Odhiambo,[1] Hanika Patel,[2] Anderson Mutuiri,[3] Fazal Yakub,[1] and Ahmed Sokwala[3]

[1]*Internal Medicine, The Aga Khan University Hospital, Nairobi, Kenya*
[2]*Radiology, The Aga Khan University Hospital, Nairobi, Kenya*
[3]*The Aga Khan University Hospital, Nairobi, Kenya*

Correspondence should be addressed to John Odhiambo; johnotieno1991@gmail.com

Academic Editor: Yoshihide Fujigaki

This was a case of a 39-year-old gentleman known to have diabetes mellitus since February 2021 on insulin glargine (Lantus) 16 units nocte and sitagliptin/metformin 50/500 mg once a day who presented to a tertiary teaching hospital in Kenya in May 2021 with a three-week history of vomiting and diarrhea. He had been previously admitted to a different facility with acute alcoholic pancreatitis. His examination was nonremarkable except for mild dehydration and pallor. He had moderate metabolic acidosis and deranged renal function. Prior to this, his creatinine was normal. As part of the evaluation for the rapid deterioration of renal function, a kidney biopsy performed revealed oxalate nephropathy. He was started on renal replacement therapy with hemodialysis.

1. Background

Oxalate nephropathy is a rare condition associated with excess oxalate in the system. This can be either from increased absorption from the gastrointestinal tract or endogenously from the liver because of glyoxylate metabolism. These are referred to as secondary and primary hyperoxaluria, respectively. Primary hyperoxaluria ensues in the background of reduced or absent activity of enzymes involved in the glyoxylate metabolism [1, 2]. In secondary hyperoxaluria, there is either increased exposure to dietary sources of oxalate or any pathological conditions that increase intestinal absorption of oxalic acid. These conditions are associated with fat malabsorption. Excess oxalate results in hyperoxaluria since it is primarily excreted by the kidneys [3]. This causes renal dysfunction, which is diagnosed primarily on kidney biopsy [4].

2. Case Presentation

This is a case of a 39-year-old male known to have diabetes mellitus since February 2021 on Lantus 16 units nocte and sitagliptin/metformin 50/500 mg once daily. He presented to the hospital in May 2021 with a three-week history of postprandial, nonbilious vomiting and a four-day history of watery, nonbloody diarrhea, associated with reduced appetite, progressive generalized body malaise, and reduced urine output. He had also noted decreasing insulin requirements with the last injection 2 weeks prior to presentation. The past medical history was remarkable for an admission 3 months prior to presentation and managed for acute alcoholic pancreatitis. At presentation, he was moderately pale and dehydrated, with a PR at – 87 bpm and raised BP at 157/90 mmHg. Systemic examination was nonremarkable. The initial laboratory parameters are highlighted in Tables 1 and 2.

Table 1: Laboratory parameters.

Initial laboratory work-up		
Laboratory test	Results	Reference range
White blood cells (total)	6.59×10^9/L	4–10
Hemoglobin	5.8 g/dl	13–18
Platelet count	241×10^9/L	150–400
Creatinine	1206 μmol/L	62–115
Potassium	5.78 mmol/L	3.5–5.5
Urea	36.7 mmol/L	3.2–8.2

Table 2: Blood gas results.

Arterial Blood Gas		
	Results	Reference range
pH	7.18	7.35–7.45
Bicarbonate	10 mmol/L	22–29
Potassium	5.7 mmol/L	3.5–4.5

An impression of acute kidney injury likely due to rapidly progressive glomerulonephritis with high anion gap metabolic acidosis, symptomatic uremia, and microcytic hypochromic anemia in the diabetic patient was made.

2.1. Initial Management. He was admitted to a high dependency unit where he underwent urgent hemodialysis, transfusion with two units of packed red blood cells, intravenous fluid resuscitation, and insulin therapy.

He also underwent lower and upper gastrointestinal endoscopy as evaluation for the anemia, which revealed gastric erosions and hemorrhoids. Table 3 shows the results of the additional tests carried out.

2.2. Imaging. Kidney ureter and bladder ultrasound showed bilateral renal parenchymal disease. Contrast-enhanced computed tomography revealed features consistent with chronic pancreatitis; moderately edematous kidneys with moderate periphrenic stranding. The impression was revised to nondiabetic kidney disease with possibility of oxalosis because of chronic pancreatitis seen on the contrast-enhanced CT abdomen. Figures 1 and 2 show the images of the CT scans.

2.3. Histopathology. Kidney biopsy was performed in view of the above results. This showed 1 core with 28 glomeruli, one of which was globally sclerosed. There were no segmental scars. The mesangium showed normal cellularity with a marked increase in the matrix and focal nodule formation. There was no endocapillary hypercellularity. The capillary walls showed mild thickening without spikes or double contours on silver stain. The tubules showed diffuse acute on chronic tubular injury and numerous oxalate casts on polarized light microscopy. There were severe (50%) interstitial fibrosis and tubular atrophy with chronic inflammation present in fibrotic areas. There were moderate hyaline arteriolosclerosis and arteriosclerosis. Immunofluorescence microscopy, referred out, was reported as follows: 8 glomeruli negative for immunoglobulin and complement deposits. Electron microscopy was not performed. The diagnosis was severe acute on chronic tubular injury with calcium oxalate deposits and nodular diabetic glomerulosclerosis (see Figures 3 and 4).

Table 3: Additional laboratory workup.

Test	Results	Reference range
Urine albumin creatinine ratio	3.37	<3.5 mg/mmol
Transferrin saturation	14.7%	15–45%
Parathyroid hormone level	101 pg/ml	15–65 pg/ml
Vitamin	11	30–100 ng/ml
Complement 3 (C3)	Normal	
Complement 4 (C4)	Normal	
Antinuclear antibody	Negative	
Lipid profile	Normal	
Urinalysis	No hematuria/proteinuria	

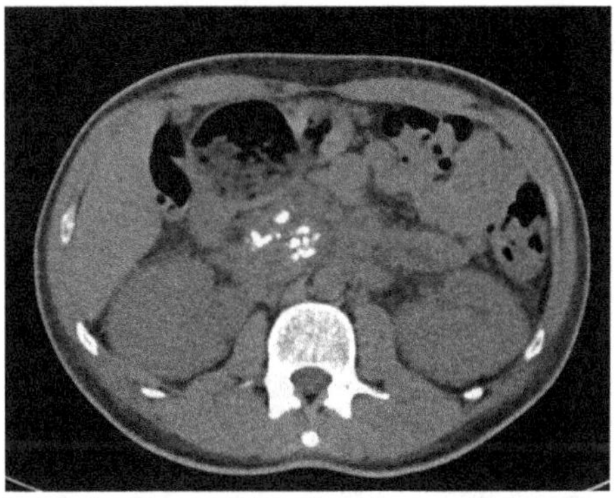

Figure 1: Axial noncontrast CT through the head of the pancreas shows coarse calcifications within the pancreatic parenchyma more pronounced in the head and uncinate process and are also seen in bilateral perinephric fat stranding.

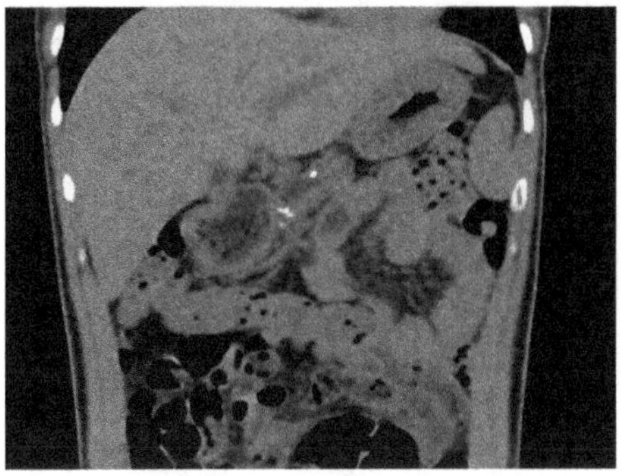

Figure 2: Coronal noncontrast CT through the upper abdomen shows calcifications along the body of the pancreas and mild dilatation of the pancreatic duct measuring up to 9.7 mm.

3. Discussion and Conclusion

At presentation, the aforementioned patient's renal dysfunction would have been attributed to diabetes that had been diagnosed three months before presentation. However, everything else pointed towards a possibility of nondiabetic kidney disease. He had no proteinuria, no hematuria, or any

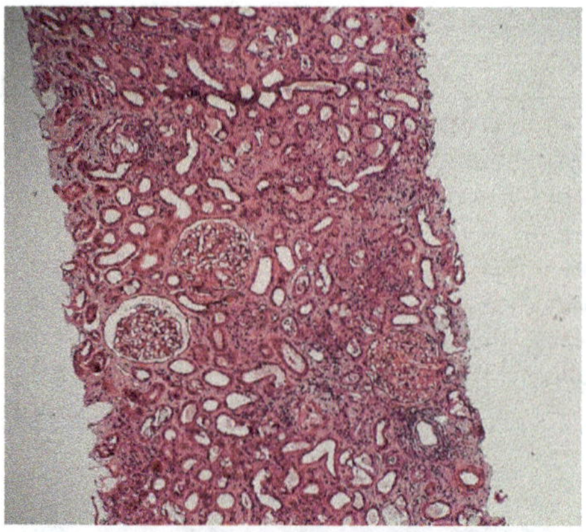

Figure 3: H&E (X200): diffuse acute tubular injury characterized by tubular epithelial simplification and dilation with numerous pale refractile intratubular casts.

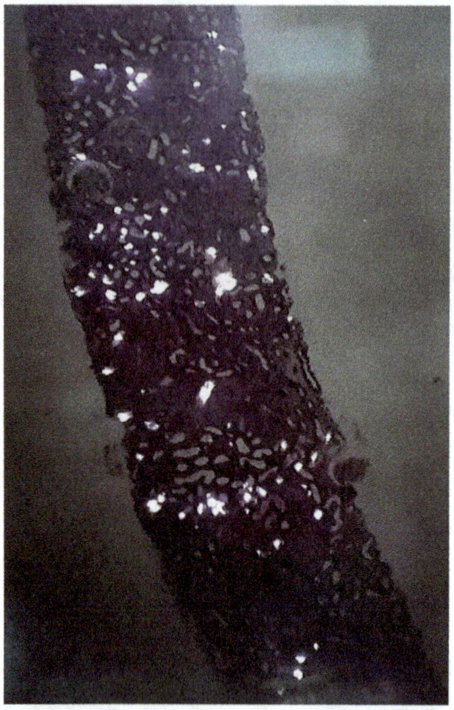

Figure 4: Partially polarized light microscopy (X100) shows diffuse birefringent intratubular casts.

other microvascular complications and had a rapid decline of renal function, therefore, meeting the criteria for renal biopsy [5]. These, together with a previous history of acute pancreatitis and abdominal CT scan findings, raised a possibility of secondary hyperoxaluria with oxalate nephropathy. This diagnosis was confirmed on histology.

Oxalate nephropathy results from excess oxalate in the system. This can be because of increased absorption from the gastrointestinal tract, ascorbic acid administration (intravenously or orally), or increased endogenous production from defects in the enzymes involved in the glyoxylate metabolism.

Normally, oxalate present in the gastrointestinal tract is bound to calcium preventing its absorption and increasing its excretion. However, impaired exocrine function, in acute or chronic pancreatitis, leads to reduced digestion of fatty acids, hence resulting in fat malabsorption. The free fatty acids bind calcium instead, leaving the oxalate unbound and increasing its absorption into the bloodstream from the colon [4]. The excess oxalate is excreted via the kidneys causing renal damage. Mechanisms of renal damage include recurrent nephrolithiasis from calcium oxalate complexes and crystals, nephrocalcinosis, and interstitial fibrosis [6].

A systemic review on secondary nephropathy showed that 35% of the patients present with acute kidney injury followed by 29% presenting with acute on chronic kidney disease [7]. The aforementioned patient presented with acute kidney injury.

In conclusion, one needs to have a high index of suspicion for possibility of nondiabetic kidney disease in diabetic patients with rapidly deteriorating renal function, especially in the absence of other microvascular complications of diabetes.

References

[1] A. Weigert, C. Martin-Higueras, and B. Hoppe, "Novel therapeutic approaches in primary hyperoxaluria," *Expert Opinion on Emerging Drugs*, vol. 23, no. 4, pp. 349–357, 2018.

[2] R. Belostotsky and Y. Frishberg, "Novel therapeutic approaches for the primary hyperoxalurias," *Pediatric Nephrology*, vol. 36, no. 9, pp. 2593–2606, 2021.

[3] S. F. Garrelfs, G. Rumsby, H. Peters-Sengers et al., "Patients with primary hyperoxaluria type 2 have significant morbidity and require careful follow-up," *Kidney International*, vol. 96, no. 6, pp. 1389–1399, 2019.

[4] S. Makkapati, V. D. D'Agati, and L. Balsam, ""Green smoothie cleanse" causing acute oxalate nephropathy," *American Journal of Kidney Diseases*, vol. 71, no. 2, pp. 281–286, 2018.

[5] N. Oliva-Damaso, J. M. Mora-Gutiérrez, and A. S. Bomback, "Glomerular diseases in diabetic patients: implications for diagnosis and management," *Journal of Clinical Medicine*, vol. 10, no. 9, p. 1855, 2021.

[6] B. Hoppe, B. B. Beck, and D. S. Milliner, "The primary hyperoxalurias," *Kidney International*, vol. 75, no. 12, pp. 1264–1271, 2009.

[7] N. Lumlertgul, M. Siribamrungwong, B. L. Jaber, and P. Susantitaphong, "Secondary oxalate nephropathy: a systematic review," *Kidney International Reports*, vol. 3, no. 6, pp. 1363–1372, 2018.

18

Mycoplasma pneumoniae Infection Associated C3 Glomerulopathy Presenting as Severe Crescentic Glomerulonephritis

Lalani De Silva, Dinesha Jayasinghe, and Priyani Amarathunga

Department of Pathology, Faculty of Medicine, University of Colombo, Colombo, Sri Lanka

Correspondence should be addressed to Lalani De Silva; lalanidesilva7@gmail.com

Academic Editor: Phuong Chi Pham

C3 glomerulopathy (C3GP) is a group of diseases caused by a deregulated complement system, which encompasses both dense deposit disease and C3 glomerulonephritis. Renal manifestations of C3GP are primarily of proliferative glomerulonephritis, and only a few case reports of crescentic glomerulonephritis (CGN) in association with C3GP are available. Here is a case of an adult South-Asian female, who was diagnosed as seropositive acute *Mycoplasma pneumoniae* infection, with associated systemic manifestations, including immune-type extravascular haemolysis and nephrotic range proteinuria. Subsequent renal biopsy revealed CGN with disrupted Bowman's capsules and necrotizing lesions. Immunofluorescence showed coarse granular mesangial C3 deposits with negative IgM, IgG, IgA, and C1q. The immunomorphological phenotype raised two possibilities including C3GP and infection-related glomerulonephritis (IRGN). Persistent proteinuria with no evidence of resolution even after 6 months of follow-up favoured C3GP over IRGN. The patient proceeded to end-stage renal failure requiring renal replacement despite aggressive immunosuppression. This case illustrates the rare association of CGN with C3GP induced by *Mycoplasma pneumoniae* infection, highlighting the importance of correct diagnosis as well as timely identification of triggering factors in CGN on patient outcome.

1. Introduction

Complement deposits are seen in virtually all types of glomerulonephritis [1]. Most of the complement-mediated renal diseases are caused as a secondary event following immune complex-mediated injury, such as membranoproliferative glomerulonephritis, lupus nephritis, antiphospholipid syndrome, IgA nephropathy, and cryoglobulinaemic glomerulonephritis. Primary complement-mediated injury is seen in C3 glomerulopathy (C3GP) and some infection-related glomerulonephritis (IRGN) including atypical haemolytic uremic syndrome (HUS) [1, 2]. C1q disease, although diagnosed based on dominant C1q deposits in immunofluorescence, is considered as a disease mediated by immune complexes rather than a disease of complement deregulation; thus, immune complexes are invariably identified in immunofluorescence studies [1–3]. CGN with isolated C3 deposits in immunofluorescence is a rare type of pauci-immune CGN. This incorporates most of the C3 glomerulopathy cases and occasional cases of resolving IRGN [4].

Herein is a case with severe crescentic glomerulonephritis showing isolated C3 deposits in immunofluorescence induced by *Mycoplasma pneumoniae* lung infection.

2. Case Presentation

A 58-year-old lady presented to a medical unit in a tertiary-care hospital with a four-day history of fever with chills and cough, associated with vomiting and loss of appetite. She denied any symptoms related to renal dysfunction prior to this admission. Basic investigations (full blood count, urine full report, ECG, serum creatinine, and AST/ALT) done a few years back for a medical checkup were within normal limits.

On examination, she was pale and had mild icterus and bilateral ankle oedema. Her hemodynamic parameters were normal (pulse rate: 86 beats/min, regular, good volume; blood pressure: 130/90 mmHg). There was mild splenomegaly with no hepatomegaly or free fluid. Chest examination revealed bilateral basal end-inspiratory crackles.

Initial investigations showed anaemia (hemoglobin: 7.5 g/dl), neutrophil leukocytosis (total leukocyte count: 25000/mm^3; neutrophils: 90%), elevated C-reactive protein (28 U/l) and ESR (170 mm/1st hour), indirect hyperbilirubinaemia (total bilirubin: 22.3 mg/l; direct fraction: 5.8 mg/l), and high serum creatinine (174 mmol/l). Urine examination revealed nephrotic range proteinuria and microscopic haematuria. Chest X-ray showed diffuse, reticular, ground-glass opacity in the bilateral lung bases, more in the left side, suggestive of interstitial pneumonia. She was started on a second-generation cephalosporin, in addition to basic supportive care and antipyretic therapy.

Based on the findings of pallor, icterus, splenomegaly, anaemia, and indirect hyperbilirubinaemia, an extravascular haemolytic anaemia was suspected. A subsequent blood picture revealed normochromic normocytic red blood cells with cold-type autoagglutination, neutrophil leukocytosis with toxic change, and normal platelets. Positive Coombs test turned the diagnosis towards immune-type haemolytic anaemia. Prednisolone 40 mg daily was started on the 6th day of admission as a treatment for immune haemolytic anaemia.

Despite antibiotic treatment, general supportive care, and transfusion of three pints of red cell concentrate, the patient continued to deteriorate with progressive leukocytosis (total leukocyte count: 25000/mm^3 to 48000/mm^3), anaemia (hemoglobin: 7.5 g/dl to 6.2 g/dl), and rising serum creatinine (174 mmol/l to 214 mmol/l) over 10 days. Additional laboratory workup revealed progressive nephrotic range proteinuria (561 mg/dl, urine protein/creatinine ratio: 837 mg/mmol) and positive mycoplasma IgM antibody titer (1/320). Antinuclear antibody, DsDNA, antistreptolysin O titer (ASOT), hepatitis B and C, VDRL, and HIV serology were negative. Both antimyeloperoxidase ANCA and antiproteinase-3 ANCA were negative. Bacteriological cultures of urine and blood were sterile. 2D-echocardiogram was performed to exclude the possibility of infective endocarditis and was compatible with mild myocarditis and global ventricular dysfunction with no evidence of infective endocarditis. A macrolide was added in view of positive mycoplasma serology, and her respiratory symptoms were markedly improved in a few days.

Because of persistent nephrotic range proteinuria and rising serum creatinine, a percutaneous renal biopsy was performed on the 12th day of hospital admission. The biopsy showed diffuse endocapillary proliferative glomerulonephritis with crescents. These crescents expanded beyond the limit of Bowman's capsule disrupting the glomerular outline (Figure 1). There were focal leukocyte infiltration, karyorrhexis, and necrotizing lesions. No evidence of capillary microthrombi or vasculitis. A few tubules showed red cell casts. Immunofluorescence examination revealed isolated C3 deposits in the mesangium with negative IgA, IgG, IgM, and C1q. It was concluded as ANCA-negative pauci-immune CGN with isolated C3 deposits (Figure 2).

As the patient did not respond to oral prednisolone, she was started on intravenous methylprednisolone with which her serum creatinine level became normal. However, she continued to have nephrotic range proteinuria and the clinical decision was to start her on cyclophosphamide pulse therapy. During the follow-up, she continued to have proteinuria even with cyclophosphamide therapy for more than 6 months. As the possibility of IRGN is unlikely to be continued more than 8-week duration, the clinical diagnosis of C3GP was made. However, the unavailability of specific genetic testing to identify the defect in the complement cascade precluded further narrowing down of possibilities in arriving at a specific definitive diagnosis.

3. Discussion

C3 glomerulopathy was identified as a specific pathological entity in 2012 by a group of experts emphasizing that it is a heterogeneous group of diseases with isolated/dominant C3 deposits. It requires further evaluation to identify the specific complement defects in the cascade, if any, to approach a specific anticomplement targeted therapy; meanwhile, these targeted complement inhibitors are being developed [4].

The term C3GP incorporates two specific entities including dense deposit disease (DDD) and C3 glomerulonephritis. Distinction of these two is solely based on the morphology of the deposits on electron microscopy (EM) as the clinical and light microscopic features are almost identical. The light microscopy of these two entities ranges from mesangioproliferative, membranoproliferative, and endocapillary proliferative to severe CGN [4, 5]. The typical EM findings of DDD are the presence of highly electron-dense, osmophilic deposits within glomerular basement membranes forming band-like or "sausage-like" shapes with punctated skipped areas of more normal looking glomerular basement membranes. When the EM appearance of C3 deposits fails to achieve those specific features, by means of being less electron-dense, ill-defined, more confluent, or more rounded, the disease is classified as C3 glomerulonephritis [4–6].

Differentiation of these two entities in CGN is prognostically important [7]. As observed in one study, patients with C3 glomerulonephritis presented with severe necrotizing and crescentic glomerulonephritis showed more stable renal function following immunosuppressive therapy, compared with more patients with DDD presented with crescents progressed to end-stage renal failure requiring renal transplant, despite various immunosuppressive modalities. Two of them had recurrence of DDD in the grafted kidney [8].

The pathogenic mechanism of C3GP is the uncontrolled activation of the complement cascade through an alternative pathway, which can be either inherited/familial or acquired [9]. Genetic alterations leading to familial forms of C3GP include mutations in complement regulatory proteins such as factor H, factor I, and CD46, gain-of-function mutation of complement activating proteins such as factor B and C3, and genomic rearrangement within complement factor H related

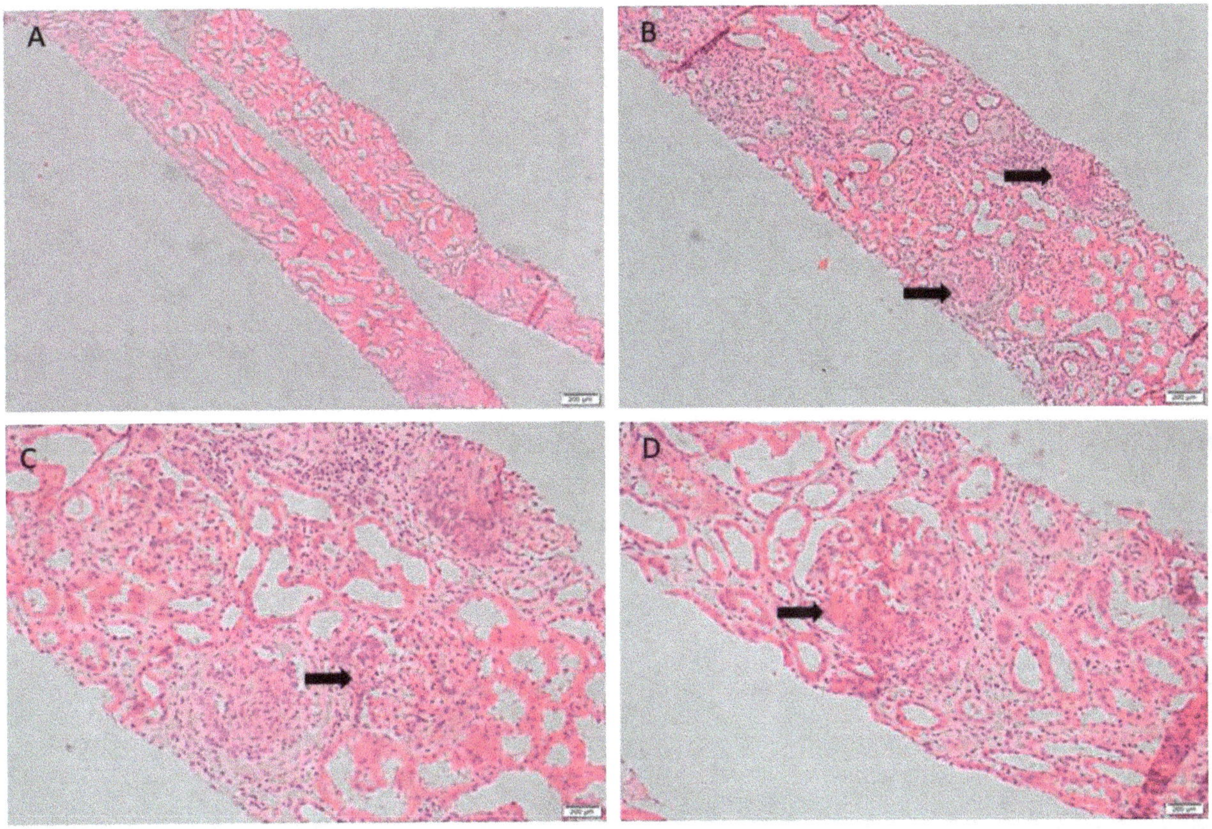

FIGURE 1: Microscopic images of the renal biopsy (H&E). (a) The biopsy was composed of two cores of renal tissue (40x). (b) It showed diffuse endocapillary proliferative glomerulonephritis with epithelial crescents (arrow) (100x). (c) Some glomeruli showed neutrophil infiltration (arrow) (400x) and (d) necrotizing lesions (arrow) (400x).

genes which includes five separate genes, namely, CFHR1, CFHR2, CFHR3, CFHR4, and CFHR5 [9]. The acquired form is resulted from uncontrolled activation of complement mostly through autoimmune mechanisms. C3 nephritic factor, an autoantibody stabilizing alternative pathway C3 convertase C3bBb, anti-factor B autoantibody, and anti-factor H autoantibody are some of the identified autoantibodies [9]. In addition, monoclonal gammopathy also plays a role in the acquired form of C3GP [4, 9].

Genetic and serological testing to identify defects in the complement cascade requires highly specialized laboratory facilities and expert interpretation which are not available in most of the developing countries. Therefore, in most of the instances, evaluation of patients suspecting C3GP is halted at this level due to a lack of resources [4].

Current approach to specific treatment for C3GP is controversial due to the lack of adequate data on therapeutic trials. Steroid therapy, although a common practice, fails to show an effective response especially in DDD. Anti-C5 therapy (e.g., eculizumab) has shown some beneficial effects. Future therapeutic approach is heading towards the development of targeted therapy for specific complement defects, thereby achieving a complete remission of the disease [10, 11].

Clinical presentation of this patient raised the possibility of IRGN. Although the usual presentation of IRGN is an acute nephritic syndrome, approximately a third of patients can be presented with nephrotic range proteinuria [12]. In addition, the associated extrarenal manifestation and serum hypocomplementaemia also favoured IRGN. The possibility of IRGN due to mycoplasma infection is raised based on clinical symptoms of pulmonary (interstitial pneumonia) and extrapulmonary (myocarditis and extravascular haemolysis) manifestations and positive mycoplasma IgM antibodies together with supportive serological evidence (neutrophil leukocytosis, high CRP/ESR, positive direct Coombs test, cold-type autoimmune haemolytic anaemia, and hypocomplementaemia).

Renal manifestations of mycoplasma infection include a spectrum of tubulointerstitial nephritis and glomerulonephritis, including mesangioproliferative glomerulonephritis and endocapillary proliferative glomerulonephritis [13, 14]. Although rare, a few cases of CGN are also reported [15, 16]. CGN with isolated C3 deposition as seen in this patient is extremely rare, with only a single case reported in the literature [17]. As reported by Mao et al., an 8-year-old girl presented with a one-week history of oedema, haematuria, and anaemia with positive serology for both mycoplasma and ASOT. The renal biopsy showed CGN with isolated C3 deposition and subepithelial dense material deposition on EM. She was successfully treated with immunosuppressive therapy with methylprednisolone and cyclophosphamide and showed an excellent clinical outcome [17]. However, the possibility of IRGN due to streptococcus infection should also be considered in this scenario.

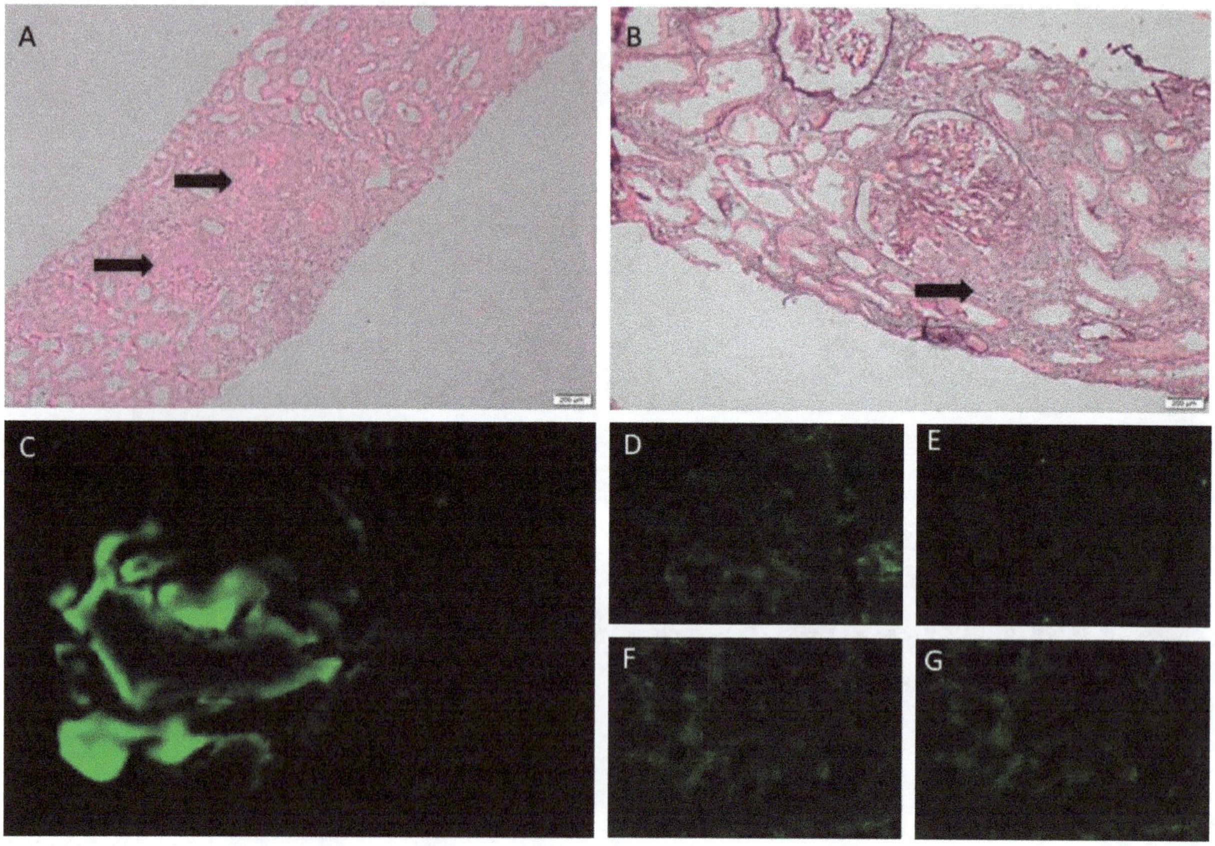

Figure 2: Periodic acid-Schiff (a) and silver (b) stained sections showed disruptive crescents extending beyond the limit of Bowman's capsule (arrows) (400x). (c) Immunofluorescence of C3 showed coarse granular mesangial deposits (400x). Immunofluorescence was negative for IgG (d), IgA (e), IgM (f), and C1q (g).

Resolving stage of IRGN can show isolated C3 deposits in immunofluorescence similar to the findings of C3GP. Therefore, the differentiation of these two is solely based on clinical follow-up. Patients with IRGN are expected to be completely recovered from renal derangement in 8–12 weeks, while patients with C3GP show persistent proteinuria even with immunosuppressive therapy [4]. Considering the fact that this patient is having persistent heavy proteinuria over 6-month duration, even with advanced immunosuppressive therapy, C3GP is considered the most possible diagnosis over IRGN.

Extravascular haemolysis associated with acute kidney injury can be seen in atypical HUS. Atypical HUS contributes approximately 10% of all HUS and includes cases which are not related to Shiga toxins of enteric bacteria [18]. Both C3GP and atypical HUS are related to defects in the alternative pathway of complement cascade and show similar pathogenesis. Over 40% of atypical HUS patients show genetic mutations in the genes of complement proteins and of its regulatory proteins or autoantibodies to factor H, which makes it is practically impossible to differentiate atypical HUS from C3GP even with extensive genetic analysis [18, 19]. However, atypical HUS is unlikely in this patient because of the positive Coombs test (atypical HUS is a nonimmune haemolytic disease and in turn Coombs negative), absence of thrombocytopaenia (a key presenting feature), and absence of capillary microthrombi in the renal biopsy.

Considering overall clinical and immunomorphological features, C3GP was considered as the most possible diagnosis in this patient. We suggest that mycoplasma infection would have triggered the activation of immunosusceptibility of C3 complement pathway in this patient. However, limited resources precluded the detection of specific defects in complement cascade.

In conclusion, CGN is a disease process rather than a specific disease, due to a variety of causative agents. Identification of specific aetiology early in the process is important therapeutically to make clinical decisions on treatment modality and thereby to achieve a better outcome. Although biopsy diagnosis with basic light microscopic categorization of CGN is fundamental, supplementary evidence by immunofluorescence and EM is invaluable in arriving at a specific diagnosis. Knowledge on the genetic basis of the disease and its practical application for diagnostic and therapeutic process is important nowadays in evaluating patients with CGN, although the required facilities are not well established in most places.

Authors' Contributions

The authors equally contributed for histopathological diagnosis, evaluation of patient's clinical data, and preparation of manuscript. All authors read and approved the final manuscript.

References

[1] D. Turnberg and H. T. Cook, "Complement and glomerulonephritis: new insights," *Current Opinion in Nephrology and Hypertension*, vol. 14, no. 3, pp. 223–228, 2005.

[2] K. A. Vernon and H. T. Cook, "Complement in glomerular disease," *Advances in Chronic Kidney Disease*, vol. 19, no. 2, pp. 84–92, 2012.

[3] R. J. Popat and M. G. Robson, "Complement and glomerular diseases," *Nephron Clinical Practice*, vol. 128, no. 3-4, pp. 238–242, 2014.

[4] M. C. Pickering, V. D. D'agati, C. M. Nester et al., "C3 glomerulopathy: consensus report," *Kidney International*, vol. 84, no. 6, pp. 1079–1089, 2013.

[5] S. Thomas, D. Ranganathan, L. Francis, K. Madhan, and G. T. John, "Current concepts in C3 glomerulopathy," *Indian Journal of Nephrology*, vol. 24, no. 6, pp. 339–48, 2014.

[6] T. D. Barbour, M. C. Pickering, and H. Terence Cook, "Dense deposit disease and C3 glomerulopathy," *Seminars in Nephrology*, vol. 33, no. 6, pp. 493–507, 2013.

[7] National Institute for Health and Care Excellence, *Prevention of Recurrence of C3 Glomerulopathy Post-Transplant: Eculizumab*, National Institute for Health and Care Excellence, London, UK, 2015.

[8] A. Ravindran, F. C. Fervenza, R. J. H. Smith, and S. Sethi, "C3 glomerulonephritis with a severe crescentic phenotype," *Pediatric Nephrology*, vol. 32, no. 9, pp. 1625–1633, 2017.

[9] V. Master Sankar Raj, R. Gordillo, and D. H. Chand, "Overview of C3 glomerulopathy," *Frontiers in pediatrics*, vol. 4, p. 45, 2016.

[10] C. Lebreton, J. Bacchetta, F. Dijoud, L. Bessenay, V. Fremeaux-Bacchi, and A. L. Sellier-Leclerc, "C3 glomerulopathy and eculizumab: a report on four paediatric cases," *Pediatric Nephrology*, vol. 32, no. 6, pp. 1023–1028, 2017.

[11] T. Welte, F. Arnold, J. Kappes et al., "Treating C3 glomerulopathy with eculizumab," *BMC Nephrology*, vol. 19, no. 1, p. 7, 2018.

[12] S. H. Nasr, J. Radhakrishnan, and V. D. D'Agati, "Bacterial infection-related glomerulonephritis in adults," *Kidney International*, vol. 83, no. 5, pp. 792–803, 2013.

[13] R. Watanabe, K. Kaira, and A. Takise, "Acute renal failure and nephrotic syndrome associated with mycoplasma pneumoniae pneumonia," *Kitakanto Medical Journal*, vol. 55, no. 1, pp. 41–44, 2005.

[14] H. Lee, K. C. Moon, and S. Kim, "Cutaneous vasculitis and renal involvement inMycoplasma pneumoniaeinfection," *The Korean Journal of Internal Medicine*, vol. 30, no. 3, p. 402, 2015.

[15] A.-L. Adra, M.-G. Vigue, F. Dalla Vale et al., "Favorable outcome in a case of Mycoplasma pneumoniae-associated crescentic glomerulonephritis," *Pediatric Nephrology*, vol. 25, no. 9, pp. 1765–1769, 2010.

[16] H. Wang, X. Chen, W. Xu, and J. Du, "Acute postinfectious glomerulonephritis with a large number of crescents caused by Mycoplasma pneumoniae," *Indian Journal of Pathology & Microbiology*, vol. 58, no. 3, p. 374, 2015.

[17] S. Mao, X. Xuan, Y. Sha, S. Zhao, A. Zhang, and S. Huang, "Crescentic acute glomerulonephritis with isolated C3 deposition: a case report and review of literature," *International Journal of Clinical and Experimental Pathology*, vol. 8, no. 2, pp. 1826–1829, 2015.

[18] T. H. J. Goodship, H. T. Cook, F. Fakhouri et al., "Atypical hemolytic uremic syndrome and C3 glomerulopathy: conclusions from a "kidney disease: improving global outcomes" (KDIGO) controversies conference," *Kidney International*, vol. 91, no. 3, pp. 539–551, 2017.

[19] L. A. Trouw, M. A. Seelen, and M. R. Daha, "Complement and renal disease," *Molecular Immunology*, vol. 40, no. 2–4, pp. 125–134, 2003.

19

A Case of Acute Colonic Pseudo-Obstruction (Ogilvie's Syndrome) in a Nonsurgical Patient with Plasma Cell Leukemia

Akbar Hamid,[1,2] Jacob Sabu,[1,2] Omar Elhawary,[1,2] Isha Puri,[1,2] Moro Salifu,[1,2] Man Oh,[1] and Mary Mallappallil[1,2]

[1]*Division of Nephrology, Department of Medicine, SUNY Downstate Health Sciences University, Brooklyn, NY, USA*
[2]*Division of Nephrology, Department of Medicine, Kings County Hospital Center, Brooklyn, NY, USA*

Correspondence should be addressed to Akbar Hamid; akbar.hamid@downstate.edu

Academic Editor: Phuong Chi Pham

Ogilvie's syndrome, also known as acute colonic pseudo-obstruction (ACPO), is a rare, nonobstructive dilation of the colon of unclear etiology. We present the case of a patient who presented with Ogilvie's syndrome and significant hypokalemia due to colonic loss despite repletion. This case report demonstrates the difficulty in diagnosis, treatment, and outcome.

1. Introduction

Ogilvie's syndrome refers to pathologic dilation of the colon without underlying mechanical obstruction, occurring primarily in patients with significant comorbidities. The diagnosis is based on clinical and radiologic grounds [1]. The incidence of the disease is frequently cited as approximately 100 cases per 100,000 hospital admissions per year, with a higher prevalence in men. The average age at presentation is approximately 60 years. Surgical patients are more likely to be diagnosed on postoperative days 3–5 [2].

2. Case Presentation

A 69-year-old African American woman with a history of type 2 diabetes mellitus, hypertension, hyperlipidemia, and elite control HIV infection (not on antivirals and with an undetectable viral load) presented with worsening lower back pain for a month. The laboratory tests showed marked leukocytosis, anemia, mild renal impairment, and a paraprotein gap. On skeletal survey, she was noted to have lytic lesions, and an MRI of the spine showed extensive compression, deformities, and epidural extension. A bone biopsy showed more than 80% blast cells with a marked increase in circulating plasma cells. She was diagnosed with plasma cell leukemia. In addition, she was also noted to have cauda equina syndrome. An abdominal CT scan showed a markedly dilated ascending colon, suggestive of obstruction, but she continued to have bowel movements. The patient successfully underwent chemotherapy induction and was discharged. When the patient was readmitted for the second cycle of chemotherapy (cisplatin and bortezomib), serum potassium was noted to be 1.8 mmol/L with a U wave on the electrocardiogram. However, serum magnesium levels were never below the normal range. She also complained of abdominal distension, diarrhea, and bilateral lower extremity edema. Multiple stool studies, including those for *Clostridioides difficile*, were negative. Several abdominal CT scans with intravenous contrast revealed dilated loops of the bowel without obstruction (Figure 1). She developed acute kidney injury, and the differential diagnosis included abdominal compartment syndrome; bladder pressure measured was noted to be elevated at 29 mmHg and decreased to 21 mmHg with the placement of a rectal tube. She became anuric, developed bacteremia with *Escherichia coli*, and subsequently died. See Table 1 for serum, urine, and stool electrolytes.

3. Discussion

A systematic review found that there was no uniform identification of ACPO in the literature, and inconsistent terminology prevented reliable data synthesis [3]. ACPO is

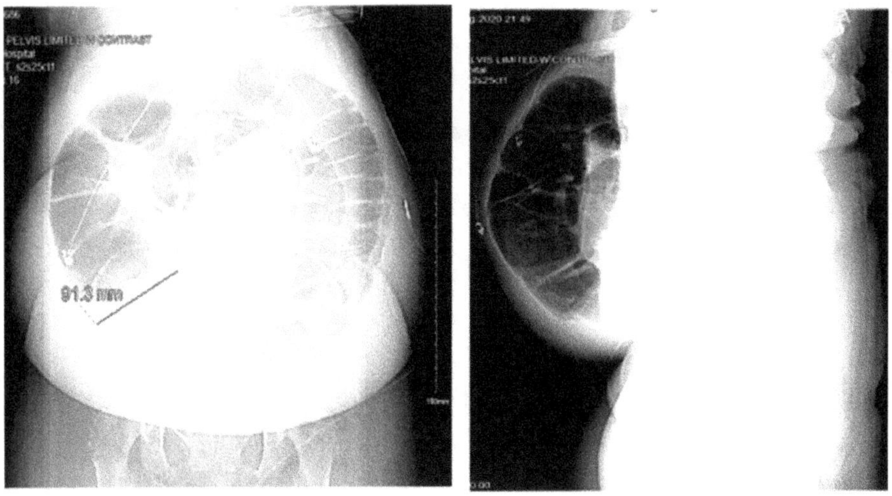

FIGURE 1: CAT scan with intravenous contrast showing dilated loops of bowel.

TABLE 1: Hypokalemia with significant stool loss of potassium and relatively low urine potassium.

Date	Serum potassium (mmol/L)	Urine osmolarity (mOsm/kg)	Urine potassium (mmol/L)	Urine sodium (mmol/L)	Urine chloride (mmol/L)	Urine magnesium (mg/dL)	Stool potassium (mmol/L)	Stool sodium (mmol/L)	Stool osmolarity (mOms/kg)
8/09/20	1.8								
8/11/20	2.6		23	<20	63		>100	42	
8/12/20	3.2	212	17	39					
8/15/20	2.7		18						
8/19/20	3.1		46	88	174				
8/20/20	3.4		45	37	134	10.4			
8/25/20	3.4		32	65	121		95.9	41	413
8/28/20	2.8		5	133	122			<20	
8/29/20	2.9		14	66	77				
9/1/20	3.8		14	110	75				

a diagnosis of exclusion made by excluding infectious causes such as *Clostridium difficile*. Delays in diagnosis may result in ineffective supportive treatment and may risk unnecessary aggressive therapies. Our patient had findings consistent with ACPO on imaging and a negative gastrointestinal infectious workup.

While the exact pathophysiology is unclear, the current hypothesis suggests an imbalance of autonomic regulation in the distal colon [4]. Sympathetic innervation to the distal colon comes from T9–L2, whereas parasympathetic innervation is from S2–S4 sacral segments of the spinal cord [5]. Moreover, neurogenic bowel dysfunction can also result from medications, spinal trauma, and immobility. Our patient had morbidity that would increase systemic sympathetic expression due to the spinal cord and immobility.

Potassium homeostasis is maintained by the kidney and the gut. The big potassium (BK) channels, also called Maxi-K channels, are large conductance, voltage-gated, flow-mediated channels that are found in various tissues and widely expressed in the kidney and the distal intestinal colon crypts [6]. BK channels are associated with one of the four subunits (BKβ1–β4) and are responsible for flow-induced K secretion [7].

Significant loss of fluid in diarrhea with hypokalemia is reported to be common [8]. The secretory diarrhea in ACPO is driven by potassium secretion, in contrast to the inhibition of sodium reabsorption or chloride secretion, which are the more common pathophysiologic mechanisms of other forms of secretory diarrhea [9]. It is common that patients may lose more than 100 millimoles of potassium daily. The source of hypokalemia appears to be gastrointestinal potassium loss. The kidney response to hypokalemia is compensatory potassium conservation with a low amount of potassium lost in urine. Our patient had an initial urine potassium of 23 mmol/L, and it peaked at 45.8 mmol/L; the first stool potassium was >100 mmol/L with a stool volume of 900 milliliters. A repeat stool study after a week showed stool potassium of 95.9 mmol/L and stool sodium of 42 mmol/L. Our patient received more than 200 mEq of potassium supplement a day, but her serum potassium level persistently remained below 3.5 mmol/L.

Imaging, including an abdominal x-ray on admission, showed distension of the colon, which measured up to 11.4 cm in diameter at the cecum and 8.2 cm at the transverse level. The difference in distension between the transverse and distal colon supports the autonomic dysfunction hypothesis since the splenic flexure is the point where innervation sources change [10]. Serial

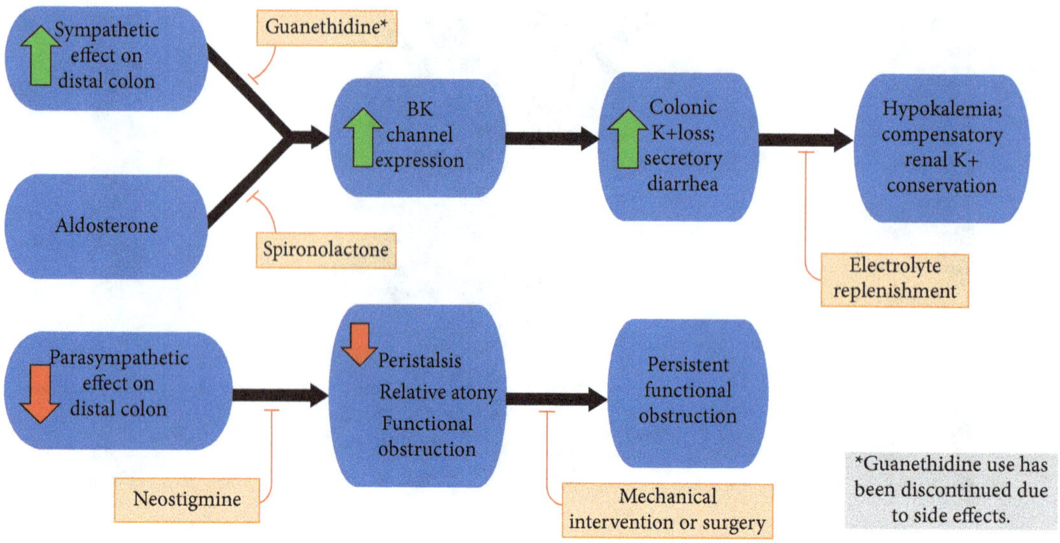

Figure 2: Pathophysiology and treatment options for acute colonic pseudo-obstruction.

imaging of the bowel showed worsening diffused colonic dilation.

Once a diagnosis is made, it is important to determine the pace of the treatment plan (Figure 2). Urgency in treatment includes a diameter of more than 12 cm, which is often considered less responsive to conservative therapy, and decompression may be needed to reduce the risk of colonic perforation [4].

If less pressing, conservative therapy with electrolyte replacement and pharmacologic therapy may be used. In an attempt to restore balance, historical studies on the treatment of ACPO have used the adrenergic blocker guanethidine, followed by neostigmine, which inhibits acetylcholinesterase and is a parasympathomimetic [11]. Questionable efficacy and side effects of postural hypotension led to discontinuation of the use of guanethidine. Neostigmine was tested successfully and is still prescribed in the management of ACPO [12]. As aldosterone upregulates the BK channels, a case report of aldosterone inhibition with spironolactone has also been tried with success [13].

Mechanical interventions may include rectal tubes, needle decompression, epidural anesthesia, percutaneous cecostomy, and various options for surgery. Surgery, which is usually considered as a final option, is associated with high rates of morbidity and mortality [14].

4. Conclusion

ACPO is a diagnosis of exclusion in patients with abdominal symptoms often accompanied by hypokalemia, which has high morbidity, but timely determination of the cause can prevent inadvertent surgery and complications.

References

[1] M. Haj, M. Haj, and D. C. Rockey, "Ogilvie's syndrome: management and outcomes," *Medicine*, vol. 97, no. 27, e11187 pages, 2018.

[2] S. Conner, A. Nassereddin, and C. Mitchell, StatPearls Publishing, 2021, https://www.ncbi.nlm.nih.gov/books/NBK526102/.

[3] C. I. Wells, G. O'Grady, and I. P. Bissett, "Acute colonic pseudo-obstruction: a systematic review of aetiology and mechanisms," *World Journal of Gastroenterology*, vol. 23, no. 30, pp. 5634–5644, 2017.

[4] V. W. Vanek, M. Al-Salti, L. Al-Salti, and M. D. Musbah, "Acute pseudo-obstruction of the colon (Ogilvie's syndrome)," *Diseases of the Colon & Rectum*, vol. 29, no. 3, pp. 203–210, 1986.

[5] A. Krassioukov, F. Biering-Sørensen, W. Donovan et al., "Autonomic standards committee of the American spinal injury association/international spinal cord society i," *J Spinal Cord Med*, vol. 35, no. 4, pp. 201–210, 2012.

[6] M. Sausbier, J. E. Matos, U. Sausbier et al., "Distal colonic K(+) secretion occurs via BK channels," *Journal of the American Society of Nephrology*, vol. 17, no. 5, pp. 1275–1282, 2006.

[7] J. D. Holtzclaw, P. R. Grimm, and S. C. Sansom, "Role of BK channels in hypertension and potassium secretion," *Current Opinion in Nephrology and Hypertension*, vol. 20, no. 5, pp. 512–517, 2011.

[8] N. Sunnoqrot and R. F. Reilly, "Hypokalemia associated with colonic pseudo-obstruction (Ogilvie's Syndrome)," *Case Rep Nephrol Dial*, vol. 5, no. 2, pp. 118–123, 2015.

[9] J. R. Thiagarajah, M. Donowitz, and A. S. Verkman, "Secretory diarrhoea: mechanisms and emerging therapies," *Nature Reviews Gastroenterology & Hepatology*, vol. 12, no. 8, pp. 446–457, 2015.

[10] J. S. Choi, J. S. Lim, H. Kim et al., "Colonic pseudoobstruction: CT findings," *American Journal of Roentgenology*, vol. 190, no. 6, pp. 1521–1526, 2008.

[11] R. Hutchinson and C. Griffiths, "Acute colonic pseudo-obstruction: a pharmacological approach," *Annals of the Royal College of Surgeons of England*, vol. 74, no. 5, pp. 364–367, 1992.

[12] R. J. Ponec, M. D. Saunders, and M. B. Kimmey, "Neostigmine for the treatment of acute colonic pseudo-obstruction," *New England Journal of Medicine*, vol. 341, no. 3, pp. 137–141, 1999 Jul 15.

[13] P. Ram, A. Goyal, M. Lu, J. Sloan, and W. McElhaugh, "Use of Aldosterone Antagonist to Treat Diarrhea and Hypokalemia of Ogilvie's Syndrome," *Case Reports in Gastrointestinal Medicine*, vol. 2016, pp. 1–3, Article ID 1207240, 2016.

[14] P. Pereira, F. Djeudji, P. Leduc, F. Fanget, and X. Barth, "Ogilvie's syndrome-acute colonic pseudo-obstruction," *Journal of Visceral Surgery*, vol. 152, no. 2, pp. 99–105, 2015.

20

Evaluation and Transplantation of a SARS-CoV-2 Seropositive Kidney Candidate

Maya C. Graves,[1] Sapna A. Mehta ,[1,2] Bonnie E. Lonze,[1,2] and Nicole M. Ali[1,2]

[1]New York University Grossman School of Medicine, New York, NY, USA
[2]New York University Langone Transplant Institute, New York, NY, USA

Correspondence should be addressed to Sapna A. Mehta; sapna.mehta@nyulangone.org

Academic Editor: David Mudge

The COVID-19 pandemic affected transplant center activity in areas with high number of cases such as New York City and prompted reevaluation of patients awaiting organ transplant diagnosed with SARS-CoV-2 infection. To resume safe transplantation at our center, we found it necessary to (1) identify transplant candidates with possible exposure to or history of COVID-19 infection, (2) outline a clinical and laboratory assessment to determine adequate clinical recovery from COVID-19 for transplantation, and (3) determine whether the possibility of perioperative COVID-19 transmission from the patient to staff would pose unacceptable risk. Here, we describe our center's approach to proceeding with transplantation in a SARS-CoV-2 seropositive living donor kidney transplant recipient and describe early posttransplant outcomes.

1. Introduction

Kidney transplantation is a lifesaving treatment for many patients with end-stage renal disease (ESRD). The spread of the SARS-CoV-2 pandemic in areas such as New York City, where a surge in COVID-19 cases occurred, created a need to suspend solid organ transplantation when COVID-19-safe pathways for postoperative care were not available. While dialysis can be a temporary treatment option available to patients with kidney failure, this surrogate option is costlier and leads to higher morbidity and mortality rates than kidney transplantation [1]. Currently, there is limited guidance for safely transplanting patients during this COVID-19 era [2]. Additionally, kidney transplant candidates are at risk for exposure to COVID-19 while awaiting organ transplantation, particularly patients undergoing community-based hemodialysis. As the ability to safely resume transplantation from a hospital resource standpoint was regained, a new pretransplant framework was required to assess risk for patients exposed to or recovered from COVID-19. We describe a case of a living donor kidney transplant (LDKT) candidate found to be SARS-CoV-2 seropositive and the protocol we (Figure 1) utilized to assess the COVID-19 related risk to the recipient, donor, and provider care team which informed decision-making regarding timing of transplantation.

2. Case Report

A 30-year old female with a past medical history of hypertension, hyperlipidemia, polycystic ovarian syndrome, and focal segmental glomerulosclerosis presented with Stage IV chronic kidney disease (CKD) for an LDKT. Roughly, one year prior to presentation for the LDKT, she was evaluated by the transplant review committee to assess candidacy for a deceased donor kidney transplant (DDKT). She was approved and listed as active on the kidney transplant waiting list. During her waiting period, she never initiated dialysis. One year later, her kidney function was poor with creatinine elevated to 5.02 mg/dl, urine protein elevated to 265 mg/dL, BUN elevated to 43 mg/dl, and estimated GFR was 11 ml/min/1.73^2. She was in imminent need for either transplantation or initiation of community-based hemodialysis. A living donor candidate was evaluated and approved to donate just prior to the outbreak of the COVID-19 pandemic. Months later, during routine

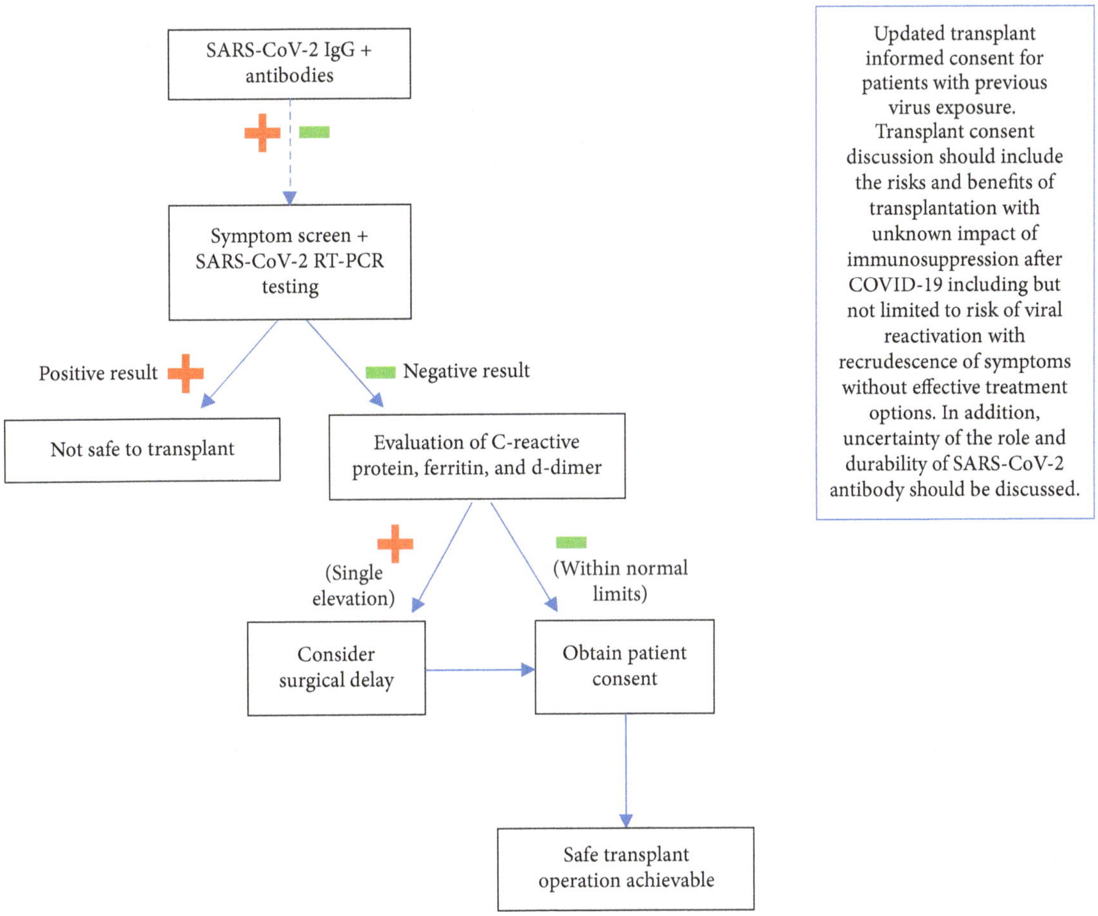

Figure 1: Protocol for transplant pre-operative evaluation for all transplant candidates during COVID-19 pandemic.

preoperative evaluation, she underwent a complete COVID-19 symptom screen via telemedicine visit which was normal. During routine preoperative laboratory testing, the patient underwent SARS-CoV-2 IgG testing at an outside laboratory using the Abbott assay which resulted positive (23.88 UA/mL). Upon repeat discussion with the patient, she recalled that two months prior she had experienced 2 days of body aches and one day of fever with Tmax 38.6°C followed by two weeks of poor appetite. However, at the time of her symptoms, SARS-CoV-2 RT-PCR testing was not widely available and the patient had been tested only for influenza virus by nasopharyngeal swab which was negative. Her prolonged poor appetite was attributed to mild uremic symptoms from ESRD but improved without renal replacement therapy. The transplant team concluded that the patient had experienced a self-limited febrile illness during a period of known SARS-CoV-2 transmission in the New York City that was consistent with COVID-19 and that she had likely been infected.

Two days prior to scheduled transplant surgery, the patient underwent repeat symptom screen, reported no symptoms of COVID-19, and underwent SARS-CoV-2 RT-PCR testing by nasopharyngeal sample. In addition, as a further measure to assess potential patient-to-staff transmission risk, SARS-CoV-2 RT-PCR testing was performed on the patient's stool specimen and also resulted negative. The Cepheid Xpert Xpress SARS-CoV-2 assay was validated for both nasopharyngeal and stool samples by our institution's clinical laboratory. She was admitted for scheduled living donor kidney transplant surgery. She had normal vital signs, an unremarkable lung exam, and an admission chest X-ray showing clear lungs without signs of pneumonia. Repeat SARS-CoV-2 RT-PCR testing by nasopharyngeal swab was negative and laboratory values for inflammatory markers (ferritin, d-dimer, and C-reactive protein) were all within normal limits. The patient had an uncomplicated intra- and postoperative course. The kidney was flushed, per surgeon standard practice, with porcine heparin (2500 units in 500 mL normal saline), and the patient was given standard venous thromboembolism (VTE) prophylaxis. She was administered high-dose methylprednisone intraoperatively followed by basiliximab (20 mg) for induction therapy. Induction immunosuppression for transplant surgery was not modified based on the history of COVID-19. The patient was ambulating on postoperative day 1, serum creatinine continued to improve to normal, and urine output was excellent. She was discharged on postoperative day 4 on an immunosuppressive regimen of tacrolimus, mycophenolate mofetil, and prednisone. At the time of this report, she has completed 6 months of outpatient follow up with no signs or symptoms of infection, rejection, or other complications. She has undergone surveillance SARS-CoV-2 PCR testing at 0, 2, 4, 6, and 22 weeks after transplant, and the results have remained negative.

3. Discussion

This is the first reported case of kidney transplantation in a SARS-CoV-2 seropositive patient in the United States with 6 months of posttransplant follow-up. Transplant candidates with a history of clinical COVID-19 or seropositivity for SARS-CoV-2 are increasingly common as we move forward in the COVID-19 era [3–5]. As a transplant center located in the initial epicenter at the onset of the COVID-19 outbreak in the United States, we found it critical to create a systematic approach (Figure 1) to (1) identify whether transplant candidates had evidence of SARS-CoV-2 infection, (2) determine when the patient was adequately clinically recovered to proceed with transplantation and use of immunosuppression, and (3) assess risk of SARS-CoV-2 transmission from the patient to the clinical care team.

Three cardinal concerns were identified:

(1) Confirmation of prior SARS-CoV-2 infection and assessment for active viral infection with transmission potential

(2) Consideration of risk of recrudescence of COVID-19 symptoms or potential for SARS-CoV-2 reactivation with onset of immunosuppression, given the limited data to date

(3) Adequate precautions for our surgeons, physicians, and all healthcare personnel caring for a seropositive patient in the peritransplant period

We addressed the first concern by thorough history including the review of any prior laboratory testing, COVID-19 symptom screening, use of validated SARS-CoV-2 serologic assay, and SARS-CoV-2 RT-PCR testing. Our patient was found to be seropositive for SARS-CoV-2 first at an outside laboratory which was utilized until a validated COVID-19 serologic assay was available at our hospital. Subsequently, when serologic testing became available at our transplant center, the test was performed on sera stored from the same date as the sample tested with the Abbott assay and was found to be positive, increasing our confidence in a true positive serology result. We assessed transmission potential by SARS-CoV-2 RT-PCR testing on nasopharyngeal and stool samples. Our rationale for utilizing both nasopharyngeal and stool RT-PCR testing was based on data in adults and children showing SARS-CoV-2 RT-PCR positivity in stool for a longer duration (>4 weeks) than nasopharyngeal or respiratory samples [6]. Given that 2 months had lapsed since our patient's COVID-19 compatible symptoms, our suspicion for positive nasopharyngeal RT-PCR testing was low. The RT-PCR Cepheid Xpert Xpress SARS-CoV-2 Assay was validated by our institution's clinical laboratory for both nasopharyngeal and stool samples. The utility of the RT-PCR SARS-CoV-2 assay under the Food and Drug Administration's Emergency Use Authorization in our institution's core-laboratory facilitated prompt turn-around times (<5 hours) amidst the pandemic, allowing for time sensitive decision-making regarding transplantation [7]. All transplant candidates at our center undergo SARS-CoV-2 PCR by nasopharyngeal swab testing prior to transplant surgery, regardless of the presence of COVID-19 symptoms or whether prior SARS-CoV-2 serology testing has been performed.

The third element of laboratory data reviewed which provided confidence that our patient was clinically recovered from COVID-19 were inflammatory markers. C-reactive protein, d-dimer, and ferritin were reviewed as numerous studies, and meta-analyses have identified abnormalities in these values as dominant biomarkers for COVID-19 disease progression and poor outcome [8]. All values were within normal limits at the time of preoperative evaluation (Figure 2).

The long-term natural history of SARS-CoV-2 remains to be fully characterized, and the risk associated with induction immunosuppression soon after infection is unclear. While prolonged SARS-CoV-2 PCR positivity has been reported in patients following clinical recovery from COVID-19, persistence of replicative virus regardless of serial nasopharyngeal PCR results and risk of recrudescence of symptoms remains unclear. We felt it was prudent and ethically necessary to address this unknown and potential risk with the patient through a modification of informed consent for kidney transplantation. The risk versus benefit analysis when discussing the option to move forward with transplantation and initiation of life-long immunosuppression required patient acknowledgement of the unknown risks of a novel pathogen including, but not limited to, reactivation or recrudescence of COVID-19 symptoms, impact on the kidney allograft, and potential for poor long-term outcome. Additionally, the unknown durability and immunologic role of SARS-CoV-2 IgG were discussed.

During the kidney transplant procedure, safety precautions taken by the operating room team members included the use of an N95 or Delta mask for all operating room staff and face shields for those performing the orotracheal intubation. In accordance with algorithmic precautions for operating members during the COVID-19 pandemic set forward by Forrester et al., our risk assessment performed by symptomology, measurement of inflammatory markers, and utilization of repeat RT-PCR testing provided confidence that patient did not have evidence of ongoing nasopharyngeal viral shedding and that use of an N95 or Delta mask in combination with eye protection would be sufficient for healthcare worker protection [9].

Given the atypical nature of respiratory disease presentation in immunocompromised populations [10], close clinical surveillance for the recrudescence of COVID-19 symptoms in our patient remains important. Case series of kidney transplant recipients with COVID-19 have described variable initial clinical presentations, including gastrointestinal symptoms, vomiting, fever, cough, generalized

Laboratory marker	Patient	Reference
C-reactive protein	0.3 mg/L	0–5 mg/L
Ferritin	53 ng/mL	5–204 ng/mL
D-dimer	106 ng/mL	<230 ng/mL

FIGURE 2: Inflammatory markers used to evaluate COVID-19 clinical recovery in SARS-CoV-2 seropositive transplant candidate.

fatigue, or chills [11–14]. To our knowledge, no cases of recrudescence of COVID-19 symptoms following organ transplantation have been described. After transplantation, our patient's clinical care has been managed via telemedicine every 2–4 weeks by transplant nephrology and with routine posttransplant weekly laboratory testing (complete blood count with differential, complete metabolic panel, magnesium, phosphorus, tacrolimus level, BK virus, and Epstein–Barr Virus, and a urinalysis). In addition, SARS-CoV-2 RT-PCR testing was repeated at weeks 0, 2, 4, 6, and most recently, 22 weeks after transplant. As recommended by the Centers for Disease Control and Prevention (CDC), the use of telemedicine has allowed for active monitoring of our patient while mitigating increased risk of repeat COVID-19 exposure for both patient and provider [15]. At 6 months of posttransplant follow-up, our patient has not encountered any complications suggestive of SARS-CoV-2 symptom recurrence, rejection, or other complications. We report favorable early outcomes after kidney transplantation in a recipient with recent SARS-CoV-2 infection and suggest development of a systematic risk assessment for organ transplantation after COVID-19. Further long-term data on posttransplant outcomes in COVID-19 recovered patients are needed.

Abbreviations

CDC: Centers for Disease Control and Prevention
COVID-19: Coronavirus disease 2019
CKD: Chronic kidney disease
ESRD: End-stage renal disease
LDKT: Living donor kidney transplant
RT-PCR: Real-time reverse transcription polymerase chain reaction
SARS-CoV-2: Severe acute respiratory syndrome coronavirus 2.

Consent

Written informed consent for this paper to be published was obtained from the patient.

References

[1] R. Fu, N. Sekercioglu, W. Berta, and P. C. Coyte, "Cost-effectiveness of deceased-donor renal transplant versus dialysis to treat end-stage renal disease," *Transplantation Direct*, vol. 6, no. 2, p. e522, 2020.
[2] N. T. N. Galvan, N. F. Moreno, J. E. Garza et al., "Donor and transplant candidate selection for solid organ transplantation during the COVID-19 pandemic," *American Journal of Transplantation*, vol. 20, no. 11, pp. 3113–3122, 2020.
[3] C. Clarke, M. Prendecki, A. Dhutia et al., "High prevalence of asymptomatic COVID-19 infection in hemodialysis patients detected using serologic screening," *American Society of Nephrology*, vol. 31, no. 9, pp. 1969–1975, 2020.
[4] R. W. Corbett, S. Blakey, D. Nitsch et al., "Epidemiology of COVID-19 in an urban dialysis center," *Journal of the American Society of Nephrology*, vol. 31, no. 8, pp. 1815–1823, 2020.
[5] V. Schwierzeck, J. C. König, J. Kühn et al., "First reported nosocomial outbreak of severe acute respiratory syndrome coronavirus 2 (SARS-CoV-2) in a pediatric dialysis unit," *Clinical Infectious Diseases*, vol. 72, no. 2, pp. 265–270, 2020.
[6] W. A. Szymczak, D. Y. Goldstein, E. P. Orner et al., "Utility of stool PCR for the diagnosis of COVID-19: comparison of two commercial platforms," *Journal of Clinical Microbiology*, vol. 58, no. 9, Article ID e01369, 2020.
[7] T. A. Paczos, "Mounting a regional response to the COVID-19 pandemic: another reason to "keep" your lab," *Archives of Pathology & Laboratory Medicine*, vol. 144, no. 11, pp. 1321–1324, 2020.
[8] I. Huang, R. Pranata, M. A. Lim, A. Oehadian, and B. Alisjahbana, "C-reactive protein, procalcitonin, D-dimer, and ferritin in severe coronavirus disease-2019: a meta-analysis," *Therapeutic Advances in Respiratory Disease*, vol. 14, 2020.
[9] J. D. Forrester, A. K. Nassar, P. M. Maggio, and M. T. Hawn, "Precautions for operating room team members during the COVID-19 pandemic," *Journal of the American College of Surgeons*, vol. 230, no. 6, pp. 1098–1101, 2020.
[10] J. H. Shelhamer, G. B. Toews, H. Masur et al., "Respiratory disease in the immunosuppressed patient," *Annals of Internal Medicine*, vol. 117, no. 5, pp. 415–431, 1992.
[11] E. Guillen, G. J. Pineiro, I. Revuelta et al., "Case report of COVID-19 in a kidney transplant recipient: does immunosuppression alter the clinical presentation?" *American Journal of Transplantation*, vol. 20, no. 7, pp. 1875–1878, 2020.
[12] E. Seminari, M. Colaneri, M. Sambo et al., "SARS Cov-2 infection in a renal-transplanted patient: a case report," *American Journal of Transplantation: Official Journal of the American Society of Transplantation and the American Society of Transplant Surgeons*, vol. 20, no. 7, pp. 1882–1884, 2020.
[13] L. Ning, L. Liu, W. Li et al., "Novel coronavirus (SARS-CoV-2) infection in a renal transplant recipient: case report," *American Journal of Transplantation*, vol. 20, no. 7, pp. 1864–1868, 2020.
[14] A. Imam, S. A. Abukhalaf, R. Imam, S. Abu-Gazala, H. Merhav, and A. Khalaileh, "Kidney transplantation in the times of COVID-19 - a literature review," *Ann Transplant*, vol. 25, Article ID e925755, 2020.
[15] F. Aziz, M. R. Jorgenson, N. Garg et al., "The care of kidney transplant recipients during a global pandemic: challenges and strategies for success," *Transplantation Reviews*, vol. 34, no. 4, Article ID 100567, 2020.

21

Refractory Acute Interstitial Nephritis in the Setting of Nivolumab Therapy

Antonio Faieta[1] **and Tavis Dancik**[2]

[1]Department of Internal Medicine, Beaumont Health System, Royal Oak, MI, USA
[2]Department of Nephrology, Beaumont Health System, Royal Oak, MI, USA

Correspondence should be addressed to Antonio Faieta; antonio.faieta@beaumont.org

Academic Editor: Hern n Trimarchi

A 65-year-old male patient with metastatic CCRCC developed steroid-dependent, grade 3 AIN secondary to nivolumab weeks after its initiation that resulted in 3 hospitalizations with acute renal failure. The patient was started on MM and his AIN was successfully controlled after a 2-year period of follow-up. Refractory renal AIN resulting from PD-1 inhibitor use is rare, and its successful treatment with mofetil mycophenolate with a 2-year follow-up in a patient with metastatic CCRCC has not been reported. This case is important because not only was his renal irAEs controlled but also long-term treatment with MM did not result in progression of metastatic disease.

1. Introduction

A 65-year-old male with a past medical history of essential hypertension, type 2 diabetes mellitus, obesity with a BMI of 31.65 kg/m^2, stage 2 chronic kidney disease (CKD), COPD, paroxysmal atrial fibrillation, dyslipidemia, and history of urinary retention secondary to benign prostate hyperplasia was found to have a $9.5 \times 6 \times 7.1$ cm enhancing mass in the left kidney after an abdominal CT scan with intravenous contrast done for an R renal cyst follow-up. A high-resolution CT scan of the chest (HRCT) revealed numerous nodules suspicious for metastases. A CT scan-directed lung biopsy revealed metastatic clear cell renal cell carcinoma (CCRCC). One month later, the patient underwent a left nephrectomy and lymphectomy followed by sequential therapy with sunitinib, everolimus, and bevacizumab, which overall controlled the disease for a total period of 31 months. However, his disease eventually progressed, and new brain metastasis was found. The patient underwent gamma knife radiosurgery and was started on nivolumab, a checkpoint inhibitor (CPI). Two months later, around his fourth cycle of nivolumab, the patient's creatinine was found to be 1.6 mg/dl, from his baseline of 1.0–1.2 mg/dl. Four months after nivolumab was started, following his 8th cycle of nivolumab, the patient was admitted to the hospital because a creatinine level of 4 mg/dl was noted. The patient had recently completed a course of cephalexin for a throat infection and was on omeprazole, but not NSAIDs or ACEi. On admission, creatinine was 6.09 mg/dl and BUN was 68 mg/dl, and there were metabolic acidosis and hyperkalemia. There was evidence of urinary retention on kidney and bladder ultrasound based on a PVR of 450 cc. Urinalysis revealed few eosinophils, 3–10 leukocytes, and subnephrotic range proteinuria. Complement levels were normal. The patient was started on intravenous hydration, omeprazole was discontinued, and a Foley catheter was placed. However, his renal function did not improve. The patient was subsequently started on 45 mg of prednisone orally twice daily for presumptive acute interstitial nephritis (AIN) secondary to nivolumab. He was discharged on a prednisone taper and his renal function continued to improve.

Two months later, close after ending his prednisone taper, the patient presented to the ER complaining of 2 weeks of worsening shortness of breath and 20-pound weight gain. On admission, physical examination revealed jugular venous distension and 4+ lower extremity pitting edema up to the knee, but no lung rales. Creatinine was 7.79 mg/dL, BUN 81 mg/dL, and potassium 6.4 mg/dL. Urinalysis revealed eosinophiluria, subnephrotic range proteinuria, and leukocyturia >50. Urinary retention was ruled out. Urine cultured grew 100,000 CFU of *E. coli*. Chest X-rays revealed signs of lung congestion and new small bilateral pleural effusions. A transthoracic echo demonstrated severely enlarged left atrium, mild to moderate tricuspid regurgitation, evidence of mildly elevated right ventricular systolic pressure, and trace pulmonary regurgitation that were not present on a TTE done 2 years prior. Left ventricular chamber size was normal, there were no distinct wall motion abnormalities, and a visually estimated ejection fraction was 55%. He was started on furosemide and antibiotics, but his renal function continued to worsen. The presumptive diagnosis of recurrent AIN secondary to nivolumab was made, and the patient was started on a pulse IV methylprednisolone followed by oral prednisone. After creatinine peaked to 8.29 mg/dL, the patient was discharged one week later with a creatinine level of 3.74 mg/dL on a prednisone taper and his creatinine continued to improve weeks later.

Few weeks after ending his second steroid taper, the patient was hospitalized for the third time because of a creatinine level of 8.27 mg/dL. There were eosinophiluria, proteinuria, significant leukocyturia, metabolic acidosis, and hyperkalemia with peak T waves on EKG. The patient was deemed to be steroid-dependent, and consideration to a steroid-sparing drug was given. The patient was started once again on pulse 500 mg IV methylprednisolone and 1 gram of mofetil mycophenolate (MM) twice daily. Renal biopsy was finally done and showed moderate interstitial inflammation mainly composed of lymphocytes along with secondary acute tubular injury. In addition, trichrome staining revealed a moderate amount of interstitial fibrosis and tubular atrophy. No evidence of glomerulonephritis or crescent formation was present. On immunofluorescence, glomeruli were negative for IgG, IgA, IgM, C3, kappa, lambda, and C1q. Renal function improved, and the patient was discharged on a prednisone taper and mofetil mycophenolate. In the following months, the patient was able to complete his prednisone taper and his creatinine remained stable on his new baseline, 2 mg/dL, and proteinuria, leukocyturia, and proteinuria resolved. The entire course of his acute kidney injury and response to treatment is depicted in Figure 1. His dose of mofetil was eventually weaned to 250 mg twice daily which he is presently on. Overall, the patient only received 8 cycles of nivolumab. PET CT after 3 years off nivolumab and while receiving MM revealed no new or progressive lesion, decreased avidity in the only avid lesion in a subcarinal lymph node, and stable brain lesion. The patient is currently doing well.

2. Discussion

Nivolumab, a checkpoint inhibitor, is a human IgG4 anti-PD-1 antibody that selectively blocks the interaction between PD-1 expressed in activated Th lymphocytes and its ligands, PD-L1 and PD-L2, expressed in tissues and cancer cells [1]. PD-L1 and PD-L2 expressions in tissues are one of the major determinants of peripheral immune tolerance. PD-L1 is overexpressed in tissues via lymphokines during states of T-cell activation as a means to safeguard themselves from being "attacked." Furthermore, some tumors constitutively express PD-L1 which dampens the activation of tumor-infiltrating lymphocytes. By blocking the interaction between PD-1 and PD-L1, the T-cell response is unleashed against the tumor. CCRCC expresses PD-L1 and there lies the rationale for nivolumab use. Nivolumab was approved by the FDA for its use in metastatic CCRCC in 2015 after demonstrating a significantly superior objective response rate and overall survival compared to everolimus in patients previously treated with bevacizumab [2].

Sometimes, T cells turn against a person's own tissues due to loss of peripheral tolerance induced by CPIs, resulting in immune-related adverse events (irAEs). Overall, irAEs are common in patients on CPIs and can affect almost any organ. CPIs are indicated for the treatment of several metastatic cancers. As cancer is more common with increasing age, the typical patient receiving CPIs is in the elderly age group and has numerous comorbidities and thus limited organ reserve, as the patient in this case vignette. IrAEs' timing of presentation and severity are vastly heterogeneous but more frequently occur between 21 and 245 days after they are initiated [3]. Commonly, irAEs present grade 1-2 events (at most requiring only symptomatic management), but grade 3 or 4 events (organ- or life-threatening) can occur in up to 15% of the patients that merits discontinuation of CPIs [4]. However, there are not practical ways for clinicians to predict the degree of an irAE's severity and refractoriness early on its course, when the affected organ is at its best chance of recovery. In addition, most of the irAEs are reversible with treatment.

Renal irAEs can occur with CPIs. The patient can present with variable elevation in creatinine, leukocyturia, and subnephrotic range proteinuria [5, 6]. Case reports and series of renal irAEs, including this case vignette, patients commonly had numerous risk factors for and/or an already established CKD. Furthermore, they were frequently receiving medications typically associated with drug-related AIN, such as proton pump inhibitors or first-generation cephalosporins. CKIN recommends monitoring creatinine frequently early in the initiation of CPIs as irAEs tend to occur more frequently during this period [7]. AIN is the most common renal irAE [6]. However, pathologic specimens have shown that renal irAEs are histologically heterogeneous and may inform about renal outcomes and treatment response. A higher degree of interstitial lymphocytic infiltrate and acute tubular damage may predict loss of renal function while a higher degree of granulomatous necrotizing vasculitis and glomerulonephritis (GN) seems to portend better renal outcomes [3, 6]. Furthermore, in a case series of 16 patients with renal irAEs, who were treated initially with a course of steroids and CPI discontinuation, none of the 5 AIN cases had complete renal function recovery and 2 of them ended up in permanent hemodialysis. Those with GN had a variable response to treatment depending on the type of GN. Those with granulomatous GN had complete recovery while IgA GN did not

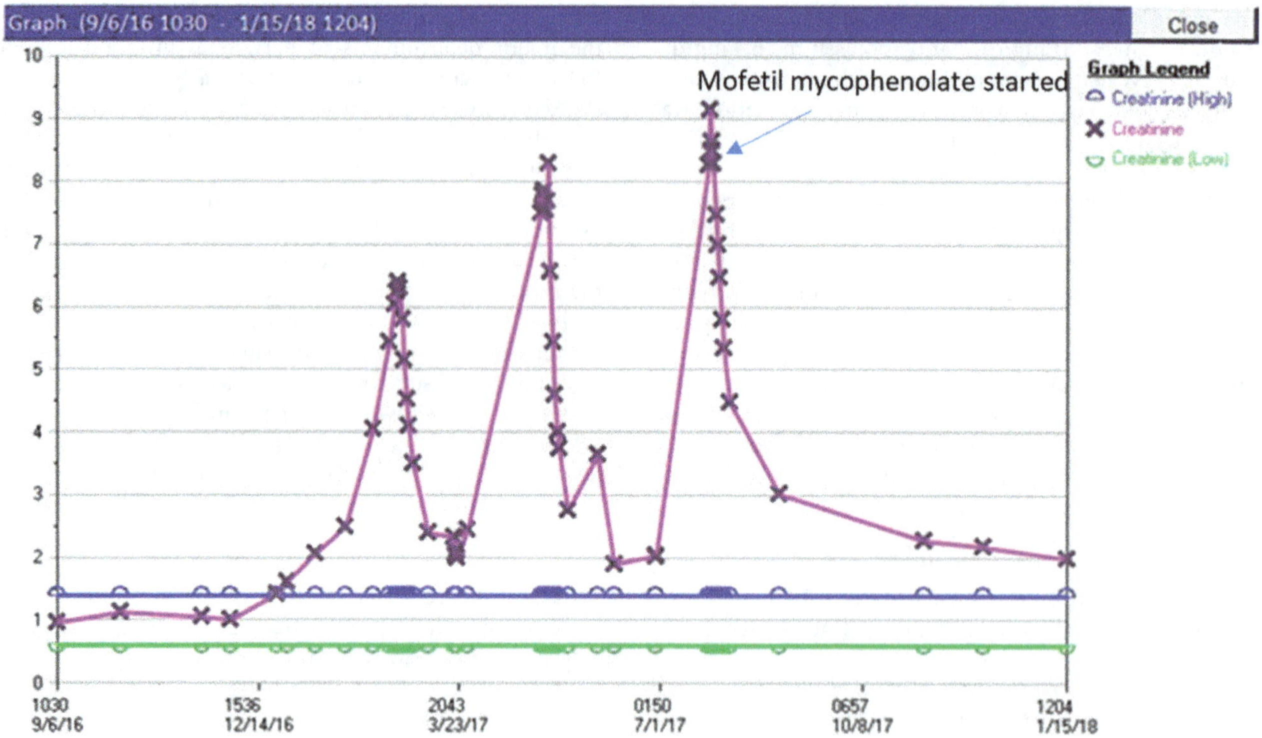

FIGURE 1: Patient's acute kidney injury course. The first 2 creatinine peaks represent acute kidney injury during steroid tapering. Note that when mofetil mycophenolate was initiated, the patient's renal function improved and eventually stabilized, and complete steroid weaning was possible.

respond to steroids or MM [6]. Because of the severe renal irAEs' rareness, there are no guidelines for their management. Most of the information about the management of renal irAEs comes from case reports and series in which glucocorticoids were favored as front-line therapy [3, 6, 8, 9]. Overall, it seems that patients who were older, who developed AIN close to the start of CPIs, who had a high creatinine elevation peak, had metastatic disease, and those undergoing concurrent treatment with nivolumab and ipilimumab, present with more aggressive AIN phenotype characterized by severe lymphocytic AIN and tubular injury that may benefit from early and prolonged steroid-sparing immunosuppression. In addition, long-term use of immunosuppressive medication to treat CPI high-grade adverse effects has not been associated with worse prognosis or overall survival [5]. On the other hand, the prognosis of a patient with CKD stage 2 that progresses to stage 4 (our patient) after an irAE may potentially be worse. Thus, early biopsy and immunosuppression may decrease the risk of irreversible kidney damage, particularly in patients with grade 3-4 renal irAEs and those with low physiological reserve such as the elderly or patients with comorbidities. It is important to notice that, in this case, biopsy was delayed under the presumption of nivolumab-induced interstitial nephritis which missed the severity of the histologic phenotype and other potential differential diagnoses. The duration of immunosuppression is unknown, but our patient did well 3 years on MM and off nivolumab.

Also, it is unknown whether immunosuppressive medication can be used concomitantly with CPIs to control irAEs. Interestingly, a report of an elderly patient with metastatic anal melanoma was treated with a sequential use of ipilimumab followed by nivolumab after which she developed severe steroid-dependent AIN. This patient was kept on nivolumab concurrently with maintenance prednisone at a dose of 10 mg, and her renal function improved and stabilized. When prednisone was stopped, she developed a recurrence of AIN and nivolumab had to be discontinued. Of note, most of her metastatic lesions demonstrated ongoing regression except for new brain lesions treated with stereotaxic radiation after nivolumab was discontinued [9]. Some patients will only need a course of steroids and discontinuation of CPIs to treat their AIN [10]. In a series of 13 cases of AKI secondary to CPIs, AIN was the most common histological finding; the most common cancer treated was metastatic melanoma; AIN was more common in patients treated with nivolumab alone, ipilimumab alone, and twice as common with nivolumab and ipilimumab combination compared to pembrolizumab; half of the patients partially recovered their renal function with steroids, less than a quarter had a complete response, and one patient showed TMA and did not respond to steroids [3]. In this case series, those patients treated conservatively did not have an improvement in renal function. One patient required mofetil mycophenolate because of worsening renal function on methylprednisolone.

CPIs have proven to be effective in the management of some advanced cancer, so their use is expected to increase as well as the incidence of irAEs and physicians will have a major role in diagnosing and treating them with the goal of preventing irreversible organ damage that can increase morbidity and affect prognosis. This case is relevant because it presents a patient with a refractory grade 3 renal irAEs that was effectively controlled with long-term use of mofetil mycophenolate with ongoing regression of his metastases. Finally, to change the current steroid-centered paradigm, there is a need for randomized trials that compare initial treatment with long-term treatment with steroid-sparing immunosuppressants with tapering courses of steroids in a patient with grade 3-4 irAEs and high comorbidity burden.

References

[1] E. Mashima, A. Inoue, Y. Sakuragi et al., "Nivolumab in the treatment of malignant melanoma: review of the literature," *OncoTargets and Therapy*, vol. 8, pp. 2045–2051, 2015.

[2] R. J. Motzer, B. Escudier, D. F. McDermott et al., "Nivolumab versus everolimus in advanced renal-cell carcinoma," *New England Journal of Medicine*, vol. 373, no. 19, pp. 1803–1813, 2015.

[3] F. B. Cortazar, K. A. Marrone, M. L. Troxell et al., "Clinicopathological features of acute kidney injury associated with immune checkpoint inhibitors," *Kidney International*, vol. 90, no. 3, pp. 638–647, 2016.

[4] B. L. Maughan, E. Bailey, D. M. Gill, and N. Agarwal, "Incidence of immune-related adverse events with program death receptor-1- and program death receptor-1 ligand-directed therapies in genitourinary cancers," *Frontiers in Oncology*, vol. 7, p. 56, 2017.

[5] T. Z. Horvat, N. G. Adel, T.-O. Dang et al., "Immune-related adverse events, need for systemic immunosuppression, and effects on survival and time to treatment failure in patients with melanoma treated with ipilimumab at Memorial Sloan Kettering Cancer Center," *Journal of Clinical Oncology*, vol. 33, no. 28, pp. 3193–3198, 2015.

[6] O. Mamlouk, U. Selamet, S. Machado et al., "Nephrotoxicity of immune checkpoint inhibitors beyond tubulointerstitial nephritis: single-center experience," *Journal for ImmunoTherapy of Cancer*, vol. 7, no. 1, 2019.

[7] R. Wanchoo, S. Karam, N. N. Uppal et al., "Adverse renal effects of immune checkpoint inhibitors: a narrative review," *American Journal of Nephrology*, vol. 45, no. 2, pp. 160–169, 2017.

[8] J. Belliere, N. Meyer, J. Mazieres et al., "Acute interstitial nephritis related to immune checkpoint inhibitors," *British Journal of Cancer*, vol. 115, no. 12, pp. 1457–1461, 2016.

[9] L. Bottlaender, A.-L. Breton, L. de Laforcade, F. Dijoud, L. Thomas, and S. Dalle, "Acute interstitial nephritis after sequential ipilumumab — nivolumab therapy of metastatic melanoma," *Journal for ImmunoTherapy of Cancer*, vol. 5, p. 57, 2017.

[10] J. Escandon, S. Peacock, A. Trabolsi, D. B. Thomas, A. Layka, and J. Lutzky, "Interstitial nephritis in melanoma patients secondary to PD-1 checkpoint inhibitor," *Journal for ImmunoTherapy of Cancer*, vol. 5, p. 3, 2017.

22

A 24-Year-Old Female Transplant Recipient with Type 2 Membranoproliferative Glomerulonephritis and Disseminated Shingles: A Cautionary Tale of Deferring to Primary Care

Benjamin T. Burdorf

Northeast Ohio Medical University, Rootstown, OH 44272, USA

Correspondence should be addressed to Benjamin T. Burdorf; bburdorf@neomed.edu

Academic Editor: Anja Haase-Fielitz

In this report, the case of a 24-year-old Caucasian female with type 2 membranoproliferative glomerulonephritis status-post living donor kidney transplant managed on triple regimen immunosuppressive therapy who developed shingles is discussed. With its onset, she promptly reached out to her nephrologist who deferred her to primary care. Prior to seeing her primary provider, she developed disseminated herpes zoster. She consulted emergency services where she was given inadequate care and again deferred to primary care. One day later, the dissemination included her entire torso, face, oral cavity, and all extremities. Fortunately, the patient had the insight to again reach out to her nephrologist who arranged for her to be admitted for appropriate care 6 days after her initial inquiry that carried 6 days of zoster progression. This case demonstrates how it is pertinent that specialists recognize potentially lethal complications associated with the conditions they follow. Although convenient to defer to primary care, if specialists were to take on the responsibility of providing a broader scope of care for their unique subsets of patients, it would likely result in a reduction in the 80% of serious medical errors that occur as a result of miscommunication, or lack thereof, between care providers.

1. Introduction

Type 2 membranoproliferative glomerulonephritis (MPGN 2) is a rare disease that affects primarily children and young adults at a prevalence of 2 to 3 individuals per million [1]. Its rarity is coupled with devastation. 50% of patients who incur the illness are subject to end-stage renal disease within 10 years and require dialysis as a bridge to hopeful transplantation [2]. With transplantation, the 5-year graft survival rate among patients with MPGN 2 is approximately 50.0%. It is speculated that this poor outcome is, in part, due to the high incidence of disease recurrence as shown in 67% of posttransplantation biopsies [3]. Current antirejection regimens consist of triple-agent immunosuppressive therapy that includes cyclosporin or tacrolimus, prednisone, and azathioprine or mycophenolate mofetil [4]. Although necessary, life-long immunosuppressive therapy poses a serious concern for the later development of opportunistic infections. Provided the complexity and fragility of these patients, they are inherently followed by multiple providers. As reported by the United States Joint Commission, 80% of serious medical errors occur as a result of miscommunication between care providers [5]. In this report, we will investigate how an episode of shingles eventually disseminated as a result of delayed treatment while being juggled amongst providers.

2. Case Report

A 24-year-old Caucasian female with a past medical history of hypertension, chronic kidney disease stage 3, and type 2 membranoproliferative glomerulonephritis status-post living donor kidney transplant in 2002 managed on an antirejection regimen of cyclosporin, mycophenolate mofetil, and prednisone noticed the onset of paresthesias and pain in her left lower back the evening of April 13, 2020. The morning of April 16, a grouped vesicular rash positioned along the left 3rd lumbar vertebral dermatome erupted, as shown in Figure 1. Worried about a shingles outbreak, she sent a message that evening to her nephrologist inquiring if this was something that needed to be addressed. The next morning (April 17), she received a response from a care coordinator, on behalf of the nephrologist's office, relaying that she should reach out to her primary-care provider for further work up. Unfortunately, the COVID-19 pandemic meant nonemergent visits were to be conducted via telehealth, an overwhelmed system that had yet to adequately adapt. She was unable to secure an appointment in a timely manner and upon showering the evening of April 21 found her isolated dermatomal rash evolved to include multiple pruritic, vesicular eruptions on her chest. Worried about these developments, the patient reached a nurse on the emergency health services line that informed her she needed to go to the nearest emergency room for suspected disseminated shingles. On arrival, she was afebrile (98.4°F), tachycardic (pulse 114 bpm), and hypertensive (160/107 mmHg). The emergency room physician took the photo shown in Figure 1 labeled April 21 and documented that the patient had similar eruptions in the upper chest and was immune compromised. She was diagnosed with disseminated shingles and sent home with the instructions to again follow-up with her primary doctor and to take valacyclovir 1,000 MG by mouth 3 times per day for 7 days. Despite having started the valacyclovir the night of her emergency room visit, the morning of April 22 showed worrisome progression. The vesicular eruptions that had only been on her left lower back and upper chest became diffusely distributed throughout her torso and now included the neck, face, oral mucosa, and tongue, as shown in Figure 2. Fearful of what may happen if she were to wait for a telehealth appointment with her primary-care provider, she again reached out to her nephrologists relaying her emergency-room course, the plan implemented as well as providing the photos shown in Figure 2. In review of this information, the nephrologist refuted the plan for outpatient oral valacyclovir treatment and coordinated for same day hospital admission. On admission 5 : 00 pm April 22, she was afebrile (98.1°F), tachycardic (pulse 123 bpm), and hypertensive (143/90 mmHg). Laboratory studies showed a bump in her baseline creatinine from ~1.40 mg/dL to 2.18 mg/dL indicating an acute kidney injury in the setting of viremia, hypertension, and poor oral intake. In addition, the patient's lesions had progressed to include more of her face and had invaded her proximal arms and legs. Fortunately, an ophthalmic exam did not find any involvement of the eyes. PCR analysis was conducted on lesion swabs that were negative for HSV-1 and HSV-2 but positive for varicella zoster confirming the diagnosis of disseminated shingles. She was promptly started on NaCl fluid supplementation and I.V. acyclovir 10 MG/kg twice per day for 5 days. By April 27, the patient's lesions had scabbed over and her creatinine was back to baseline. She was discharged home and instructed to take valacyclovir 1,000 MG twice per day through May 7 at which time she reported a full recovery apart from lesion scarring.

3. Discussion

This case demonstrates the importance of timely, prioritized patient management. When the patient initially reached out to her nephrologist, her zoster outbreak was isolated to one dermatome and could have been adequately managed with an outpatient oral antiviral prescription [6]. Instead of addressing the disease at that time, the wait associated with deferment to primary care allowed for the development of viremia and dissemination of the previously contained zoster virus. With dissemination in an immune compromised patient, the virus carries a mortality of 5–15% [7] and inpatient I.V. acyclovir is required as oral antivirals, such as valacyclovir, are no longer sufficient [8]. Furthermore, the delayed treatment of disseminated zoster poses an increased risk for visceral involvement. If the virus reaches this stage, it carries a more ominous outlook with an estimated mortality of 55% [9]. Fortunately, this patient had the awareness to seek care from emergency services at the first sign of dissemination. Unfortunately, she was given inadequate treatment (outpatient management with oral valacyclovir) and again deferred to primary care. As discussed, her condition continued to deteriorate as the virus wreaked havoc, manifesting within her torso, face, oral cavity, and all extremities just one day after her emergency-room visit. Thankfully, the patient again reached out to her nephrologist who took the action to have her admitted to finally receive the standard of care 6 days after her initial inquiry that carried 6 days of zoster progression. It is regrettable that, in this case, the initiative and insight to obtain adequate care continued to fall on the patient. While shingles is usually managed through primary care and the emergency-room physician provided treatment that is sufficient in most settings, a solid organ transplant recipient with recurrent type 2 membranoproliferative glomerulonephritis on triple immunosuppressive therapy falls within a unique subset of patients that often require different standards of management. Because triple immunosuppressive therapy is the standard of care, special attention should be provided to prophylactic measures for opportunistic infections. As of 2019, it is recommended that kidney transplant recipients who are varicella zoster virus seropositive receive the inactivated recombinant subunit herpes zoster vaccine, which would have likely avoided this incident entirely had it been given [10]. Provided the complexity of patients followed in an interdisciplinary manner, it is pertinent that specialists recognize potentially lethal complications associated with the conditions they follow. Although convenient to defer to primary care, if specialists were to take on the responsibility of providing a broader scope of care for their unique subsets of patients, it would likely result in a reduction in the 80% of serious medical errors that occur as a result of miscommunication, or lack thereof, between care providers.

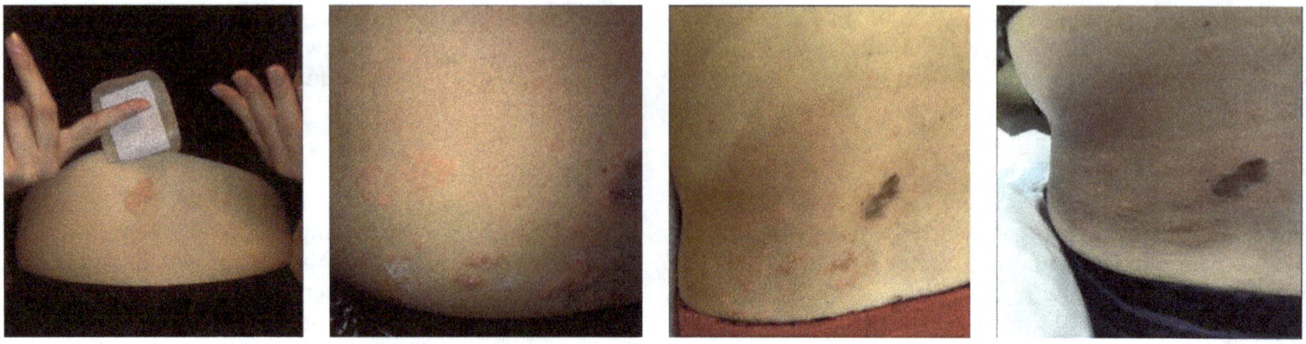

(a) (b) (c) (d)

FIGURE 1: Progression of the initial lesion from left to right. April 16 marks the first day of lesion appearance, April 21 marks her emergency room visit, And April 22 and 23 mark just prior to hospital admission and the following day. (a) April 16, 2020. (b) April 21, 2020. (c) April 22, 2020. (d) April 23, 2020.

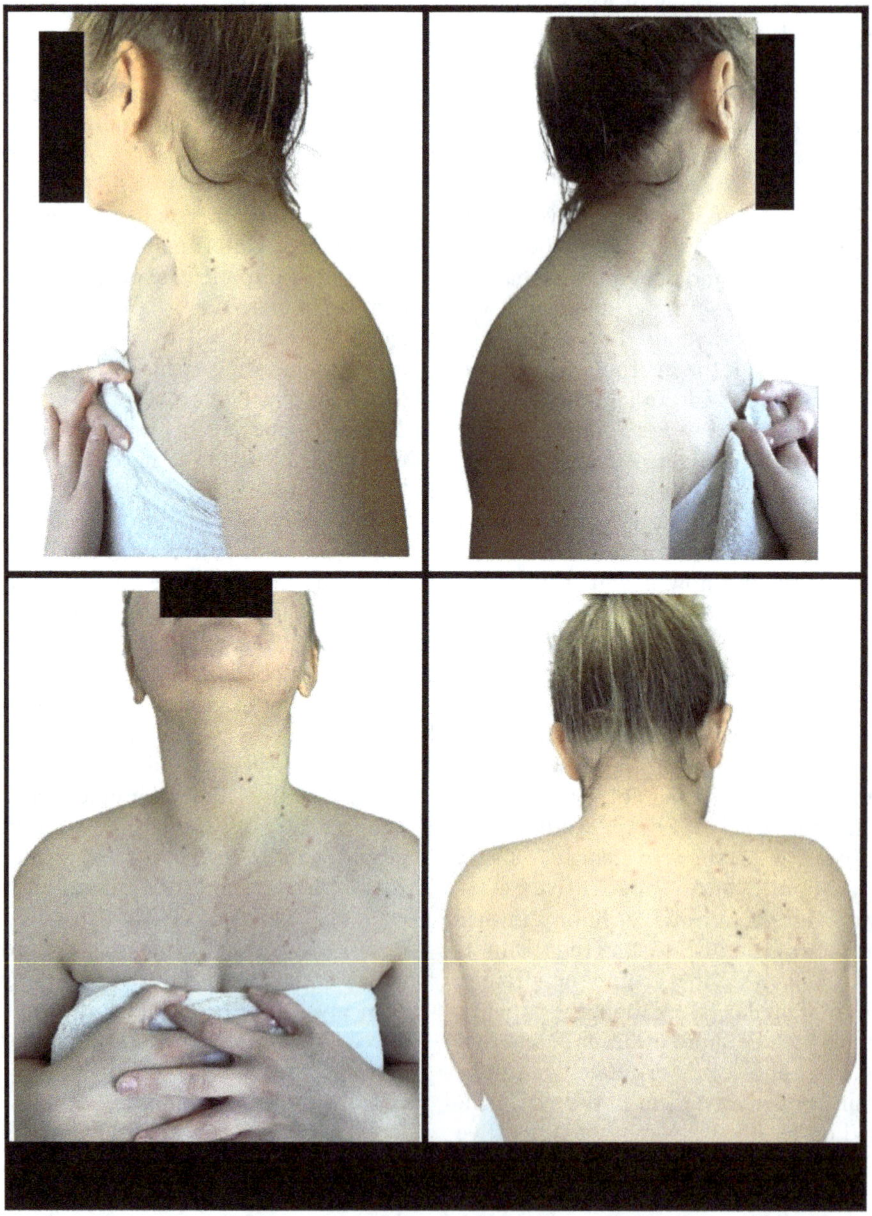

FIGURE 2: Montage of images portraying the extent of zoster dissemination and progression on April 22, despite having started oral valacyclovir the night prior during her emergency-room visit.

References

[1] T. D. Barbour, M. C. Pickering, and H. Terence Cook, "Dense deposit disease and C3 glomerulopathy," *Seminars in Nephrology*, vol. 33, no. 6, pp. 493–507, 2013.

[2] Genetic and Rare Diseases Information Center, *Dense Deposit Disease*, Genetic and Rare Diseases Information Center, Gaithersburg, MD, USA, 2014, https://rarediseases.info.nih.gov/diseases/8555/dense-deposit-disease.

[3] M. C. Braun, D. M. Stablein, L. A. Hamiwka, L. Bell, S. M. Bartosh, and C. F. Strife, "Recurrence of membranoproliferative glomerulonephritis type II in renal allografts: the north American pediatric renal transplant cooperative study experience," *Journal of the American Society of Nephrology*, vol. 16, no. 7, pp. 2225–2233, 2005.

[4] K. Hardinger and D. C. Brennan, *Kidney Transplantation in Adults: Maintenance Immunosuppressive Therapy*, UpToDate, Waltham, MA, USA, 2020, http://www.uptodate.com/contents/kidney-transplantation-in-adults-maintenance-immunosuppressive-therapy?search=kidney+transplant.

[5] L. A. Riesenberg, "Shift-to-shift handoff research: where do we go from here?" *Journal of Graduate Medical Education*, vol. 4, no. 1, pp. 4–8, 2012.

[6] J. S. Dummer and G. G. Miller, "Herpes simplex and varicella zoster viruses: forgotten but not gone," *American Journal of Transplantation*, vol. 7, no. 4, pp. 741–747, 2007.

[7] T. Jethwa, R. A. O. Bertasi, L. Kieneker, S. Pattanaik, and G. Pujalte, "Bullous disseminated herpes zoster: an atypical presentation," *Cureus*, vol. 12, no. 7, p. e9293, 2020.

[8] J. W. Gnann Jr., "Antiviral therapy of varicella-zoster virus infections," *Human Herpesviruses: Biology, Therapy, and Immunoprophylaxis*, US National Library of Medicine, Bethesda, MD, USA, 1970.

[9] Y. Furuto, M. Kawamura, A. Namikawa, H. Takahashi, and Y. Shibuya, "Successful management of visceral disseminated varicella zoster virus infection during treatment of membranous nephropathy: a case report," *BMC Infectious Diseases*, vol. 19, no. 1, p. 625, 1970.

[10] S. R. Jain and D. Kumar, "Vaccination for the post-kidney transplant population," *Current Opinion in Nephrology and Hypertension*, vol. 28, no. 6, pp. 581–586, 2019.

23

Listeria monocytogenes Peritonitis in a Patient Receiving Continuous Ambulatory Peritoneal Dialysis: A Case Report and Review of the Literature

Ho-Kwan Sin[1] **Au Cheuk,**[2] **William Lee,**[2] **Ka-Fai Yim,**[2] **Clara Poon,**[2] **Ivy Wong,**[2] **Bosco Lam,**[2] **Hon-Lok Tang,**[2] **and Samuel K. Fung**[2]

[1]*Kwong Wah Hospital, Hong Kong*
[2]*Princess Margaret Hospital, Hong Kong*

Correspondence should be addressed to Ho-Kwan Sin; kenhksin@gmail.com

Academic Editor: Yoshihide Fujigaki

Listeria monocytogenes is a rare cause of peritoneal dialysis-related peritonitis. Only a handful of cases have been reported, and the optimal management is still uncertain. We present a case of *Listeria monocytogenes* peritonitis and perform a review of the literature to elucidate optimal antibiotic therapy.

1. Introduction

Listeria monocytogenes is a Gram-positive bacillus that causes self-limiting disease in healthy subjects [1]. Risk factors for invasive infection include immunocompromised states, old age, malignancy, liver cirrhosis, pregnancy, diabetes mellitus, and alcoholism [2]. Rarely, *Listeria monocytogenes* can cause peritoneal dialysis- (PD-) related peritonitis. Optimal management of *Listeria* peritonitis in PD patients is uncertain.

2. Case Report

We present a case of a 49-year-old male patient with end-stage renal disease due to lupus nephritis who had undergone continuous ambulatory PD for 1 year, without previous episodes of peritonitis. He had concomitant ischemic heart disease and was taking prednisolone 10 mg daily and aspirin 80 mg daily. His dialysis prescription was three 2 L exchanges of 2.5% dextrose bags per day with a calcium concentration of 3.5 mEq/L (Ultrabag, Baxter International Inc.). He achieved an average weekly KT/V of over 1.7, and peritoneal equilibration testing showed that he was a "high" transporter. He produced 500 ml of urine a day. He presented to us in August 2015 with fever, abdominal pain, and turbid dialysis effluent. Physical examination revealed a blood pressure of 140/80 mmHg and a pulse rate of 90 beats/minute. His body surface area was 1.61 square meters. The abdomen was diffusely tender. The exit site was clean and healthy-looking.

Blood work on admission was unremarkable for liver function, electrolytes, and blood counts. Microscopic examination of the effluent revealed more than 1000 leucocytes/mm^3 (our laboratory did not give absolute values for counts over 1000), predominantly neutrophils (90%). Gram staining of the effluent did not reveal organisms. Blood culture was negative.

Empirical cefazolin (1 g/2 L dialysate loading and then 250 mg/2 L dialysate three times per day) and gentamicin (40 mg/2 L dialysate daily) were given via the intraperitoneal (IP) route. Owing to a lack of clinical response on as late as the third day of admission, empirical IP vancomycin (2 g/2 L dialysate, or 35 mg/kg body weight/2 L dialysate, once weekly), IP ceftazidime (1 g/2 L dialysate loading and then 250 mg/2 L dialysate three times per day), and IP amikacin (120 mg/2 L dialysate, or 2 mg/kg/2 L dialysate, once daily) were given to achieve broader antimicrobial coverage. In addition, fungal prophylaxis was given in the form of oral

TABLE 1: Nineteen reported cases of CAPD-related peritonitis caused by *Listeria monocytogenes.*

Year	Presenting symptoms	Immunocompromise/ details (if any)	Antibiotic therapy	Duration of treatment	Outcome	References
1983	Abdominal pain	Immune thrombocytopenic purpura	IV and IP erythromycin and IV trimethoprim/ sulphamethoxazole	Unknown	Resolution	[3]
1989	Abdominal pain	SLE on prednisolone and azathioprine	Ampicillin and gentamicin (route unknown)	4 weeks	Resolution	[4]
1989	Abdominal pain	SLE	Vancomycin (route unknown) and then IV ampicillin	N/A	Resolution (vancomycin failure)	[5]
1990	Abdominal pain	Wegener's granulomatosis on cyclophosphamide 25 mg daily	IP ampicillin and oral pivampicillin	3 weeks	Resolution	[6]
1991	Abdominal pain and fever	Chronic lymphocytic leukaemia on prednisolone	Oral amoxicillin and IV gentamicin	4 weeks	Resolution (vancomycin failure)	[7]
1991	Abdominal pain	Cirrhosis	Ampicillin (route unknown)	Unknown	Resolution (vancomycin failure)	[8]
1992	Abdominal pain, diarrhea, and nausea	History of kidney transplantation	IV tobramycin and IP ampicillin	2 weeks	Resolution	[9]
1994	Abdominal pain	Polymyositis	IP ampicillin and gentamicin	N/A	Resolution (vancomycin failure)	[10]
2002	Abdominal pain and nausea	SLE	IP cephalosporins and ampicillin	3 weeks	Resolution	[11]
2003	Septic shock	SLE on prednisolone 5 mg daily and azathioprine 50 mg daily	IV ampicillin and amikacin	4 weeks	Resolution	[12]
2008	Abdominal pain, cloudy effluent, and fever	Congestive heart failure	Vancomycin and netilmicin	N/A	Resolution of peritonitis but death from heart failure (after prolonged therapy)	[13]
2011	N/A	Hypertension	IV amoxicillin	N/A	Resolution	[14]
2011	N/A	Chronic glomerulonephritis	IP amoxicillin	N/A	Resolution	[14]
2011	N/A	Congestive heart failure	Vancomycin and cetazidime and IP gentamycin	N/A	Resolution (vancomycin failure)	[15]
2016	Abdominal pain, fever, nausea, and vomiting	Intake of Faroese salmon	Oral amoxicillin and IP vancomycin	Amoxicillin for 2 weeks and vancomycin for 3 weeks	Resolution	[16]
2016	Septic shock	Congestive heart failure	IP ampicillin and gentamicin	N/A	Resolution	[17]
2017	Abdominal pain, diarrhea, anorexia, and fatigue	HIV	IP ampicillin	2 weeks	Resolution	[18]
2017	Fever, cloudy effluent, and meningitis	Diabetes mellitus	Failure to respond to IP vancomycin and ceftazidime and trimethoprim-sulphamethoxazole	N/A	Vancomycin failure and death	[19]
2017	Septic shock	Chronic glomerulonephritis, alcoholic cirrhosis; intake of goat curd	IP vancomycin and amikacin	N/A	Vancomycin failure and death	[20]

CAPD, continuous ambulatory peritoneal dialysis; IV, intravenous; IP, intraperitoneal; SLE, systemic lupus erythematosus; HIV, Human Immunodeficiency Virus.

nystatin syrup at a dose of 500,000 units four times a day. Vancomycin levels were not checked. Clinical remission was achieved two days later as evidenced by clearing of the effluent and the disappearance of leucocytes on microscopy. Later, effluent bacterial culture came back with *Listeria monocytogenes*, for which the minimum inhibitory concentration of penicillin was 0.5 μg/ml. Our microbiology laboratory reported susceptibility to only penicillin for *Listeria* strains.

Accordingly, the antibiotic regime was changed to IP ampicillin (250 mg/2 L dialysate three times per day) and amikacin for 4 weeks despite clinical resolution at the time of starting IP ampicillin.

3. Discussion

Peritoneal dialysis-related peritonitis caused by *Listeria monocytogenes* is rare. To date, only 19 cases have been reported (Table 1) [3–20]. A high index of suspicion is required for timely diagnosis, especially in patients who are immunocompromised or have other risk factors [2]. As regards to treatment for *Listeria* infections in general, ampicillin is considered first-line therapy [21]. Trimethoprim/sulphamethoxazole can be considered if contraindications to ampicillin exist, such as allergies [3, 22]. Adding an aminoglycoside can enhance bacterial clearance because ampicillin alone is bacteriostatic [23]. Cephalosporins are generally ineffective [24]. While vancomycin is effective against Gram-positive bacteria, its limited ability to penetrate the eukaryote cell membrane makes it ineffectual against intracellular bacteria, such as *Listeria* species. Indeed, vancomycin failure in the context of *Listeria monocytogenes* PD-related peritonitis has been widely reported: In 6 of the reported cases where vancomycin was part of the primary regime, the only case that ended in resolution used amoxicillin as well. Vancomycin failed to clear the infection in the remaining 5 cases, even when used in combination with an aminoglycoside, a cephalosporin, or trimethoprim-sulphamethozazole (Table 1). On the other hand, the reported cases are strongly in favour of ampicillin/amoxicillin as either primary or salvage therapy: intraperitoneal ampicillin/amoxicillin with or without an aminoglycoside resulted in cure in 7 of the reported cases. Oral or intravenous ampicillin or amoxicillin resulted in cure in 5 cases. It is for the abovementioned reasons that we substituted ceftazidime and vancomycin with ampicillin while keeping the amikacin despite clinical resolution of the peritonitis following therapy with vancomycin, ceftazidime, and amikacin.

There is some concern regarding the use of ampicillin through the intraperitoneal route, as some authors have shown that ampicillin has little in vitro antibacterial activity against Enterococci when added to common peritoneal dialysates [25]. In another study, Szeto et al. showed that oral amoxicillin could effectively treat Enterococcal PD-related peritonitis [26]. Whether this holds true for *Listeria monocytogenes* peritonitis remains to be proven.

In conclusion, *Listeria monocytogenes* PD-related peritonitis should be treated with an ampicillin- or amoxicillin-based regime with or without the addition of an aminoglycoside. While the majority of reported cases used the intraperitoneal route of administration, it is as yet uncertain whether oral or intravenous administration of ampicillin or amoxicillin might be an equal or better alternative.

References

[1] V. Ramaswamy, V. M. Cresence, J. S. Rejitha et al., "Listeria—review of epidemiology and pathogenesis," *Journal of Microbiology, Immunology and Infection*, vol. 40, no. 1, pp. 4–13, 2007.

[2] C. Charlier, É. Perrodeau, A. Leclercq et al., "Clinical features and prognostic factors of listeriosis: the MONALISA national prospective cohort study," *The Lancet Infectious Diseases*, vol. 17, no. 5, pp. 510–519, 2017.

[3] J. P. Myers, G. Peterson, and A. Rashid, "Peritonitis due to Listeria monocytogenes complicating continuous ambulatory peritoneal dialysis," *Journal of Infectious Diseases*, vol. 148, no. 6, p. 1130, 1983.

[4] A. Korzets, M. Andrews, A. Campbel, J. Feehally, J. Walls, and M. Prentice, "Listeria monocytogenes peritonitis complicating CAPD," *Peritoneal Dialysis International: Journal of the International Society for Peritoneal Dialysis*, vol. 9, no. 4, p. 351, 1989.

[5] J. M. Allais, S. J. Cavalieri, M. H. Bierman, and R. B. Clark, "Listeria monocytogenes peritonitis in a patient on continuous ambulatory peritoneal dialysis," *The Nebraska Medical Journal*, vol. 74, no. 10, pp. 303–305, 1989.

[6] W. I. Al-Wali, R. Baillod, J. M. Hamilton-Miller, M. S. Kyi, and W. Brumfitt, "Listeria monocytogenes peritonitis during continuous ambulatory peritoneal dialysis (CAPD)," *Postgraduate Medical Journal*, vol. 66, no. 773, p. 252, 1990.

[7] M. S. Dryden, N. F. Jones, and I. Phillips, "Vancomycin therapy failure in Listeria monocytogenes peritonitis in a patient on continuous ambulatory peritoneal dialysis," *Journal of Infectious Diseases*, vol. 164, no. 6, p. 1239, 1991.

[8] K. A. Hart, E. A. Reiss-Levy, and P. A. Trew, "Listeria monocytogenes peritonitis associated with CAPD," *Medical Journal of Australia*, vol. 154, no. 1, pp. 59-60, 1991.

[9] N. M. Lunde, J. M. Messana, and R. D. Swartz, "Unusual causes of peritonitis in patients undergoing continuous peritoneal dialysis with emphasis on Listeria monocytogenes," *Journal of the American Society of Nephrology: JASN*, vol. 3, no. 5, pp. 1092–1097, 1992.

[10] C. Banerji, D. C. Wheeler, and J. R. Morgan, "Listeria monocytogenes CAPD peritonitis: failure of vancomycin therapy," *Journal of Antimicrobial Chemotherapy*, vol. 33, no. 2, pp. 374-375, 1994.

[11] M. Ahmad, A. Krishnan, E. Kelman, V. Allen, and J. M. Bargman, "Listeria monocytogenes peritonitis in a patient on peritoneal dialysis: a case report and review of the literature," *International Urology and Nephrology*, vol. 40, no. 3, pp. 815–819, 2008.

[12] K. C. Tse, F. K. Li, T. M. Chan, and K. N. Lai, "Listeria monocytogenes peritonitis complicated by septic shock in a patient on continuous ambulatory peritoneal dialysis," *Clinical Nephrology*, vol. 60, no. 1, pp. 61-62, 2003.

[13] K. Stylianou, A. Passam, A. Papoutsakis, K. Perakis, N. Kroustalakis, and E. Daphnis, "Listeria monocytogenes peritonitis in a peritoneal dialysis patient with severe heart failure," *Kidney*, vol. 17, no. 5, pp. 238–240, 2008.

[14] M. Bierhoff, E. Krutwagen, E. F. van Bommel, and C. A Verburgh, "Listeria peritonitis in patients on peritoneal

dialysis: two cases and a review of the literature," *The Netherlands Journal of Medicine*, vol. 69, no. 10, pp. 461–464, 2011.

[15] O. Benjelloum, J. E. Sánchez Álvarez, C. Rodríguez Suárez et al., "Listeria monocytogenes: an infrequent cause of peritonitis in peritoneal dialysis," *Nefrologia*, vol. 31, no. 3, pp. 362–365, 2011.

[16] H. B. Poulsen, T. A. Steig, J. T. Björkman, and S. Gaini, "Peritonitis with Listeria monocytogenes in a patient on automated peritoneal dialysis," *BMJ Case Reports*, vol. 2018, 2018.

[17] A. Moscovici, M. Kogan, I. Kliers, O. Kukuy, and G. Segal, "Listeria peritonitis in a patient treated with peritoneal dialysis," *The Israel Medical Association Journal: IMAJ*, vol. 18, no. 2, pp. 129-130, 2016.

[18] C. Sia, S. Wilson, M. Ananda-Rajah, J. Mills, and A. K. Aung, "Listeria monocytogenes peritonitis in an HIV-infected patient," *Clinical Nephrology*, vol. 87, no. 5, pp. 267–270, 2017.

[19] W. Beckerleg, V. Keskar, and J. Karpinski, "Peritonitis as the first presentation of disseminated listeriosis in a patient on peritoneal dialysis-a case report," *Peritoneal Dialysis International: Journal of the International Society for Peritoneal Dialysis*, vol. 37, no. 2, pp. 239-240, 2017.

[20] M. Mitrović, P. Đurić, A. Janković et al., "Unusual Listeria monocytogenes peritonitis in peritoneal dialysis patient with liver cirrhosis: a case report and review of literature," *CEN Case Reports*, vol. 6, no. 1, pp. 115–117, 2017.

[21] E. M. Jones and A. P. MacGowan, "Antimicrobial chemotherapy of human infection due to Listeria monocytogenes," *European Journal of Clinical Microbiology & Infectious Diseases*, vol. 14, no. 3, pp. 165–175, 1995.

[22] P. G. Spitzer, S. M. Hammer, and A. W. Karchmer, "Treatment of Listeria monocytogenes infection with trimethoprim-sulfamethoxazole: case report and review of the literature," *Clinical Infectious Diseases*, vol. 8, no. 3, pp. 427–430, 1986.

[23] P. H. Azimi, K. Koranyi, and K. D. Lindsey, "Listeria monocytogenes: synergistic effects of ampicillin and gentamicin," *American Journal of Clinical Pathology*, vol. 72, no. 6, pp. 974–977, 1979.

[24] A. Krawczyk-Balska and Z. Markiewicz, "The intrinsic cephalosporin resistome of Listeria monocytogenes in the context of stress response, gene regulation, pathogenesis and therapeutics," *Journal of Applied Microbiology*, vol. 120, no. 2, pp. 251–265, 2016.

[25] M. Kussmann, L. Schuster, M. Zeitlinger et al., "The influence of different peritoneal dialysis fluids on the in vitro activity of ampicillin, daptomycin, and linezolid against Enterococcus faecalis," *European Journal of Clinical Microbiology & Infectious Diseases*, vol. 34, no. 11, pp. 2257–2263, 2015.

[26] C. C. Szeto, J. K.-C. Ng, K. M. Chow et al., "Treatment of enterococcal peritonitis in peritoneal dialysis patients by oral amoxicillin or intra-peritoneal vancomcyin: a retrospective study," *Kidney and Blood Pressure Research*, vol. 42, no. 5, pp. 837–843, 2017.

24

Renal Tubular Acidosis in the Postpartum Period: A Case Report and Literature Review

Carlos E. Duran,[1] Mayra Estacio,[2] Fredy Lozano,[3] Esteban Echeverri,[4] Maria Juliana Riascos,[4] Juan Guillermo Posada,[1] and Johanna Schweineberg[1]

[1]*Department of Nephrology, Fundacion Valle del Lili, Cali, Colombia*
[2]*Health Sciences Faculty, Universidad CES, Cali, Colombia*
[3]*Health Sciences Faculty, Universidad del Valle, Cali, Colombia*
[4]*Health Sciences Faculty, Universidad ICESI, Cali, Colombia*

Correspondence should be addressed to Mayra Estacio; mayraestacio1@gmail.com

Academic Editor: Yoshihide Fujigaki

Case Presentation. Distal renal tubular acidosis (dRTA) is characterized by impaired hydrogen ion secretion in the distal nephron resulting either from decreased net activity of the proton pump or from increased luminal membrane hydrogen ion permeability. Typical complications of dRTA include severe hypokalemia, normal anion gap metabolic acidosis, nephrolithiasis, and nephrocalcinosis. The patient is a 25-year-old woman in immediate puerperium with hypokalemia leading to paralysis, and the laboratory findings in this patients were concerning for dRTA. It is rare to encounter this entity during pregnancy, and the impact of this pathology is unknown.

1. Case Presentation

A 25-year-old woman in immediate puerperium was admitted to the hospital with proximal weakness that has been increasing progressively until difficulty in mobility and subsequent prostration that occurs seven hours after cesarean.

There were no personal or family history diseases, current medications include ferrous sulfate, and she denied alcohol or recreational drugs. She had one previous pregnancy without complication. This pregnancy was normal, and a cesarean section was performed at 37 weeks for pelvic dystocia.

On physical examination, she was alert and oriented, and her vital signs were normal in the neurological examination with findings of proximal weakness, without alteration in the tendon reflexes and findings of alteration in long tracts or focal neurologic deficit.

Initial laboratory showed normal blood cell counts, severe hypokalemia (potassium, 1.91 mEq/L), and pH of 7.24, bicarbonate at 7.7 mmol/L with normal plasma anion gap (anion GAP: 12, 5 mEq/L) Table 1.

Urine studies showed urinalysis was normal with a pH of 6.5, without urine active sediment. Urinary K: Cr 83.7 mEq/g, urinary anion gap: 24 mmol/L, and urinary osmolar gap is positive Table 2.

Serologic testing was negative for autoimmune causes.

A renal ultrasound revealed normal-sized kidneys with marked increase in the echogenicity in the region of the renal pyramids bilaterally and symmetric consistent with nephrocalcinosis.

Treatment: She received potassium chloride initial by the peripheral vein, and 6 hours after admission, his serum potassium level increased to 2.1 mEq/L with improvement of weakness.

2. Discussion

The findings in this patients were concerning for dRTA complicated with severe symptomatic hypokalemia. Distal

Table 1: Laboratory findings on admission.

Parameter	Result	Reference range
Sodium, mmol/L	146.3	136–145
Potassium, mmol/L	1.9	2.5–5.1
Chloride, mmol/L	128.6	98–107
BUN, mg/dL	8.9	6–20
Creatinine, mg/dL	1.2	0.5–0.95
Calcium ionized, mmol/L	1.43	1.15–1.33
Phosphorus, mg/dL	2.44	2.5–4.5
Magnesium, mg/dL	1.78	1.59–2.56
Arterial blood gas		
pH	7.249	7.35–7.45
PCO2, mm Hg	17.9	35–45
PO2, mm Hg	189.1	83–108
Bicarbonate, mEq/L	7.7	21–28
Osmalality, mOsm/kgH20	313	275–300

Table 2: Urine studies.

Parameter	Result
Spot urine chemistry	
Osmolality, mOsm/kg H20	325
Sodium, mmol/L	113.5
Potassium, mmol/L	17.59
Chloride, mmol/L	106.3
Creatinine, mg/dL	21.13
Urea nitrogen, mg/dL	169.30
24-hour urine chemistry	
Volume, mL/24 h	4244
Sodium, mEq/24 h	447.74
Potassium, mEq/24 h	80.51
Chloride, mEq/24 h	451.14
Calcium, mg/24 h	273.74
Magnesium, mg/24 h	87.4

RTA, also known as type 1 RTA, is characterized by impaired hydrogen ion secretion in the distal nephron for a decreased net activity of the proton pump or increased hydrogen ion permeability of the luminal membrane [1].

The distal renal tubular acidosis should be considered in any patient with an otherwise unexplained normal anion gap metabolic acidosis and hypokalemia. The potassium wasting is generated by the reduction in distal hydrogen ion secretion via several mechanisms such as increase in aldosterone levels due to sodium wasting, as well as metabolic acidosis [1, 2].

This pathology can be associated with nephrocalcinosis, urinary calculi, citraturia, calciuria, osteopenia, osteomalacia, and secondary hyperparathyroidism. It can be seen in the context of immunologic diseases such as Sjögren, systemic lupus erythematosus and rheumatoid arthritis, medications (ifosfamide, amphotericin B, lithium carbonate, and ibuprofen), hypercalciuric conditions (hyperparathyroidism, vitamin D intoxication, and sarcoidosis), and others, including familial causes (medullary sponge kidney and Wilson's disease) [1, 2].

During pregnancy, there are alterations in the way the kidney manages solutes and filtration of solutes looking for an optimal environment for fetal development. The glomerular filtration rate (GFR) increases about 40–50% by week 9 [3]. There is an increase in the urea excretion and, in some cases, variable glycosuria due to a diminished glucose-absorption capacity in the distal tubule. Additionally, low-grade-level proteinuria that generally will not exceed 300 mg/24h is observed [3]. There is also a change in the osmostat, which leads to a decrease in the normal osmolality to 270 mOsm/kg, at which level the secretion of antidiuretic hormone would start, with a concomitant reduction of sodium level of around 4 to 5 mEq/L in normal pregnancy.

Pregnancy is a vasodilated state with an important grade of water retention which also contributes to the plasma sodium reduction [3]. Additionally, in most pregnancies, the rate of potassium excretion is constant with changes in tubular reabsorption that adapt to the GFR [3]. This is accompanied by a physiological compensated respiratory alkalosis due to hyperventilation which is asymptomatic, but poses a disadvantage if metabolic acidosis ensues [4].

The presence of hypokalemia in pregnancy is unusual. There are reported cases of severe hypokalemia in pregnancy associated with renal tubular acidosis in patients with a diagnosis before the pregnancy [5–7]. The impact of dRTA for the mother and child is unknown. The physiological changes in pregnancy could worsen dRTA, and it is believed that due to the increase in GFR during pregnancy, this can lead to an increase of electrolyte loss in urine, including potassium. Women without tubular alterations should be capable of dealing with the increased demand for potassium absorption in the distal tubule. Yet, if symptomatic or asymptomatic alterations exist, the state of increased renal and metabolic demand can overcome the renal potassium absorption renal capacity and lead to an increased kaliuresis and concomitant symptomatic hypokalemia [8]. Additionally, the potassium loss can be understood as a compensatory mechanism for the metabolic acidosis generated by the renal distal tubular acidosis [8].

All cases of hypokalemia in pregnant patients and during the puerperium should be investigated making emphasis in the acid-base balance, the renin/aldosterone axis, and in identifying renal or extrarenal potassium losses. Additionally, the use of certain medications such as steroids, diuretics, insulins, and beta-agonists should be discarded [9]. There are also reports of renal proximal tubular acidosis during pregnancy associated with toluene intoxication due to inhalants abuse, so drug use must always be questioned [5].

Distal tubular acidosis in pregnancy is rare. In some cases, the acid-base and potassium status during follow-up will normalize [5], so it is important to obtain serial potassium and blood gas measurements to determine their behavior in this patient. Generally, these patients are treated with bicarbonate supplementation, potassium citrate, and education for an increased awareness of the delicate and unstable balance of acid-base and potassium homeostasis in people living with renal tubular acidosis.

References

[1] R. Mustaqeem and A. Arif, *Renal Tubular Acidosis*, StatPearls

Publishing, Treasure Island, FL, USA, 2020, http://www.ncbi.nlm.nih.gov/pubmed/30085586.

[2] M. Soleimani and A. Rastegar, "Pathophysiology of renal tubular acidosis: core curriculum 2016," *American Journal of Kidney Diseases*, vol. 68, no. 3, pp. 488–498, 2016.

[3] K. L. Cheung and R. A. Lafayette, "Renal physiology of pregnancy," *Advances in Chronic Kidney Disease*, vol. 20, no. 3, pp. 209–214, 2013.

[4] V. Lim, A. Katz, and M. Lindheimer, "Acid-base regulation in pregnancy," *American Journal of Physiology-Legacy Content*, vol. 231, no. 6, pp. 1764–1769, 1976.

[5] D. Narcisse, M. Agarwal, and A. Kumar, "A rare case of transient proximal renal tubular acidosis in pregnancy," *Case Reports in Nephrology*, vol. 2017, Article ID 1342135, 4 pages, 2017.

[6] H. Seeger, P. Salfeld, R. Eisel, C. A. Wagner, and N. Mohebbi, "Complicated pregnancies in inherited distal renal tubular acidosis: importance of acid-base balance," *Journal of Nephrology*, vol. 3, 2017.

[7] O. Fikri Benbrahim, F. Cazalla Cadenas, A. Valentín Martín, and E. D. Valladares Molleda, "Acidosis tubular renal distal en una gestante de siete semanas: diagnóstico, complicaciones y tratamiento," *Nefrologia*, vol. 31, no. 6, pp. 761–763, 2011.

[8] C. J. Firmin, T. F. Kruger, and R. Davids, "Proximal renal tubular acidosis in pregnancy: a case report and literature review," *Gynecologic and Obstetric Investigation*, vol. 63, no. 1, pp. 39–44, 2007.

[9] M. Kulkarni, T. V. Srividya, and N. Gopal, "Hypokalemia paraplegia in pregnancy," *Journal of Clinical Diagnostic Research*, vol. 8, no. 6, pp. 13-14, 2014.

25

Treatment of Severe Tumoral Calcinosis with Teriparatide in a Dialysis Patient after Total Parathyroidectomy

Ho-Kwan Sin, Ping-Nam Wong, Kin-Yee Lo, Man-Wai Lo, Shuk-Fan Chan, Kwok-Chi Lo, Yuk-Yi Wong, Lo-Yi Ho, Wing-Tung Kwok, Kai-Chun Chan, Andrew Kui-Man Wong, and Siu-Ka Mak

Department of Medicine and Geriatrics, Kwong Wah Hospital, 25 Waterloo Road, Kowloon, Hong Kong

Correspondence should be addressed to Ho-Kwan Sin; kenhksin@gmail.com

Academic Editor: Hern n Trimarchi

Tumoral calcinosis is a rare but debilitating condition that can affect dialysis patients. Optimal management is largely unknown. We report the clinical course, treatment, and outcome of a peritoneal dialysis (PD) patient who developed tumoral calcinosis refractory to conventional treatment but improved with teriparatide therapy. A 26-year-old lady on PD for 2 years presented to us with tumoral calcinosis involving bilateral hands. Response to surgical excision, parathyroidectomy, and conversion to hemodialysis failed to result in sustained remission, and tumoral calcinosis progressed. After total parathyroidectomy, the patient had transient but partial remission in which her calcinosis deposits remained but were asymptomatic without pain or clinical signs of inflammation. However, she later experienced a relapse with involvement of the left elbow, right shoulder, right hip, and right thigh. Tumoral calcinosis remained uncontrolled resulting in debilitation, likely attributable to poor calcium and phosphate control because of adynamic bone disease after parathyroidectomy despite treatment of superimposed tuberculosis and therapy with sodium thiosulphate and pamidronic acid. Clinical improvement was however evident after the use of teriparatide. Asymptomatic hypocalcemia occurred after teriparatide therapy but resolved after 2 months. In conclusion, teriparatide appears to be useful for treating tumoral calcinosis in the presence of adynamic bone disease. Hypocalcemia can occur in the initial months of therapy.

1. Introduction

Tumoral calcinosis is a rare but debilitating condition that can affect dialysis patients. It is characterized by the deposition of calcium phosphate crystals in the soft tissue and periarticular areas leading to complications such as rupture, infection, and systemic inflammation [1–11]. Treatment is guided by limited evidence but involves restoration of calcium and phosphate balance by an assortment of measures that include intensification of dialysis [2–5, 10], cessation of calcium-based phosphate binders and vitamin D analogues [4, 10], use of non-calcium phosphate binders [1–5, 10], low dialysate calcium [3, 4, 10], use of cinacalcet [6], and parathyroidectomy [6, 11]. Peritoneal dialysis (PD) patients may benefit from a switch to hemodialysis [2]. The use of sodium thiosulphate (STS) and bisphosphonates has been reported [7, 9].

2. Case Report

A 26-year-old Chinese lady with end-stage renal failure (ESRD) of unknown cause presented to us in February 2009 with multiple subcutaneous nodules involving the left wrist, left little finger, and right thumb. She had been on continuous ambulatory peritoneal dialysis (CAPD) for 2 years. Her medical history was significant for gout and chronic hepatitis B infection. She had significant hyperphosphatemia and was taking oral calcium carbonate 2 g twice daily as a phosphate binder (Table 1). Radiographs showed calcified soft tissue deposits in periarticular areas of the hands. Magnetic resonance imaging showed T2-inhomogeneous hyperintense calcified deposits around the left wrist joint (Figure 1). The nodules were excised, and histological examination revealed amorphous calcified material deposited

Table 1: Medications and biochemical values at different time points.

	At diagnosis	Before parathyroidectomy	After parathyroidectomy	Recurrence of tumoral calcinosis	Persistent hypercalcemia	After teriparatide therapy
iPTH (pmol/L)	27.3	64.9	0.3	0.3	0.3	0.3
Calcium (mmol/L)	2.46	2.66	2.44	3.88	2.73	1.62
Phosphate (mmol/L)	4.0	2.8	2.3	2.0	1.8	2.2
ALP (IU/L)	92	103	91	144	152	52
Weekly KT/V from CAPD	2.0	2.4	2.4	2.4	N/A	N/A

iPTH, intact parathyroid hormone; ALP, alkaline phosphatase; CAPD, continuous ambulatory peritoneal dialysis. Calcium is corrected for serum albumin level.

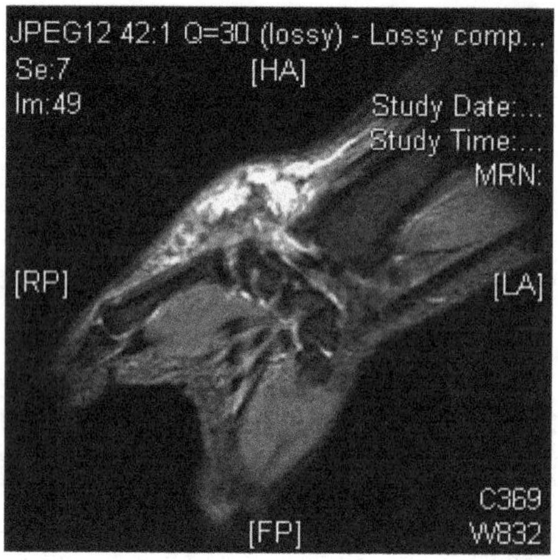

Figure 1: Magnetic resonance imaging (T2-weighted) of the left wrist.

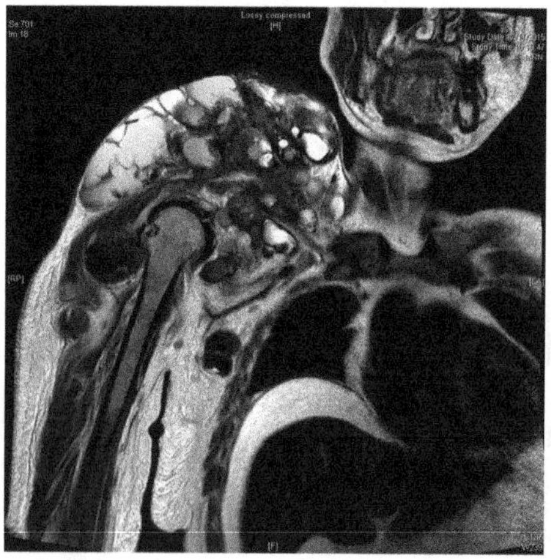

Figure 2: Magnetic resonance imaging (T2-weighted) of the right shoulder.

in the fibroadipose tissue with surrounding granulomata consistent with tumoral calcinosis. Lanthanum 500 mg thrice daily was given in place of calcium carbonate to lower phosphate, and the CAPD regime was intensified, but tumoral calcinosis persisted over the ensuing months requiring further surgical excision. In view of uncontrolled tumoral calcinosis in the face of worsening secondary hyperparathyroidism (SHPT) (Table 1), she underwent total parathyroidectomy without reimplantation in December 2011 and became largely asymptomatic save for the presence of the tumoral deposits. The parathyroid glands, 4 in total, weighed 0.99 g altogether. Three years later, she had recurrence of tumoral calcinosis, with extensive involvement of the right shoulder (Figure 2), right thigh, and right hip

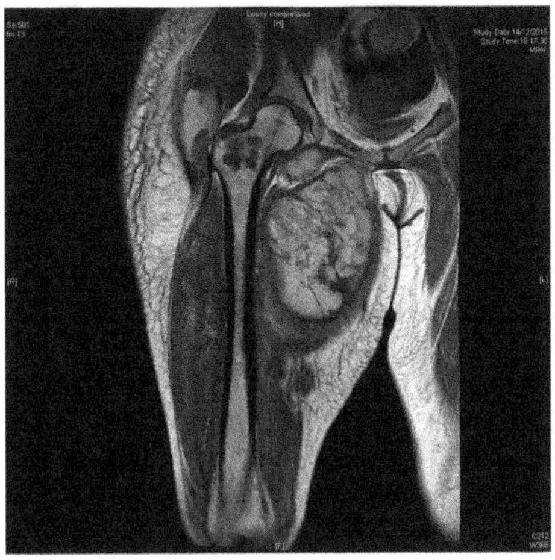

FIGURE 3: Magnetic resonance imaging (T2-weighted) of the right hip.

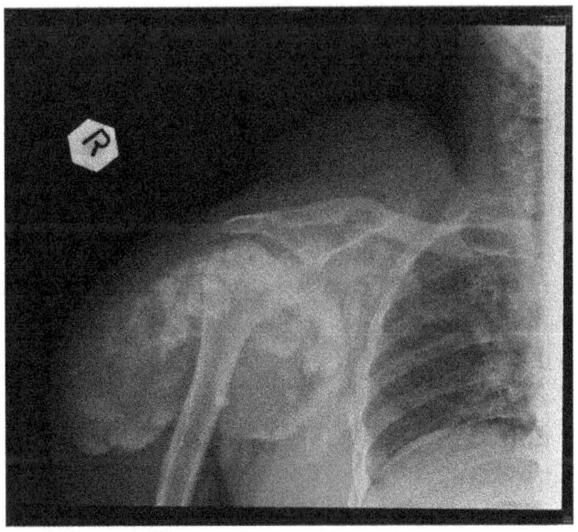

FIGURE 4: Radiograph of the right shoulder before teriparatide therapy.

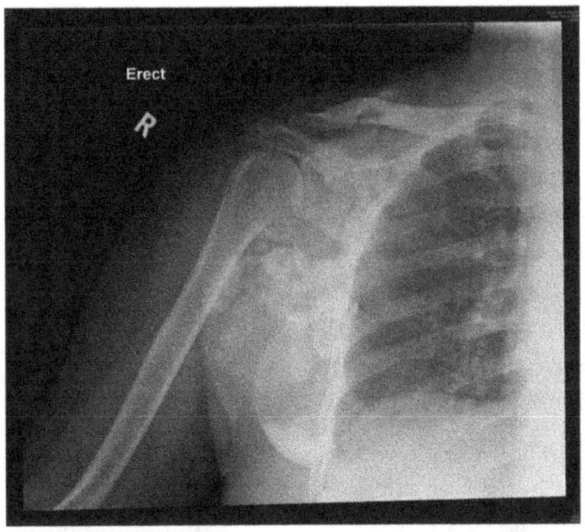

FIGURE 5: Radiograph of the right shoulder 1 year after teriparatide therapy.

(Figure 3). Despite sodium thiosulphate given at a dose of 25 g thrice weekly via the intraperitoneal route and the cessation of calcium carbonate and alfacalcidol, clinical response was absent. One 30 mg dose of pamidronic acid was then given intravenously to no effect. The huge right shoulder mass, which subsequently became infected and ruptured, revealing chalky calcified material within, was excised with histological confirmation of tumoral calcinosis. She was systemically upset at the time with anorexia, weight loss, and pyrexia. Serum calcium level was also exceedingly high up to 3.88 mol/L. Culture of the postoperative surgical drain fluid yielded *Mycobacterium tuberculosis*. A full course of antituberculosis therapy was then given which resolved her febrile response, but the tumoral calcinosis did not clear.

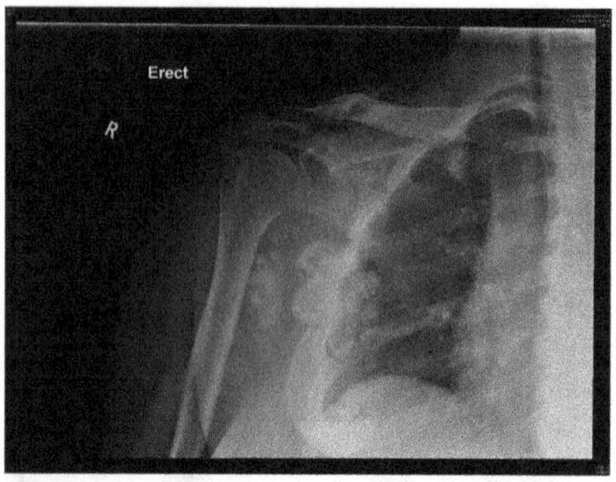

Figure 6: Radiograph of the right shoulder 2 years after teriparatide therapy.

We changed the patient over from CAPD to thrice weekly in-centre hemodialysis (HD) to enhance phosphate clearance, but the tumoral calcinosis worsened over the next year. There was also persistent hypercalcemia (serum Ca 2.73 mmol/L) in the face of low parathyroid hormone levels (iPTH 0.3 pmol/L), normal levels of parathyroid hormone-related protein (PTHrp), and 1,25-hydroxyvitamin D and the absence of paraproteinemia (Table 1). Finally, in view of the likely presence of adynamic bone disease related to antecedent total parathyroidectomy and poor response to the aforementioned efforts to lower calcium and phosphate, teriparatide was given at a dose of 20 micrograms subcutaneously every other day starting January 2017. Since the commencement of teriparatide, there had been progressive reduction in size of the tumoral deposits over the following 2 years, and the patient remained asymptomatic (Figures 4–6). Asymptomatic hypocalcemia with serum calcium dropping to 1.62 mmol/L developed (Table 1) but responded well to the use of oral calcium carbonate and a reduction of teriparatide to 20 micrograms thrice weekly with normalization of serum calcium without ongoing need for calcium carbonate supplementation 2 months later.

3. Discussion

We presented a case of refractory tumoral calcinosis developing in a PD patient. The case was difficult to tackle as we had exhausted all conventional therapeutic measures aimed at restoring calcium and phosphate balance. Parathyroidectomy was performed to address worsening SHPT which led to only transient and partial respite. While hypercalcemia and the local inflammation in association with superimposed tuberculous infection of the shoulder lesions might have aggravated the progression of calcified deposits during the first relapse after total parathyroidectomy, the persistent and otherwise unexplained hypercalcemia after the treatment of tuberculous infection was most likely due to the presence of adynamic bone disease, given the low PTH and normal serum 1,25-hydroxyvitamin D levels. Even though a bone biopsy was not performed, we endeavored to exclude secondary causes of hypercalcemia such as multiple myeloma and malignancy. In retrospect, bone metabolism markers and measurement of bone density would have been informative of status of bone turnover, but these were not available at our centre. Our decision to embark on teriparatide therapy was based on a recent report of its use in the treatment of hypercalcemia associated with ABD [12]. There was clinically significant regression of tumoral calcinosis after teriparatide therapy. Severe but asymptomatic hypocalcemia persisted for about 2 months into therapy but responded to oral calcium carbonate. We hypothesize that the intermittent administration of teriparatide increased bone turnover and formation and allowed extraosseous calcium to redistribute back into the skeleton, causing transient hypocalcemia before a new equilibrium occurred. This case report also raises the question of whether parathyroid tissue should be routinely reimplanted at the time of total parathyroidectomy, a procedure that is variably performed across centers.

In conclusion, teriparatide appears to be useful for treating tumoral calcinosis in the presence of adynamic bone disease. Hypocalcemia can occur in the initial months of therapy. More studies are needed regarding the effectiveness and safety of this drug in treating tumoral calcinosis.

Consent

Informed consent was obtained from all individual participants included in the study.

References

[1] D. L. Raja, T. Podymow, and P. Barre, "Tumoral calcinosis in a peritoneal dialysis patient," *Kidney International*, vol. 70, p. 1887, 2006.

[2] M. C. Kai, C. S. Cheuk, and Y. M. Wang, "Uraemic tumoral calcinosis," *Nephrology Dialysis Transplantation*, vol. 19, pp. 505-506, 2004.

[3] P. Binnani, V. Aggarwal, M. Bahadur, and N. Fulara, "*Tumoral calcinosis* (Teutschlander disease) in a dialysis patient," *Indian Journal of Nephrology*, vol. 18, no. 3, pp. 122–124, 2008.

[4] G. Jones, E. Kingdon, P. Sweny, and A. Davenport, "Tumoral calcinosis and calciphylaxis presenting in a dialysis patient," *Nephrology Dialysis Transplantation*, vol. 18, no. 12, pp. 2668–2670, 2003.

[5] S. Takashima, T. Sakamoto, and M. Ota, "Tumoral calcinosis in chronic renal failure," *The Lancet Diabetes & Endocrinology*, vol. 2, no. 10, p. 852, 2014.

[6] J. Floege, "When man turns to stone: extraosseous calcifica-

tion in uremic patients," *Kidney International*, vol. 65, no. 6, pp. 2447–2462, 2004.

[7] K. Mysore, R. Rommel, and M. Tom, "Tumoral calcinosis associated with pyrexia and systemic inflammatory response in hemodialysis patients: successful treatment using intravenous pamidronate," *Nephrology Dialysis Transplantation*, vol. 15, pp. 1691–1693, 2000.

[8] D. McGregor, J. Burn, K. Lynn, and R Robson, "Rapid resolution of tumoral calcinosis after renal transplantation," *Clinical Nephrology*, vol. 51, no. 1, pp. 54–58, 1999.

[9] J. T. Papakadis, A. Patrikarea, G. E. Digenis et al., "Sodium thiosulphate in the treatment of tumoral calcifications in a hemodialysis patient without hyperparathyroidism," *Nephrology Dialysis Transplantation*, vol. 72, pp. 308–312, 1996.

[10] Y. Kim, E. Hwang, and S. Park, "Resolution of uremic tumoral calcinosis in a patient on peritoneal dialysis with long-term low-calcium dialysate treatment," *Kidney Research and Clinical Practice*, vol. 33, no. 4, pp. 226–228, 2014.

[11] H.-Y. Chu, P. Chu, Y.-F. Lin, H.-K. Chou, and S.-H. Lin, "Uremic tumoral calcinosis in patients on peritoneal dialysis: clinical, radiologic, and laboratory features," *Peritoneal Dialysis International: Journal of the International Society for Peritoneal Dialysis*, vol. 31, no. 4, pp. 430–439, 2011.

[12] J. Peugh, A. Khalil, M. R. Chan et al., "Teriparatide treatment for hypercalcemia a ssociated with adynamic bone disease," *Journal of Bone and Mineral Research*, vol. 3, no. 7, Article ID e10176, 2019.

Spontaneous Retroperitoneal Bleeding as a Complication of Unusual Renal Paraganglioma

Tawfeeq I. Sangey,[1] **Hamim Abdul Rusheke**,[2] **Ansaar I. Sangey**,[3] **Nimishkumar Chaya**,[4] **and Advera Ngaiza**[3]

[1]*TMJ Super Specialized Polyclinic, Dar Es Salaam, Tanzania*
[2]*School of Medicine and Dentistry, University of Dodoma, Dodoma, Tanzania*
[3]*Muhimbili National Hospital, Dar Es Salaam, Tanzania*
[4]*TMJ Hospital, Dar Es Salaam, Tanzania*

Correspondence should be addressed to Tawfeeq I. Sangey; sangeytawfeeq@gmail.com

Academic Editor: David Mudge

Spontaneous retroperitoneal bleeding is a rare occurrence that might have catastrophic implications. We present a 58-year-old male with a 4-day history of progressively worsening left-sided flank pain due to retroperitoneal hemorrhage from a non-functional renal paraganglioma. Abdominal contrast CT scan was helpful in locating the tumor, estimating tumor size and extent of bleeding, visualizing the interaction between the tumor and the surroundings, and ruling out any potential metastasis; however, it lacked specificity in identifying the origin of the mass, needing histologic investigation for a conclusive diagnosis. MRI was not available at our center. We report a rare case of spontaneous retroperitoneal bleeding as a complication of an unusual non-functional renal paraganglioma, which was initially misdiagnosed as renal cell carcinoma but later confirmed by postoperative histopathology.

1. Introduction

Extra-adrenal autonomic paragangliomas are rare neuroendocrine tumors that develop from the paraganglia. These are tiny organs made up primarily of neuroendocrine cells generated from the embryonic neural crest that can release catecholamines [1]. Paragangliomas are closely related to pheochromocytomas, and their incident rate is about 0.6 cases per 100,000 person-years [2, 3]. In 2017, the World Health Organization described the term "paraganglioma" for extra-adrenal tumors, while the term "pheochromocytoma" was restricted to adrenal origin [4]. Histologic findings are insufficient to distinguish these two tumor types; anatomical location is employed to do so [5]. The majority of paragangliomas are nonhypersecretory and are found in the head and neck as compared to the abdominal ones [6]. The kidney, bladder, and mediastinum are among the common intra-abdominal sites [7–9]. Based on the ability of catecholamine secretion, paragangliomas can be classified as functional or nonfunctional [6, 10]. Functioning tumors present with myriad symptoms such as hypertension, headaches, diaphoresis, palpitations, and tremor [6]. Intra-abdominal paragangliomas have been linked to catecholamine hypersecretion and have been found to have the classical triad of symptoms and hypertension, as well as being benign tumors [6, 11]. However, with the increasing use of high-resolution imaging techniques in the past decades more incidentalomas have been detected, but they lack specificity due to their variable imaging appearance; surgical resection may be the only way to reach a diagnosis. Histopathology and immunohistochemistry of the excised tumor are used to make the final diagnosis [12, 13].

Spontaneous retroperitoneal hemorrhage is a well-known but uncommon condition characterized by retroperitoneal bleeding without a prior history of trauma. It may strike fast and quietly, with catastrophic consequences if not diagnosed and treated on time. Clinically, it presents with acute abdominal pain, mainly in the affected flank, palpable mass, and hypovolemic shock in severe blood loss [14]. Spontaneous retroperitoneal hemorrhage from the kidney is a rare entity. The most common renal cause is angiomyolipoma and renal cell carcinoma [15, 16]. Hemorrhagic renal paraganglioma is an extremely rare entity, and to the best of our knowledge, it has not been previously reported.

2. Case Report

A 58-year-old man presented to the emergency department complaining of left-side abdominal pain for four days. The pain began suddenly and moved to the left groin and testes. However, it was only associated with constipation through passing flatus. There was no history of vomiting, sweating, palpitation, or hematuria. There was no past medical history of hypertension or diabetes.

On examination, the patient was pale (anemic), had no pedal oedema, and had normal blood pressure of 120/70 mm/Hg. There were distended abdomen and tenderness at the left hypochondrium, left lumbar fossa, and suprapubic region.

Hematology parameters were as follows: HB, 6.0 g/dl (13.0–18.0); leukocytes, 16.47 (4.0-12.0); platelets, 170 × 10(9) (150–450); ESR, 38 mm/hr [1–45]; creatinine, 143 umol/l (62–106); eGFR, 46 ml/min; sodium, 132 mmol/l (136–145); potassium, 4.3 mmol/l (3.5–5.1); and stool for *H. pylori*, negative; stool occult blood test, negative; and urine analysis, no detection of erythrocytes.

On radiological examination, ultrasound showed a left renal complex lesion that is predominantly solid with some cystic components seen at the left upper renal pole. It demonstrated mild internal vascularity on the Doppler study.

Subsequent computed tomography (CT) of abdomen and pelvis showed an exophytic upper pole cortical mass (red arrowhead) in the left kidney (red arrow) measuring 7 × 4.5 × 7.3 cm in transverse, anterior-posterior, and craniocaudal diameter, respectively (Figure 1). On contrast study, the mass was characterized by heterogeneous enhancement with solid and cystic components. An axial image showed an ill-defined margin between the mass and the kidney denoted by a curved yellow arrow (Figure 2). A focal rounded area of intense enhancement (green arrow) was seen on arterial phase images consistent with active low-intensity bleeding (Figure 3). On noncontrast study, no calcification was seen. There was a large retroperitoneal hematoma, which was isodense to the muscle located anterior to the left kidney (blue arrow). There was no sign of local invasion into the adjacent structure. No evidence of perirenal retroperitoneal lymph nodes or bony lesions was seen. Bilateral adrenal glands were reported as normal. A provisional diagnosis of spontaneous hematoma due to bleeding renal cell carcinoma was made.

The patient was then scheduled for surgery, which included a left nephrectomy with complete mass excision, and a total of 3.5 liters of blood and clots were removed from the peritoneum (Figure 4). The hilum was sealed, and

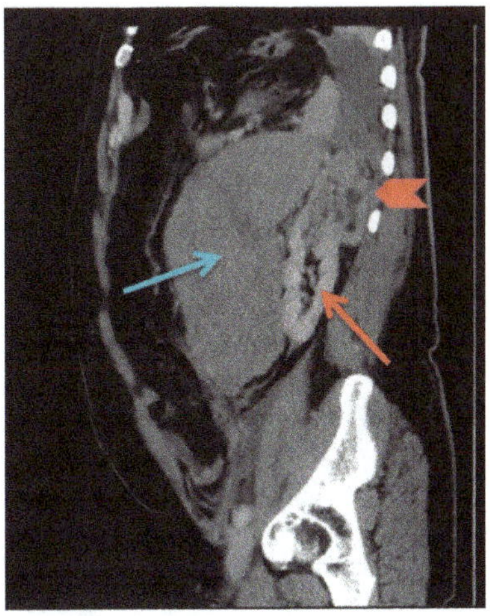

FIGURE 1: Contrast sagittal section shows a large hematoma at the left retroperitoneal region (blue arrow), the normal-appearing left kidney (thin red arrow), and an exophytic left upper pole renal mass (red arrowhead).

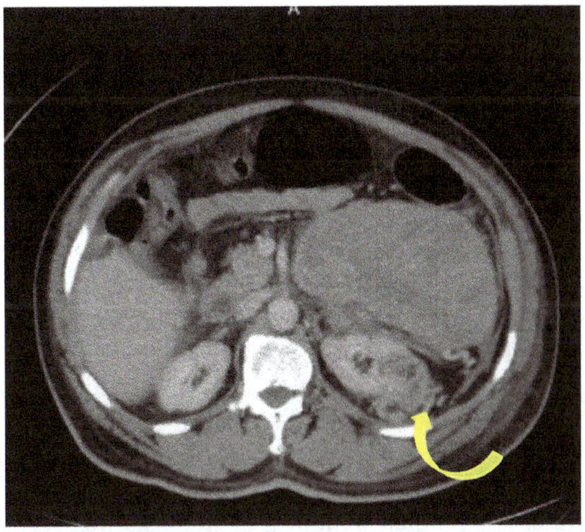

FIGURE 2: Contrast axial view section shows an ill-defined margin between the exophytic mass and the kidney (curved yellow arrow).

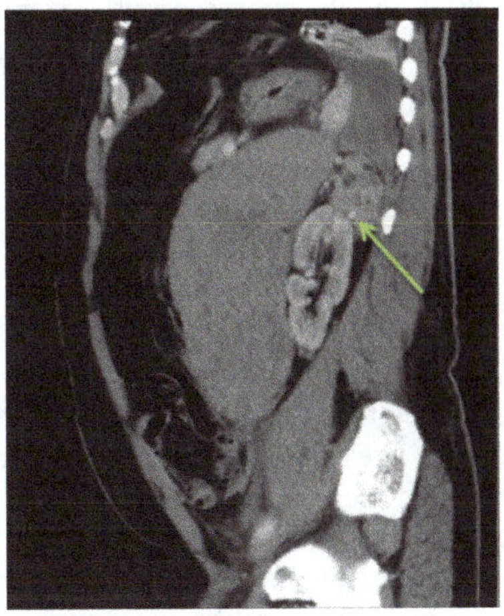

FIGURE 3: Green arrow shows a contrast extravasation consistent with active bleeding.

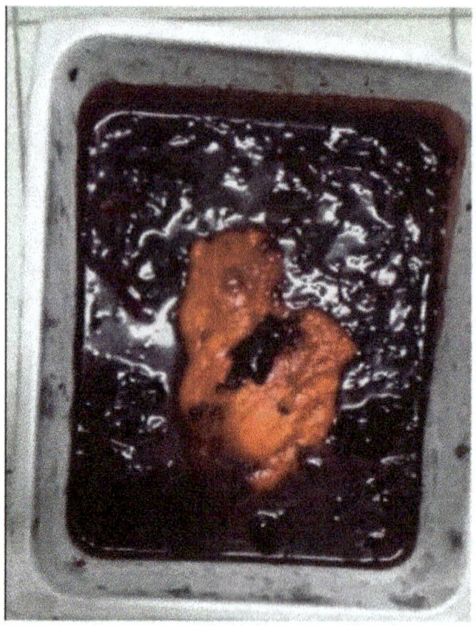

FIGURE 4: Postoperative left nephrectomy specimen with evacuated 3.5 L blood and clots.

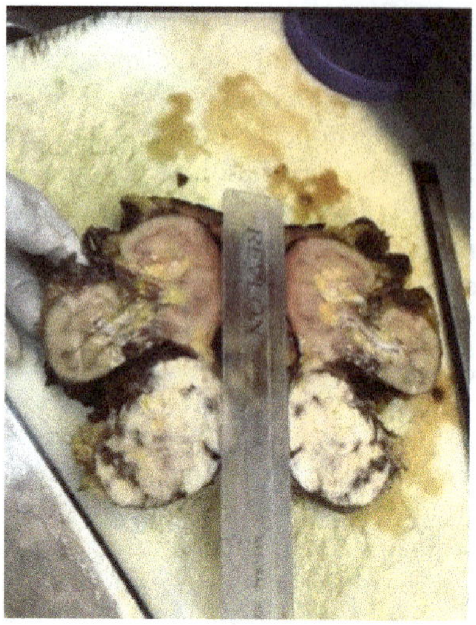

FIGURE 5: Gross anatomy specimen showing the exophytic renal cortical tumor incontinuity with the renal cortex (black arrow).

hemostasis was achieved. No intraoperative complication occurred. The excised mass was then sent for histopathologic evaluation. The patient was discharged after 3 days of stay in hospital without any postoperative complications. Gross anatomy specimen is kidney with attached tumor size of 7 cm (Figure 5). Tumor had a bright white tissue (about half) and a dirty pinkish white tissue (other half).

Histology: on low magnification, the left side shows normal-looking renal tubules and the right side shows the fatty tissue with round blue cells consistent with tumor cells (Figure 6). On high magnification, proliferating round cells with central nuclei are found. Septa separate them into vague groups and vague gland-like formations (nesting and trabecular pattern). Tumor cells had round-to-oval nuclei with abundant granular cytoplasm. Mitotic figures were not seen. Pericapsular fat shows round blue tumor cells. Cellularity is moderate. No cellular spindling or necrosis was seen (Figure 7). Ki67 activity was less than 1%. A diagnosis of pheochromocytoma was found on a conventional HE stain. PASS score was 6/21 (benign or low-grade malignant behaviour possible). A stronger scoring system (GAPP) is required to determine malignant potential, which mostly requires a combination of histologic, somatic molecular, and clinical data (urinary metanephrine/nonmetanephrine levels); the later was unfortunately not performed in our case.

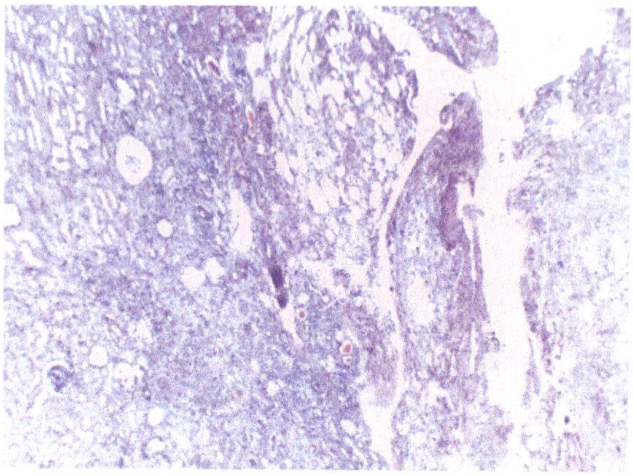

FIGURE 6: On low magnification, the left side shows normal-looking renal tubules and the right side shows the fatty tissue with round blue cells consistent with tumor cells.

3. Discussion

Paragangliomas/pheochromocytoma are rare neuroendocrine tumors arising from chromaffin cell tumors located at any extra-adrenal site along the sympathetic or parasympathetic nervous system and account for 15 to 20% of chromaffin cell tumors [1, 8]. The incidence of extra-adrenal paragangliomas is estimated to be 2–8 per million individuals and has been significantly increasing over the past two decades [17]. They can occur at any age ranging from 16 to 84 years at the time of diagnosis though they are commonly found in young adults with a median age of 30–43

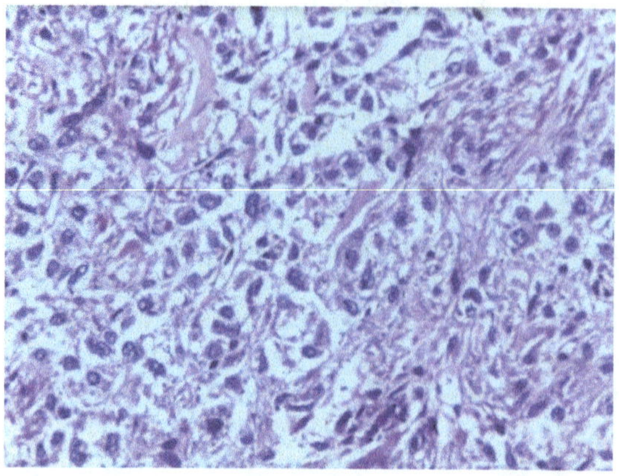

FIGURE 7: On high magnification, remarkable cellularity, granular cytoplasm, and central or slightly eccentric nuclei are observed. There are no abnormal mitosis and mild nuclear pleomorphism.

years and frequently in female patients [18, 19]. At least 30% of the patients have been shown to have certain hereditary cancer-predisposing disorders, such as multiple endocrine neoplasia, neurofibromatosis type 1, or von Hippel–Lindau syndrome [20].

Retroperitoneal extra-adrenal paragangliomas make up the majority of extra-adrenal paragangliomas, accounting for 85% of all extra-adrenal paragangliomas [21]. The renal pelvis (4.9%) is the third most common site of paragangliomas in the genitourinary tract, after the bladder (79.2%) and urethra (12.7%) [22]. Kidney paragangliomas are exceedingly rare and may develop in the hilum (32%), upper pole (26%), or lower pole (42%) within the kidney [23].

Diagnosis of paraganglioma necessitates the combination of clinical symptoms, biochemical evaluation of catecholamine production by the tumor, and tumor location [6, 24]. The patients' clinical picture can be variable from asymptomatic to a dramatic life-threatening event. The classical triad consists of headache, palpitation, and diaphoresis together with hypertension, where a diagnosis of pheochromocytoma/paraganglioma should be suspected [6] The classical triad is in fact nowadays not that common; according to a study conducted by Kopetschke, the typical triad of symptoms was found in only 10% of cases. 6.1% were normotensive, while 10% were asymptomatic [25]. Hypertension has also been linked to tumors located in the renal pelvis and hilum due to renal artery stenosis caused by the local mass effect [26]. Few studies reported paraganglioma crisis with severe life-threatening complications including cardiovascular emergencies and hypovolemic shock due to severe tumor bleeding [27–29].

The biochemical diagnosis of hyperfunctional paraganglioma or adrenal pheochromocytoma is based on excessive excretion of catecholamines and their metabolites. The 24 h urinary excretion of total metanephrine and catecholamine metabolites was determined to have a sensitivity of 74% and 89.9%, respectively [6]. The Endocrine Society Clinical Guidelines Subcommittee has also established biochemical testing recommendations for the diagnosis of paraganglioma; measurements of plasma-free or urine-fractionated metanephrines should be included in the first biochemical testing for paragangliomas. Preanalytical variables that contribute to false-positive or false-negative findings should be considered [30]. A simplified flow chart explaining the grounds for a biochemical screening procedure in a clinically suspected paraganglioma is shown in Figure 8. A threefold to fourfold increase in plasma-free normetanephrine or plasma-free metanephrine over the upper limits of the adult reference intervals indicates the likely existence of paraganglioma.

As per our case, preoperative screening for catecholamines was regrettably not performed because the patient initially presented with acute abdomen and severe anemia instead of catecholamine-related symptoms and was also normotensive. In biochemically silent abdominal paragangliomas (nonfunctional), the lack of catecholamine secretion is not related to catecholamine storage or secretion mechanisms, but rather to a deficiency in catecholamine synthesis that results in a near-complete lack of releasable reserves. The problem is caused by a lack of tyrosine hydroxylase [12, 31]. And because of the absence of clinical symptoms, nonfunctional paragangliomas are frequently misdiagnosed, posing a significant diagnostic challenge [32].

Incidental discovery of nonfunctional paragangliomas has increased over the last two decades using high-resolution abdominal imaging techniques prior to the onset of symptoms. 29.4% of the 201 total study population was diagnosed incidentally to have pheochromocytoma/paraganglioma [25]. Imaging is widely used to indicate tumor location, assess regional spread or multifocality, and exclude metastasis [33]. Paragangliomas have no pathognomonic imaging characteristics and demonstrate imaging features similar to pheochromocytomas. Enhancement characteristics on MRI are similar to CT, as Paragangliomas demonstrate rapid, avid enhancement and delayed washout, but up to one-third of pheochromocytomas have overlapping washout characteristics with adrenal adenomas [34]. A cutoff CT density of less than 10 Hounsfield units (HU) provides 100% sensitivity for diagnosing an adrenal adenoma, with a relatively low specificity of 40.5% [35]. Cystic changes, necrosis, and internal calcifications are commonly described in pheochromocytoma/paragangliomas. Internal hemorrhage can sometimes be seen within the tumor. Calcifications have been described in 10–12% of cases of pheochromocytomas and are better appreciated on non-contrast CT [36]. Pheochromocytomas/paragangliomas have a significantly more spherical shape, a sharp central necrosis, and a ring sign having a high sensitivity and specificity of 80% and 95%, respectively. An unsharp necrosis was presented as poorly defined and with a blurry margin [37]. On CT, a small size paraganglioma/pheochromocytoma is often misdiagnosed as renal cell carcinoma [23, 36] as was misdiagnosed in our case.

The classical "salt-and-pepper" appearance of paragangliomas on T1- and T2-weighted images is due to the presence of punctate areas of low signal intensity corresponding to flow voids from tumor vascularity, and hyperintense signal corresponding to areas of hemorrhage in the tumor. This sign has been described more in head and neck paragangliomas than in trunk paragangliomas, and it is also neither sensitive nor specific, as it can be seen in any hypervascularized tumor, specifically angiofibromas [38].

Spontaneous rupture of nonfunctioning retroperitoneal paraganglioma is rare and quite difficult to be diagnosed initially as it presents with severe abdominal pain that mimics other acute surgical conditions [39, 40]. Our patient was also asymptomatic until the acute abdomen discomfort caused by hemorrhagic retroperitoneal paraganglioma.

Spontaneous hemorrhage induced by paraganglioma can present as an abdominal catastrophe, which tends to be lethal. In a review of literature, so far 50–53 cases have been identified with ruptured pheochromocytoma worldwide and mortality rate of 32–34% globally [41, 42]. Although the pathophysiology of spontaneous rupture of a nonfunctioning paraganglioma is unknown, it may be related to a number of factors, such as the tumor's highly vascular nature and its potential for precarious microcirculation due to high

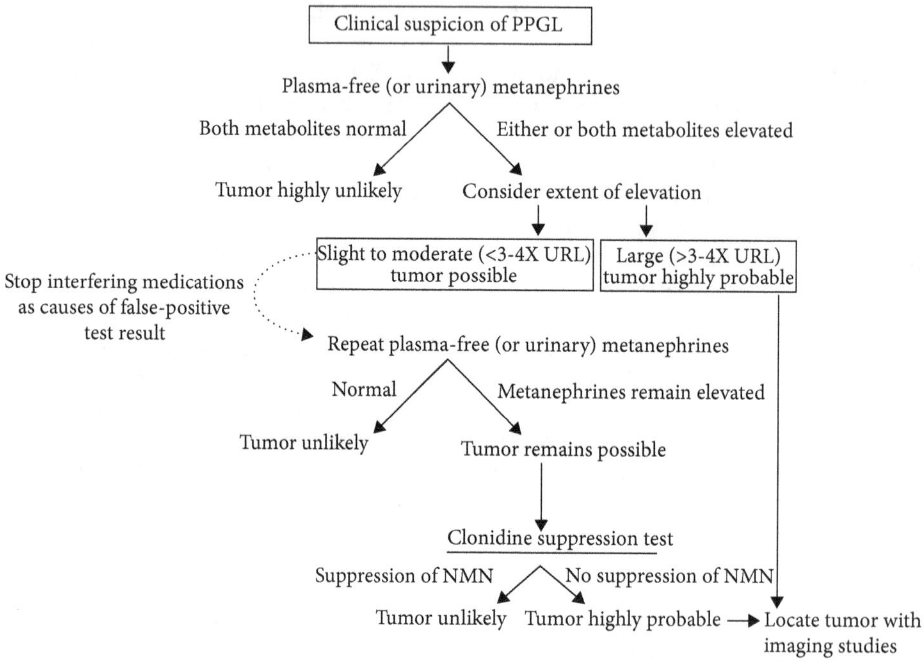

Figure 8: Flow chart illustrating the indications for the biochemical screening algorithm in a clinically suspected paraganglioma. NMN: normetanephrine. Citation: European Journal of Endocrinology 170, 3; 10.1530/EJE-13-0882.

levels of tissue vasoconstrictor substances, which could lead to spontaneously large intratumoral bleeding [43].

Histologically, paraganglioma is usually composed of solid nests known as "zellballen" of round-to-oval or elongated cells with abundant granular amphophilic or basophilic cytoplasm, within a vascular stroma, but they may also have acidophilic cytoplasm [24]. Malignant potential depends on the tumor size, level of excess catecholamine secretion, distance metastasize at time of primary tumor detection, or susceptibility to gene mutation. No cellular characteristic changes are noted in patients with a benign compared to those with a malignant tumor [42].

A concept of risk stratification is used to describe the metastatic potential of pheochromocytoma and paraganglioma [20]. Malignant pheochromocytoma has a more aggressive course than malignant paraganglioma in terms of long-term survival outcome [44] kim et al. reported 9.0% of patients with pheochromocytoma and 20.5% of those with paraganglioma developed metastatic lesions during the median 38.0 months of follow-up after primary surgical resection [45]. In 2002, Thompson designed the Pheochromocytoma of the Adrenal Gland Scaled Score (PASS) chart incorporating histologic features such as capsular or vascular invasion, mitotic rate, and necrosis [46]. Over significant possible interobserver variability, Kimura et al. introduced an alternative score chart, the Grading system for Adrenal Pheochromocytoma and Paraganglioma (GAPP), which integrates histopathologic, biochemical, and clinical data. Its scoring system is composed of six parameters that have been considered prognostic factors: histologic pattern, cellularity, comedo necrosis, capsular/vascular invasion, Ki67 labeling index, and catecholamine phenotype, with a total of 10 possible points (Table 1). A score of 0–2 is well,

Table 1: Parameters and score in the Grading system for Adrenal Pheochromocytoma and Paraganglioma (GAPP) by Noriko Kimura et al. (https://doi.org/10.3390/jcm7090242).

Parameters	Score
Histologic pattern	
Zellballen	0
Large and irregular cell nest	1
Pseudorosette (even focal)	1
Cellularity	
Low (less than 150 cells/U*)	0
Moderate (150–250 cells/U*)	1
High (more than 250 cells/U*)	2
Comedo necrosis	
Absence	0
Presence	2
Vascular or capsular invasion	
Absence	0
Presence	1
Ki67 labeling index	
Less than 1%	0
1–3%	1
More than 3%	2
Catecholamine type	
Adrenaline type (A**, or a + NA***)	0
Noradrenaline type (NA, or NA + DA****)	1
Nonfunctioning type	0
Total maximum score	10

U*: cells in the unit of 10 mm under high--power field (400); A**: adrenaline; NE***: noradrenaline; DA****: dopamine.

3–6 is moderately, and 7–10 is poorly differentiated types (Table 2). It also has an advantage of predicting metastasize and clinical prognostication [20].

Table 2: GAPP score and risk stratification by Noriko Kimura et al. (https://doi.org/10.3390/jcm7090242).

Total score (points)	Histologic grade (frequency)	Metastatic rate	5-year survival (%)	Risk stratification
0–2	Well differentiated (68%)	3.6%	100	Low
3–6	Moderately differentiated (22%)	60.0%	66.8	Intermediate
7–10	Poorly differentiated (10%)	88.2%	22.4	High

Complete surgical excision is the treatment of choice for extra-adrenal retroperitoneal paragangliomas, and recurrent or metastatic disease but should be carried out on the basis of correct drug preparation of α-receptor blocker prior to surgery [47]. In the literature, hypertension was the most common encountered as a perianesthetic risk in 31% of the 143 patients [48]; this can pose a high risk of developing intraoperative cardiac emergencies. There is also an increased risk of intraoperative massive blood loss in subjects with tumors proximal to vessels or other organs, with tumors ≥5 cm in size, or with preoperative preparation time of less than 14 days [49]. There was no intraoperative complication seen in our case study.

Furthermore, risk stratification is required to tailor the follow-up protocol after complete resection of paraganglioma. The overall rate of recurrent disease was found to be 0.98 events/100 person-years, and primary tumors larger than 5 cm have a higher risk of recurrence [50].

4. Conclusion

Retroperitoneal pheochromocytoma/paragangliomas are rare tumors that are usually benign with good prognosis. The clinical picture of the patient might range from asymptomatic to a dramatic life-threatening occurrence such as sudden acute bleeding from the tumor. Incidental discovery of the pheochromocytoma and paragangliomas on imaging is becoming an increasingly essential mode of their diagnosis. Radiological differential diagnoses are often inadequate or challenging in such cases, especially for tumors originating from kidneys. Therefore, it is important for clinicians and radiologists to be more aware of pheochromocytoma/paragangliomas and their various appearances in order to avoid potential surgical complications without further evaluation prior.

References

[1] S. G. Tevosian and H. K. Ghayee, "Pheochromocytomas and Paragangliomas," *Endocrinology and Metabolism Clinics of North America. W.B. Saunders*, vol. 48, pp. 727–750, 2019.

[2] A. M. A. Berends, E. Buitenwerf, R. R. de Krijger et al., "Incidence of pheochromocytoma and sympathetic paraganglioma in The Netherlands: a nationwide study and systematic review," *European Journal of Internal Medicine*, vol. 51, pp. 68–73, 2018.

[3] A. A. Leung, J. L. Pasieka, M. D. Hyrcza et al., "Epidemiology of pheochromocytoma and paraganglioma: population-based cohort study," *European Journal of Endocrinology*, vol. 184, no. 1, pp. 19–28, 2021.

[4] A. K. Lam, "Update on adrenal tumours in 2017 World Health Organization (WHO) of endocrine tumours," *Endocrine Pathology*, vol. 28, pp. 213–227, 2017.

[5] H. P. H. Neumann, W. F. Young, and C. Eng, "Pheochromocytoma and paraganglioma," *New England Journal of Medicine*, vol. 381, no. 6, pp. 552–565, 2019.

[6] D. Erickson, Y. C. Kudva, M. J. Ebersold, G. B. Thompson, C. S. Grant, and J. A. van Heerden, "Benign Paragangliomas: clinical presentation and treatment outcomes in 236 patients," *The Journal of Clinical Endocrinology & Metabolism*, vol. 86, 2001.

[7] L. Zhao, J. Luo, H. Zhang, and J. Da, "Pigmented paraganglioma of the kidney: a case report," *Diagnostic Pathology*, vol. 7, no. 1, p. 77, 2012.

[8] M. Song, K. Sun, T. Xia et al., "Malignant pheochromocytoma in the anterior mediastinum with sternal invasion: a case report," *Journal of Thoracic Disease*, vol. 9, no. 3, pp. E202–E209, 2017.

[9] A. Saha, K. Saha, N. Sarkar, and I. A. Geelani, "Paraganglioma of urinary bladder: an uncommon entity in uropathology," *Cureus*, vol. 13, no. 8, Article ID e17265, 2021 Aug 18.

[10] N. Aygun, *Pheochromocytoma and Paraganglioma: From Epidemiology to Clinical Findings*, SiSli Etfal Hastanesi Tip Bulteni/The Medical Bulletin of Sisli Hospital, Istanbul, Turkey, 2020.

[11] M. Al-Harthy, S. Al-Harthy, A. Al-Otieschan, S. Velagapudi, and A. S. Alzahrani, "Original Article comparison of pheochromocytomas AND abdominal AND pelvic paragangliomas with head and neck paragangliomas," *Endocrine Practice*, vol. 15, no. 194, 2009.

[12] H. Falhammar, M. Kjellman, and J. Calissendorff, "Initial clinical presentation and spectrum of pheochromocytoma: a study of 94 cases from a single center," *Endocrine Connections*, vol. 7, no. 1, pp. 186–192, 2018.

[13] R. W. Garrett, J. C. Nepute, M. E. Hayek, and S. G. Albert, "Adrenal incidentalomas: clinical controversies and modified recommendations," *American Journal of Roentgenology*, vol. 206, no. 6, pp. 1170–1178, 2016.

[14] R. D. Shah, S. Nagar, C. J. Shanley, and R. J. Janczyk, "Factors affecting the severity of spontaneous retroperitoneal hemorrhage in anticoagulated patients," *The American Journal of Surgery*, vol. 195, no. 3, pp. 410–413, 2008.

[15] O. Antonescu, M. Duhamel, B. di Giacinto, and J. Spain, "Spontaneous renal hemorrhage: a case report and clinical protocol," *Cureus*, vol. 13, no. 6, Article ID e15547, 2021.

[16] D. Durak, F. Eren, Nursel, T. İnanir, B. Eren, and S. Çetin, "Spontaneous rupture of a renal cell carcinoma associated with fatal bleeding," *Journal of Clinical Medicine Case Reports Case Reports 275 Maedica A Journal of Clinical Medicine*, vol. 9, 2014.

[17] A. Singh, "Extra-adrenal retroperitoneal paraganglioma: report of a rare case," *International Journal of Molecular Biology*, vol. 2, no. 5, 2017.

[18] S. C. FitzGerald, L. M. Gingell, C. N. Parnaby, J. M. Connell, and P. J. O'Dwyer, "Abdominal paragangliomas: analysis of

surgeon's experience," *World Journal of Endocrine Surgery*, vol. 3, no. 2, pp. 55–58, 2011.

[19] M. Hofko, B. Hergan, and F. A Fellner, "Incidental retroperitoneal paraganglioma, imaging workup and CT-guided biopsy: a case report," *Global Imaging Insights*, vol. 5, no. 2, 2020.

[20] N. Kimura, K. Takekoshi, and M. Naruse, "Risk stratification on pheochromocytoma and paraganglioma from laboratory and clinical medicine," *Journal of Clinical Medicine*, vol. 7, 2018.

[21] P. Brahmbhatt, P. Patel, A. Saleem, R. Narayan, and M. Young, "Retroperitoneal paraganglioma presenting as a chest pain: a case report," *Case Reports in Oncological Medicine*, vol. 2013, Article ID 329472, 4 pages, 2013.

[22] C. Yi, L. Han, R. Yang, and J. Yu, "Paraganglioma of the renal pelvis: a case report and review of literature," *Tumori*, vol. 103, no. 1_suppl, pp. S47–S49, 2017.

[23] L. E. Hempenstall, A. R. Siriwardana, and D. J. Desai, "Investigation of a renal mass: diagnosing renal paraganglioma," *Urology Case Reports*, vol. 21, pp. 8-9, 2018.

[24] S. L. Asa, S. Ezzat, and O. Mete, "The diagnosis and clinical significance of paragangliomas in unusual locations," *Journal of Clinical Medicine*, vol. 7, 2018.

[25] R. Kopetschke, M. Slisko, A. Kilisli et al., "Frequent incidental discovery of phaeochromocytoma: data from a German cohort of 201 phaeochromocytoma," *European Journal of Endocrinology*, vol. 161, no. 2, pp. 355–361, 2009.

[26] B. Bahar, S. E. Pambuccian, G. N. Gupta, and G. A. Barkan, "Renal paraganglioma: report of a case managed by robotic assisted laparoscopic partial nephrectomy and review of the literature," *Case Reports in Urology*, vol. 2014, Article ID 527592, 6 pages, 2014.

[27] S. Y-Hassan and H. Falhammar, "Cardiovascular manifestations and complications of pheochromocytomas and paragangliomas," *Journal of Clinical Medicine*, vol. 9, pp. 1–19, 2020.

[28] A. C. Meijs, M. Snel, and E. P. M. Corssmit, *TEACHING CASE PRESENTATIONS Pheochromocytoma/paraganglioma Crisis: Case Series from a Tertiary Referral Center for Pheochromocytomas and Paragangliomas*, 2000.

[29] B. Schifferdecker, D. Kodali, E. Hausner, and J. Aragam, "Adrenergic shock—an overlooked clinical entity?" *Cardiology in Review*, vol. 13, no. 2, pp. 69–72, 2005.

[30] J. W. M. Lenders, Q. Y. Duh, G. Eisenhofer, A. P. Gimenez-Roqueplo, S. K. G. Grebe, and M. H. Murad, "Pheochromocytoma and paraganglioma: an endocrine society clinical practice guideline," *Journal of Clinical Endocrinology and Metabolism. Endocrine Society*, vol. 99, pp. 1915–1942, 2014.

[31] H. J. L. M. Timmers, K. Pacak, T. T. Huynh et al., "Biochemically silent abdominal paragangliomas in patients with mutations in the succinate dehydrogenase subunit B gene," *The Journal of Clinical Endocrinology & Metabolism*, vol. 93, no. 12, pp. 4826–4832, 2008.

[32] E. Gannan, P. van Veenendaal, A. Scarlett, and M. Ng, "Retroperitoneal non-functioning paraganglioma: a difficult tumour to diagnose and treat," *International Journal of Surgery Case Reports*, vol. 17, pp. 133–135, 2015.

[33] R. Clifton-Bligh, "Diagnosis of silent pheochromocytoma and paraganglioma," *Expert Review of Endocrinology and Metabolism*, vol. 8, no. 1, pp. 47–57, 2013.

[34] S. Woo, C. H. Suh, S. Y. Kim, J. Y. Cho, and S. H. Kim, "Pheochromocytoma as a frequent false-positive in adrenal washout CT: a systematic review and meta-analysis," *European Radiology*, vol. 28, no. 3, pp. 1027–1036, 2018.

[35] A. H. Hamrahian, A. G. Ioachimescu, E. M. Remer et al., "Clinical utility of noncontrast computed tomography attenuation value (hounsfield units) to differentiate adrenal adenomas/hyperplasias from nonadenomas: cleveland clinic experience," *The Journal of Clinical Endocrinology & Metabolism*, vol. 90, no. 2, pp. 871–877, 2005.

[36] G. A. Motta-Ramirez, E. M. Remer, B. R. Herts, I. S. Gill, and A. H. Hamrahian, *Comparison of CT Findings in Symptomatic and Incidentally Discovered Pheochromocytomas*, https://www.ajronline.org, 2005.

[37] F. Ctvrtlik, Z. Tudos, P. Szasz et al., "Characteristic CT features of pheochromocytomas—probability model calculation tool based on a multicentric study," *Biomedical Papers*, vol. 163, no. 3, pp. 212–219, 2019.

[38] K. Y. Lee, Y. W. Oh, H. J. Noh et al., "Extraadrenal paragangliomas of the body: imaging features," *American Journal of Roentgenology*, vol. 187, no. 2, pp. 492–504, 2006.

[39] K. K. Yau, W. T. Siu, and M. Ka-Wah Li, "Unusual cause of acute abdomen-ruptured retroperitoneal paraganglioma," *Asian Journal Of Surgery*, vol. 31, 2008.

[40] Y. Yang, G. Wang, H. Lu, Y. Liu, S. Ning, and F. Luo, "Haemorrhagic retroperitoneal paraganglioma initially manifesting as acute abdomen: a rare case report and literature review," *BMC Surgery*, vol. 304, no. 1, 2020.

[41] T. Kobayashi, A. Iwai, R. Takahashi, Y. Ide, K. Nishizawa, and K. Mitsumori, "Spontaneous rupture of adrenal pheochromocytoma: review and analysis of prognostic factors," *Journal of Surgical Oncology*, vol. 90, no. 1, pp. 31–35, 2005.

[42] O. Hamidi, W. F. Young, N. M. Iñiguez-Ariza et al., "Malignant pheochromocytoma and paraganglioma: 272 patients over 55 years," *The Journal of Clinical Endocrinology & Metabolism*, vol. 102, no. 9, pp. 3296–3305, 2017.

[43] K. Suga, K. Motoyama, A. Hara, N. Kume, M. Ariga, and N. Matsunaga, "Tc-99m MIBG imaging in a huge clinically silent pheochromocytoma with cystic degeneration and massive hemorrhage," *Clinical Nuclear Medicine*, vol. 25, 2000.

[44] P. Goffredo, J. A. Sosa, and S. A. Roman, "Malignant pheochromocytoma and paraganglioma: a population level analysis of long-term survival over two decades," *Journal of Surgical Oncology*, vol. 107, no. 6, pp. 659–664, 2013.

[45] K. Y. Kim, J. H. Kim, A. R. Hong et al., "Disentangling of malignancy from benign pheochromocytomas/paragangliomas," *PLoS One*, vol. 11, no. 12, Article ID e0168413, 2016.

[46] L. D. R. Thompson, *Pheochromocytoma of the Adrenal Gland Scaled Score (PASS) to Separate Benign from Malignant Neoplasms A Clinicopathologic and Immunophenotypic Study of 100 Cases*, vol. 26, no. 5, pp. 551–566, 2002.

[47] H. Z. Li, G. Ji, Q. Mao, B. Shi, J. Wen, and W. Yan, "A decade of clinical experience with extra-adrenal paragangliomas of retroperitoneum: report of 67 cases and a literature review," *Urology Annals*, vol. 2, no. 1, p. 12, 2010.

[48] M. A. O. Kinney, M. E. Warner, J. A. Vanheerden, T. T. Horlocker, W. F. Young, and D. R. Schroeder, *Perianesthetic risks and outcomes of pheochromocytoma and paraganglioma resection Anesthesia and Analgesia*, vol. 91, 2000.

[49] H. Liu, B. Li, X. Yu, and Y. Huang, "Preoperative risk factors for massive blood loss in adrenalectomy for pheochromocytoma," 2017, https://www.impactjournals.com/oncotarget.

[50] L. Amar, C. Lussey-Lepoutre, J. W. M. Lenders, J. Djadi-Prat, P. F. Plouin, and O. Steichen, "Recurrence or new tumors after complete resection of phaeochromocytomas and paragangliomas. a systematic review and meta-analysis," *European Journal of Endocrinology*, vol. 175, no. 4, 2016.

27

The Role of Patiromer in Delaying the Onset of Renal Replacement Therapy in Patients with Advanced Renal Failure

Nand K. Wadhwa[1] **Jason A. Kline,**[2] **and Sreedhar R. Adapa**[3]

[1]*Nephrology Division, NY Health, Stony Brook, NY, USA*
[2]*Cooper Medical School of Rowan University, Camden, NJ, USA*
[3]*The Nephrology Group, Inc., Visalia, CA, USA*

Correspondence should be addressed to Nand K. Wadhwa; nwadhwa@nyhealth.com

Academic Editor: Hern N. Trimarchi

Patients with chronic kidney disease (CKD) are at an increased risk of developing hyperkalemia, which can be potentially life threatening. Hyperkalemia is frequently encountered with renin-angiotensin-aldosterone system inhibitor (RAASi) therapy use in patients with CKD and often results in the underdosing or discontinuation of these drugs. RAASi therapy has been proven to delay the progression of CKD, ameliorate proteinuria, and reduce the overall risk of cardiovascular morbidity and mortality. Patiromer is a sodium-free, potassium-binding polymer used for the treatment of hyperkalemia. We present a case series of four patients with Stage 4 or 5 CKD in whom the initiation of dialysis was delayed with the use of patiromer. For one patient, dialysis was delayed by 18 months, whereas the remaining three patients, in whom hyperkalemia was one of the main complications, remain dialysis independent to date.

1. Introduction

Patients with chronic kidney disease (CKD) are at an increased risk of developing hyperkalemia because of decreased luminal secretion of potassium (K^+) in the distal tubule [1]. Hyperkalemia is a potentially life-threatening electrolyte abnormality that can cause arrhythmias and cardiac arrest [1]. The main risk factors for developing hyperkalemia include decreased estimated glomerular filtration rate (eGFR), use of renin-angiotensin-aldosterone system inhibitors (RAASi), older age, male gender, diabetes mellitus, and metabolic acidosis [1, 2].

Treatment with RAASi has been proven to delay the progression of CKD, improve proteinuria, and decrease the overall risk of cardiovascular morbidity and mortality and is therefore recommended as a first-line treatment for hypertension in patients with CKD [3]. However, hyperkalemia is a frequent problem encountered with RAASi therapy in patients with CKD and often results in the underdosing or discontinuation of these drugs [4].

We present a case series of four patients with advanced Stage 4 or 5 CKD in which the initiation of dialysis was delayed following the use of the sodium-free potassium-binding polymer, patiromer. For one patient, initiation of dialysis was delayed by 18 months, whereas the remaining three patients are still dialysis independent. In all four patients, hyperkalemia was managed successfully with patiromer, despite the concomitant use of RAASi therapy.

2. Case Series

2.1. Patient 1. An 80-year-old woman was followed up in the outpatient nephrology clinic for the management of Stage 4 CKD and proteinuria. Other significant medical history included type 2 diabetes (T2D), hypertension, obesity, and heart failure with reduced ejection fraction (HFrEF). Her medications included irbesartan 150 mg daily, carvedilol 25 mg twice daily, torsemide 40 mg daily, and insulin. The patient's CKD and proteinuria were secondary to diabetes and had been diagnosed 5 years previously. Proteinuria was in the subnephrotic range, with a urine albumin-to-creatinine ratio (ACR) of 113–169.5 mg/mmol. She had a serum creatinine level of 221 μmol/L and an eGFR of 20–25 mL/min/1.73 m^2.

The dose of irbesartan was increased to reduce proteinuria, conserve renal function, and maximize the benefit of RAASi therapy for the management of her CHF. When irbesartan was increased to its maximum dose of 300 mg daily, K^+ levels increased from 4.5 mmol/L to 5.7 mmol/L. The K^+ level remained elevated between 5.5 mmol/L and 6.0 mmol/L on repeated testing. Patiromer 8.4 g/day was subsequently initiated, enabling the patient to continue taking the maximum dose of irbesartan (300 mg daily) without recurrence of hyperkalemia. Within a year, her urine ACR had decreased to 79.1 mg/mmol and showed further improvement, remaining around 11.3–22.6 mg/mmol.

The patient subsequently developed metastatic lung cancer and chose to spend her remaining days at home with family and under the care of home hospice services. She opted to withdraw from the management of her chronic medical conditions but remained on patiromer 8.4 g daily, with control of hyperkalemia for 3 years after the initiation of therapy. Renal function had been unchanged from the initial baseline visit when irbesartan was initially maximized, and proteinuria had remained controlled. The patient's CHF had remained stable with no HF-related hospital admissions while receiving the maximum dose of irbesartan (300 mg daily). Her serum potassium was 4.6, sodium 137 mmol/L, chloride 96 mmol/L, bicarbonate 24 mmol/L, calcium 9.3 mg/dL, phosphorus 4.3 mg/dL, and Mg 2.0 mg/dL during patiromer therapy. There were no reported complications with patiromer, such as constipation or other gastrointestinal side effects, hypokalemia, or hypomagnesemia.

2.2. Patient 2. A 70-year-old man with Stage 5 CKD due to diffuse diabetic glomerulosclerosis on kidney biopsy was referred for evaluation to assess the need to initiate peritoneal dialysis. His medical history included liver transplantation for hepatitis C–induced cirrhosis and liver cancer (managed with cyclosporine and mycophenolic acid [MPA] for immunosuppression and ledipasvir/sofosbuvir therapy for hepatitis C). Other significant medical history included nephrotic-range proteinuria, hyperkalemia, HF with preserved ejection fraction with a prior bioprosthetic aortic valve replacement, coronary artery disease with stent placement, T2D (being treated with insulin), hypertension, and gout. His medications included torsemide 100 mg once daily, metolazone 5 mg once daily, carvedilol 25 mg twice daily, cyclosporine, MPA, insulin, and allopurinol. He was clinically hypervolemic due to volume overload but was not uremic. Evaluation of laboratory parameters showed the following: serum creatinine 562.4 μmol/L, eGFR 9 mL/min/1.73 m^2, urine ACR 463.6 mg/mmol, and serum K^+ 5.0 mmol/L.

Peritoneal dialysis was not feasible because of his liver transplant. It was not possible to obtain arteriovenous (AV) fistula access because of the lack of veins in the upper extremities. It was decided to place the AV graft 2 weeks before initiating dialysis. To meet his fluid intake goals, the patient was advised to consume fruits and vegetables (4–5 servings per day) rather than only drinking water. He was also counselled to reduce his dietary intake of animal-based protein and instead consume more plant-based protein. Treatment with metolazone was discontinued, and the patient was prescribed torsemide 60 mg once daily and spironolactone 25 mg once daily (three times a week) after which his volume status improved and stabilized. The patient was also started on patiromer 8.4 g once daily (two to three times a week) in order to maintain his serum K^+ levels below 5.6 mmol/L. After clinical evaluation, he was placed on the deceased donor kidney transplant list.

Evaluation of his laboratory parameters at subsequent follow-up appointments over 18 months showed that his eGFR remained stable at 8–10 mL/min/1.73 m^2 and urine ACR decreased to 60.1 mg/mmol. Serum albumin remained between 42 and 45 g/L, whereas serum bicarbonate ranged from 20 to 23 mmol/L. Serum K^+ fluctuated between 4.7 and 5.6 mmol/L. His serum sodium 140 mmol/L, chloride 95 mmol/L, calcium 8.8 mg/dL, phosphate 4.3 mg/dL, and magnesium 2.0 mg/dL were within normal range while receiving patiromer. His liver function also remained normal, and his glycated hemoglobin (HbA_{1c}) ranged from 26.8 to 32.2 mmol/mol. After 18 months from the time he was supposed to start dialysis, he continued to remain clinically euvolemic with no signs and symptoms of uremia and was not on dialysis. There were no reports of adverse events related to patiromer. To date, he remains on the deceased donor kidney transplant list.

2.3. Patient 3. A 71-year-old man with Stage 5 CKD due to autosomal dominant polycystic kidney disease was referred for the evaluation to initiate home hemodialysis. His medical history included liver cysts, hypertension, nephrolithiasis, vitamin D deficiency, and hyperkalemia. He was on the deceased donor kidney transplant list at the time of his referral, at which time his prescribed medications included furosemide 80 mg daily, spironolactone 25 mg daily (twice a week), metoprolol succinate 50 mg daily, hydralazine 50 mg three times daily, and doxazosin 2 mg daily. He reported feeling well and had been actively pursuing his hobby of vintage car restoration, which involved frequent travel, so he questioned the need to start dialysis treatment. He was not clinically uremic and reported having a good appetite but was clinically euvolemic. Evaluation of laboratory parameters showed the following results: serum creatinine 683.5 μmol/L, eGFR 7 mL/min/1.73 m^2, and serum K^+ 5.2 mmol/L. His 24-hour urine protein was 53.9 mg/day. The left brachiocephalic AV fistula was revised to a left brachial basilic transposition due to the lack of maturation. In order to increase the likelihood of receiving a kidney transplant, his transplant status was updated to include the hepatitis C-positive deceased donor list. He was advised to increase his consumption of water to prevent further progression of kidney cysts and to reduce his sodium intake. In line with data presented in the recent Kidney Disease: Improving

Global Outcomes (KDIGO) controversies conference report [5], he was advised to decrease his intake of animal-based protein and to increase plant-based protein intake instead and also to consume more fruits and vegetables (4–5 servings a day).

The patient was started on treatment with patiromer 8.4 g once daily (2-3 times a week) to maintain his serum K^+ levels below 5.6 mmol/L. Evaluation of laboratory parameters at subsequent follow-up appointments showed that his eGFR remained between 6.5 and 7.5 mL/min/1.73 m^2, serum K^+ fluctuated between 4.9 and 5.8 mmol/L, and serum albumin remained at 43–47 g/L. His other electrolytes were serum sodium 145 mmol/L, chloride 100 mmol/L, bicarbonate 24, calcium 9.0 mg/dL, phosphate 5.7 mg/dL, and magnesium 2.3 mg/dL. His liver function remained normal. He was clinically euvolemic with no signs and symptoms of uremia and still reported having a good appetite. The patient was still not on dialysis 16 months after its proposed initiation and tolerated patiromer without adverse events. To date, he remains on the deceased donor kidney transplant list, including the hepatitis C–positive pool.

2.4. Patient 4. A 69-year-old man was followed up in the outpatient nephrology clinic for Stage 5 CKD and proteinuria. His medical history was significant for T2D, hypertension, hyperlipidemia, and diabetic neuropathy. His medications included pravastatin 20 mg daily, atenolol 50 mg daily, lisinopril 40 mg daily, gabapentin 300 mg daily, and insulin. His serum creatinine was 343.1 μmol/L with an eGFR of 15 mL/min/1.73 m^2. The patient had subnephrotic-range proteinuria with a urine ACR of 61.8 mg/mmol. Serum K^+ levels ranged from 5.3 to 6.0 mmol/L, even after repeated dietary counseling. The patient worked as a farm laborer, and his diet included predominantly fruits and vegetables, which are rich in K^+.

The patient was started on patiromer 8.4 g once daily and serum K^+ levels subsequently trended within the normal range (3.5–5.1 mmol/L). The other serum electrolytes remained within a normal range, including sodium 136 mmol/L, chloride 104 mml/L, bicarbonate 23 mmol/L, calcium 9.1 mg/dL, phosphorus 4.1 mg/dL, and magnesium 1.8 mg/dL. Proteinuria and renal function remained stable for almost 12 months, and he continued to take lisinopril 40 mg daily with no interruptions. Hyperkalemia recurred once during this period after the patient stopped taking patiromer. He received education on his medication including diet and was restarted on patiromer. No episodes of hypercalcemia noted when he was taking patiromer. Over time, his eGFR declined to 9–12 mL/min/1.72 m^2, but there was no recurrence of hyperkalemia. No gastrointestinal side effects or hypokalemia was encountered during patiromer therapy. After 18 months of follow-up, dialysis was initiated for the management of uremic symptoms.

3. Discussion

Hyperkalemia is one of the relatively common complications encountered in patients with impaired renal function. The typical Western diet contains an average daily K^+ intake of ~2600 mg [6]. The role of the kidney in maintaining K^+ homeostasis is critical [7]: it is the primary organ responsible for maintaining total body K^+ by excreting 90% of K^+ intake. The gastrointestinal tract (primarily the colon) accounts for 10% of K^+ secretion [8]. In individuals with normal kidney function, the proximal tubule and loop of Henle reabsorb 80–90% of the filtered K^+ load, and luminal secretion in the distal tubule constitutes the primary mechanism of renal K^+ excretion [1]. However, this luminal secretion of the K^+ is impaired in CKD, resulting in hyperkalemia, which can be exacerbated by RAASi treatment.

As demonstrated by the African American Study of Kidney Disease and Hypertension (AASK) trial, conducted in 1,094 nondiabetic African American patients with hypertensive CKD [9], the occurrence of hyperkalemic episodes is higher when GFR is <30 mL/min/1.73 m^2 than when GFR is >50 mL/min/1.73 m^2. In contrast to the AASK trial, a higher event rate of hyperkalemia was reported by Einhorn et al. [10] in their analysis of the United States Veterans Health study. This was due to the inclusion of patients with diabetes and of a higher proportion of elderly subjects and those with multiple comorbidities [10]. The magnitude and frequency of hyperkalemia varies depending on a multitude of factors. In particular, several studies have shown the risk of hyperkalemia increases in CKD with the use of RAASi therapy [9, 11]. Hyperkalemia can cause potentially life-threatening cardiac arrhythmias and is associated with an increased risk of major cardiovascular morbidity and mortality in various populations [12, 13].

The incidence of hyperkalemia in patients with CKD receiving dual-agent RAASi therapy is approximately 5–10%, compared with <2% in patients without CKD on RAASi monotherapy [14]. The most common approach to reduce the risk of hyperkalemia is to downtitrate the dose or discontinue the use of RAASi [4]. However, suboptimal dosing of RAASi is associated with adverse outcomes, including the increased risk of cardiac events, mortality, and earlier progression to end-stage renal disease, which in turn leads to increased health care costs [15].

Various clinical practice guidelines recommend the use of RAASi therapy in adults for the management of common comorbidities. Treatment with angiotensin-converting enzyme inhibitors (ACEi) or angiotensin II receptor blockers (ARBs) prevents the progression of CKD in both people with and without diabetes and reduces urine albumin excretion [16]. Treatment with ACEi or ARBs also improves renal outcomes in patients with hypertension and CKD [17]. Furthermore, ACEi and ARBs have been shown to reduce morbidity and mortality in patients with HFrEF and also prevent symptomatic HF [18]. Treatment with mineralocorticoid receptor antagonists (MRAs) decrease mortality and morbidity in patients with New York Heart Association (NYHA) functional Class II–IV HFrEF [18]. Given the benefits of RAASi therapy in reducing the risk of cardiovascular events and CKD progression, clinicians are commonly faced with the challenge of hyperkalemia in CKD when using RAASi.

Health benefits associated with foods enriched in K^+ are their alkalinity and fiber, micronutrient (vitamin and mineral, including K^+), and phytochemical content [19, 20]. A diet rich in K^+ reduces the risk of cardiovascular disease, stroke, nephrolithiasis, and cholesterol and improves the acid-base balance, blood pressure, and progression of chronic kidney disease, thereby reducing mortality rate [21, 22]. Patients with advanced CKD are at higher risk of developing hyperkalemia with a K^+-liberalized diet. The relationship between dietary K^+ intake and serum K^+ levels is not well established, although studies report that the restriction of dietary K^+ intake has minimal impact on reducing serum K^+ levels [4]. Recently, a KDIGO controversies conference report suggested that plant-based diets may be more suitable for patients with CKD and that they should be educated on the benefits of low-K^+ plant-based foods, particularly vegetables that can be incorporated into their diet [5]. The use of loop diuretics, either alone or in conjunction with thiazide diuretics, will aid in the urinary excretion of K^+ by increasing flow and sodium delivery to the distal nephron [14]. However, in patients with advanced CKD, diuretic therapy for the management of hyperkalemia can be inadequate [14].

Oral K^+-binding therapies can enable and facilitate the appropriate use of a K^+-rich diet and of RAASi in patients with CKD, CHF, or both. Oral K^+-binding agents like sodium polystyrene sulfonate (SPS), sodium zirconium cyclosilicate (SZC), and patiromer are approved by the United States Food and Drug Administration (FDA) for the treatment of hyperkalemia [1]. These agents work by exchanging cations for K^+ in the gastrointestinal (GI) tract, resulting in K^+ binding and the excretion of K^+ in the feces. These K^+-binding agents should not be used for emergency treatment of life-threatening hyperkalemia because of their delayed onset of action.

SPS is a sodium-K^+ exchange resin that was approved by the FDA in 1958 for the treatment of hyperkalemia [4]. However, robust clinical safety and efficacy data for SPS in hyperkalemia were lacking prior to the FDA approval. With its foul taste and consistency, and the potential risk for serious gastrointestinal injury [23], it has not been demonstrated to be an effective approach in long-term clinical studies to manage chronic hyperkalemia.

The K^+-lowering efficacy and safety profiles of the two newer K^+-binding agents, SZC and patiromer, were evaluated in phase 2 and 3 randomized controlled trials prior to their approval for use in clinical practice [4].

SZC is an inorganic, insoluble, and highly selective K^+ binder approved in the United States and European Union for the treatment of hyperkalemia in adults [24]. SZC binds K^+ and ammonium ions in GI tract in exchange for sodium and hydrogen ions, and the bound K^+ is subsequently excreted in the feces [25, 26]. Clinical studies in hyperkalemic patients have shown that most individuals treated with SZC achieve normal serum K^+ levels within 4 hours of their first 10 g dose and that normokalemia can be maintained for up to 28 days with once daily doses of 5–15 g [27, 28]. Furthermore, the tolerability profile of SZC has been shown to be comparable with that of placebo [27, 28]. Increases in serum bicarbonate have been observed during SZC treatment [25, 28], potentially due to SZC binding ammonium ions [26]. SZC should not be used as emergency treatment for life-threatening hyperkalemia because of its delayed onset of action.

Spinowitz et al. [24] evaluated the use of SZC for the control of hyperkalemia over 1 year in a study that included 746 participants with hyperkalemia, of whom the majority had an eGFR below 60 mL/min/1.73 m^2 (74%) and were receiving RAASi therapy (65%). During the 12-month maintenance phase, SZC was administered once daily dissolved in a small amount of water, taken separately from other medications by at least 2 hours. Overall, SZC was well tolerated, and common adverse events that occurred during treatment included constipation (6%), hypertension (11%), and peripheral edema (10%) [24]. In a one-year study of SZC, edema events occurred more frequently in the subgroup of patients with eGFR of <30 mL/min/1.73 m^2 compared with those with eGFR of ≥30 mL/min/1.73 m^2 (21% vs. 11%, respectively) [29]; SZC exchanges sodium for K^+, which may explain the occurrence of hypertension and edema with this medication, especially if higher doses are used. During months 3–12 of the maintenance phase, the serum K^+ level was maintained at ≤5.1 mmol/L in 88% of participants and ≤5.5 mmol/L in 99% of participants [24].

Patiromer is a sodium-free, K^+-binding polymer that exchanges calcium for K^+ in the GI tract, predominantly in the colon [2]. It is an oral suspension of spherical beads of uniform size (~100 μm) that are too large to be absorbed passively in the GI tract [30]. The drug substance consists of the active moiety, patiromer, and the calcium–sorbitol complex, the counterion that acts in K^+ exchange, resulting in the binding of K^+ and its fecal excretion [2].

Patiromer has a delayed onset of action of 4–7 hours, so it should not replace existing emergency treatments for lifethreating hyperkalemia [2]. The initial starting dose of patiromer is 8.4 g once daily, and the dose can be titrated as necessary at intervals of 1 week or longer, in increments of 8.4 g, up to a maximum dose of 25.2 g once daily [2]. No dosage adjustments are needed for patients on dialysis or with renal impairment [2]. Clinical drug–drug interaction studies of patiromer conducted in healthy volunteers showed that 9 out of 12 medications commonly used in the CKD population did not demonstrate clinically relevant drug–drug interactions when administered together with patiromer [31]. Nonetheless, it is recommended that administration of concomitant medications should occur at least 3 hours before or after administration of patiromer [31].

In the patient cases reported here, hyperkalemia treatment with patiromer was selected for several reasons. Patiromer uses calcium rather than sodium as the exchange ion, thus the risk of hypertension and edema, particularly in patients who should restrict their sodium intake or are prone to fluid overload, such as those with heart failure or hypertension, is avoided. The choice of a binder that does not contain sodium appears to be particularly important in the patient with volume overload, and the patient who is advised to restrict sodium intake.

In an exploratory analysis of phase 3 OPAL-HK study (4-week initial treatment phase of 243 patients; 8-week randomized withdrawal phase of 107 patients), patiromer was associated with a reduction in aldosterone levels independent of plasma renin activity in patients with CKD and hyperkalemia on RAAS inhibitors [32]. In addition, patiromer use was also associated with decreased systolic and diastolic blood pressure, as well as albuminuria [32]. Pharmacodynamic effects of patiromer in an animal model with chronic hyperkalemia showed a significant reduction in serum K^+ that correlated with serum aldosterone [33]. The effect of patiromer on aldosterone may be related indirectly to reduction in serum K^+ level but remains unexplained. Furthermore, the patients with CKD Stage 4 or 5 were being managed with RAAS inhibitors, either with maximally dosed ACEi or an ARB or with the mineralocorticoid receptor antagonist, spironolactone. Placebo-controlled clinical trial data suggest that treatment of hyperkalemia with patiromer may maintain RAASi therapy by reducing the risk of recurrent hyperkalemia [34] and that patiromer may prevent the development of hyperkalemia in patients initiating spironolactone, thereby allowing uptitration to optimal doses [35, 36]. More recently, the AMBER trial in patients with resistant hypertension and advanced CKD [35] showed that patiromer treatment was more effective than placebo at maintaining spironolactone treatment over 12 weeks, resulting in a statistically larger mean cumulative dose of spironolactone. A Phase-3b, multinational, double-blind, placebo-controlled, withdrawal study (DIAMOND; NCT03888066) is currently underway in HFrEF patients who develop hyperkalemia while receiving RAASi therapies, in order to evaluate the effects of patiromer compared with placebo on changes in serum K^+ levels (primary end point) and hyperkalemia events, durable enablement of MRA target dose, and hyperkalemia-related hard outcomes(key secondary end points) [37].

Finally, patiromer is an appropriate choice of treatment in the cases described here, based on its rigorous safety and tolerability profile, with data on up to 52 weeks of exposure [38]. The most common side effects with patiromer are typically related to GI, such as constipation and diarrhea [2, 39]. Because patiromer has the potential to bind magnesium in the GI tract, it is recommended that clinicians monitor magnesium in patients receiving patiromer and consider an increased dietary magnesium intake or magnesium supplementation in patients who develop low serum magnesium levels. In clinical trials, 9% of patients developed a serum magnesium level below 1.4 mg/dL, and none developed a level below 1.0 mg/dL [2]. Because patiromer uses calcium as the counterexchange ion, some of the released calcium appears to bind to intestinal phosphate. In patients with hyperphosphatemia, this binding may result in reductions in serum and urine phosphate [40]. Very rarely, cases of hypercalcemia have been reported [41]. Of note, a recent 4-year pharmacovigilance report indicates that patiromer's adverse event profile in the real-world setting is predictable and consistent with clinical trial data, with no evidence of any new safety signals to date [42].

4. Conclusion

The suboptimal dosing of RAASi secondary to hyperkalemia results in detrimental outcomes in the patients with heart failure and CKD and is associated with significant economic burden. Hyperkalemia is one of the major complications in CKD and limits complete RAAS blockade. A K^+-exchange polymer, such as patiromer, is effective in controlling hyperkalemia and maintaining normokalemia, while, at the same time, potentially maximizing the benefits of RAASi therapy and an increased consumption of a healthy plant-based diet. In the current case series, we show that patiromer was effective in controlling hyperkalemia in conjunction with dietary counselling and thereby delaying the initiation of dialysis in four patients with Stage 4 or 5 CKD. This strategy requires further study in a controlled setting.

Authors' Contributions

N.K.W., J.A.K., and S.R.A. wrote the first draft of the cases; S.R.A. wrote the first draft of the introduction and discussion; N.K.W. revised the introduction and discussion for clinical relevance and provided supporting references. All the authors reviewed and approved the final version.

References

[1] S. L. Seliger, "Hyperkalemia in patients with chronic renal failure," *Nephrology Dialysis Transplantation*, vol. 34, no. 3s, pp. iii12–iii18, 2019.

[2] H. A. Blair, "Patiromer: a review in hyperkalaemia," *Clinical Drug Investigation*, vol. 38, no. 8, pp. 785–794, 2018.

[3] Kidney Disease: Improving Global Outcomes Blood Pressure Work Group, "KDIGO 2021 clinical practice guideline for the management of blood pressure in chronic kidney disease," *Kidney International*, vol. 99, no. 3S, pp. S1–S87, 2021.

[4] B. F. Palmer, "Potassium binders for hyperkalemia in chronic kidney disease-diet, renin-angiotensin-aldosterone system inhibitor therapy, and hemodialysis," *Mayo Clinic Proceedings*, vol. 95, no. 2, pp. 339–354, 2020.

[5] C. M. Clase, J. J. Carrero, D. H. Ellison et al., "Potassium homeostasis and management of dyskalemia in kidney diseases: conclusions from a kidney disease: improving global outcomes (KDIGO) controversies conference," *Kidney International*, vol. 97, no. 1, pp. 42–61, 2020.

[6] M. E. Cogswell, Z. Zhang, A. L. Carriquiry et al., "Sodium and potassium intakes among US adults: NHANES 2003-2008," *American Journal of Clinical Nutrition*, vol. 96, no. 3, pp. 647–657, 2012.

[7] I. Lazich and G. L. Bakris, "Prediction and management of hyperkalemia across the spectrum of chronic kidney disease," *Seminars in Nephrology*, vol. 34, no. 3, pp. 333–339, 2014.

[8] B. F. Palmer, "Potassium homeostasis in chronic kidney disease," *Nephrology News & Issues*, vol. 30, no. 4, 2016.

[9] J. M. Weinberg, L. J. Appel, and G. Bakris, "Risk of hyperkalemia in nondiabetic patients with chronic kidney disease receiving antihypertensive therapy," *Archives of Internal Medicine*, vol. 169, no. 17, pp. 1587–1594, 2009.

[10] L. M. Einhorn, M. Zhan, V. D. Hsu et al., "The frequency of hyperkalemia and its significance in chronic kidney disease," *Archives of Internal Medicine*, vol. 169, no. 12, pp. 1156–1162, 2009.

[11] W. C. Winkelmayer, Z. Zhang, S. Shahinfar, M. E. Cooper, J. Avorn, and B. M. Brenner, "Efficacy and safety of angiotensin II receptor blockade in elderly patients with diabetes," *Diabetes Care*, vol. 29, no. 10, pp. 2210–2217, 2006.

[12] J. An, J. Lee, H. Jeon et al., "Severe hyperkalemia requiring hospitalization: predictors of mortality," *Critical Care*, vol. 16, no. 6, p. R225, 2012.

[13] J. Khanagavi, T. Gupta, W. S. Aronow et al., "Hyperkalemia among hospitalized patients and association between duration of hyperkalemia and outcomes," *Archives of Medical Science*, vol. 2, no. 2, pp. 251–257, 2014.

[14] C. P. Kovesdy, "Management of hyperkalaemia in chronic kidney disease," *Nature Reviews Nephrology*, vol. 10, no. 11, pp. 653–662, 2014.

[15] M. Polson, T. C. Lord, A. Kangethe et al., "Clinical and economic impact of hyperkalemia in patients with chronic kidney disease and heart failure," *Journal of managed care & specialty pharmacy*, vol. 23, pp. S2–S9, 2017.

[16] Kidney Disease: Improving Global Outcomes CKD Work Group, "KDIGO 2012 clinical practice guideline for the evaluation and management of chronic kidney disease," *Kidney International Supplements*, no. 3, pp. 1–150, 2013.

[17] P. A. James, S. Oparil, B. L. Carter et al., "2014 evidence-based guideline for the management of high blood pressure in adults," *Journal of the American Medical Association*, vol. 311, no. 5, pp. 507–520, 2014.

[18] C. W. Yancy, M. Jessup, B. Bozkurt et al., "2017 ACC/AHA/HFSA focused update of the 2013 ACCF/AHA guideline for the management of heart failure," *Journal of the American College of Cardiology*, vol. 70, no. 6, pp. 776–803, 2017.

[19] K. Kalantar-Zadeh and D. Fouque, "Nutritional management of chronic kidney disease," *New England Journal of Medicine*, vol. 377, no. 18, pp. 1765–1776, 2017.

[20] D. R. Tennant, J. Davidson, and A. J. Day, "Phytonutrient intakes in relation to European fruit and vegetable consumption patterns observed in different food surveys," *British Journal of Nutrition*, vol. 112, no. 7, pp. 1214–1225, 2014.

[21] K. J. Aaron and P. W. Sanders, "Role of dietary salt and potassium intake in cardiovascular health and disease: a review of the evidence," *Mayo Clinic Proceedings*, vol. 88, no. 9, pp. 987–995, 2013.

[22] H. J. Adrogué and N. E. Madias, "Sodium surfeit and potassium deficit: keys to the pathogenesis of hypertension," *Journal of the American Society of Hypertension*, vol. 8, no. 3, pp. 203–213, 2014.

[23] Z. Harel, S. Harel, P. S. Shah, R Wald, J Perl, and C. M Bell, "Gastrointestinal adverse events with sodium polystyrene sulfonate (Kayexalate) use: a systematic review," *The American Journal of Medicine*, vol. 126, no. 3, pp. 264–324, 2013.

[24] B. S. Spinowitz, S. Fishbane, P. E. Pergola et al., "Sodium zirconium cyclosilicate among individuals with hyperkalemia," *Clinical Journal of the American Society of Nephrology*, vol. 14, no. 6, pp. 798–809, 2019.

[25] S. R. Ash, B. Singh, P. T. Lavin, F. Stavros, and H. S. Rasmussen, "A phase 2 study on the treatment of hyperkalemia in patients with chronic kidney disease suggests that the selective potassium trap, ZS-9, is safe and efficient," *Kidney International*, vol. 88, no. 2, pp. 404–411, 2015.

[26] F. Stavros, A. Yang, A. Leon, M. Nuttall, and H. S. Rasmussen, "Characterization of structure and function of ZS-9, a K+ selective ion trap," *PLoS One*, vol. 9, no. 12, Article ID e114686, 2014.

[27] M. Kosiborod, H. S. Rasmussen, P. Lavin et al., "Effect of sodium zirconium cyclosilicate on potassium lowering for 28 Days among outpatients with hyperkalemia," *Journal of the American Medical Association*, vol. 312, no. 21, pp. 2223–2233, 2014.

[28] D. K. Packham, H. S. Rasmussen, P. T. Lavin et al., "Sodium zirconium cyclosilicate in hyperkalemia," *New England Journal of Medicine*, vol. 372, no. 3, pp. 222–231, 2015.

[29] S. D. Roger, P. T. Lavin, E. V. Lerma et al., "Long-term safety and efficacy of sodium zirconium cyclosilicate for hyperkalaemia in patients with mild/moderate versus severe/end-stage chronic kidney disease: comparative results from an open-label, phase 3 study," *Nephrology Dialysis Transplantation*, vol. 36, no. 1, pp. 137–150, 2021.

[30] L. Li, S. D. Harrison, M. J. Cope et al., "Mechanism of action and pharmacology of patiromer, a nonabsorbed cross-linked polymer that lowers serum potassium concentration in patients with hyperkalemia," *Journal of Cardiovascular Pharmacology and Therapeutics*, vol. 21, no. 5, pp. 456–465, 2016.

[31] L. J. Lesko, E. Offman, C. T. Brew et al., "Evaluation of the potential for drug interactions with patiromer in healthy volunteers," *Journal of Cardiovascular Pharmacology and Therapeutics*, vol. 22, no. 5, pp. 434–446, 2017.

[32] M. R. Weir, G. L. Bakris, C. Gross et al., "Treatment with patiromer decreases aldosterone in patients with chronic kidney disease and hyperkalemia on renin-angiotensin system inhibitors," *Kidney International*, vol. 90, no. 3, pp. 696–704, 2016.

[33] S. P. N. Iyer, L. Lee, and L. Li, "Pharmacodynamic effects of the K^+ binder patiromer in a novel chronic hyperkalemia model in spontaneously hypertensive rats," *Physiological Reports*, vol. 8, no. 18, Article ID e14572, 2020.

[34] M. R. Weir, G. L. Bakris, D. A. Bushinsky et al., "Patiromer in patients with kidney disease and hyperkalemia receiving RAAS inhibitors," *New England Journal of Medicine*, vol. 372, no. 3, pp. 211–221, 2015.

[35] R. Agarwal, P. Rossignol, A. Romero et al., "Patiromer versus placebo to enable spironolactone use in patients with resistant hypertension and chronic kidney disease (AMBER): a phase 2, randomised, double-blind, placebo-controlled trial," *The Lancet*, vol. 394, no. 10208, pp. 1540–1550, 2019.

[36] B. Pitt, S. D. Anker, D. A. Bushinsky, D. W. Kitzman, F. Zannad, and I.-Z. Huang, "Evaluation of the efficacy and safety of RLY5016, a polymeric potassium binder, in a double-blind, placebo-controlled study in patients with chronic heart failure (the PEARL-HF) trial," *European Heart Journal*, vol. 32, no. 7, pp. 820–828, 2011.

[37] "Patiromer for the management of hyperkalemia in subjects receiving RAASi medications for the treatment of heart failure (DIAMOND)," https://www.clinicaltrials.gov/ct2/show/NCT03888066.

[38] W. Ali and G. Bakris, "Evolution of patiromer use: a review," *Current Cardiology Reports*, vol. 22, no. 9, p. 94, 2020.

[39] European Medicines Agency, "Veltassa® (patiromer) summary of product characteristics," 2017, https://www.ema.europa.eu/en/documents/product-information/veltassa-epar-product-information_en.pdf.

[40] D. A. Bushinsky, D. M. Spiegel, J. Yuan, S. Warren, J. Fogli, and P. E. Pergola, "Effects of the potassium-binding polymer patiromer on markers of mineral metabolism," *Clinical Journal of the American Society of Nephrology*, vol. 14, no. 1, pp. 103–110, 2019.

[41] M. R. Wiederkehr, A. N. Mehta, and M. Emmett, "Case re-

port: patiromer-induced hypercalcemia," *Clinical Nephrology-Case Studies*, vol. 7, no. 1, pp. 51–53, 2019.

[42] P. Rossignol, L. David, C. Chan, A. Conrad, and M. R. Weir, "Safety and tolerability of the potassium binder patiromer from a global pharmacovigilance database collected over 4 Years compared with data from the clinical trial program," *Drugs-Real World Outcomes*, vol. 8, no. 3, pp. 315–323, 2021.

28

Cell-Free and Concentrated Ascites Reinfusion Therapy during Hemodialysis for Intradialytic Hypotension and Intractable Ascites

Hideyuki Hayasaka,[1] Kiyonori Ito,[2] Susumu Ookawara,[2] Masaya Kofuji,[1] Takayuki Uchida,[1] Shunto Kawamura,[3] Ayumi Gomyo,[3] Haruhisa Miyazawa,[2] Yuichiro Ueda,[2] Keiji Hirai,[2] Shun-ichi Kimura,[3] Naoki Momose,[1] Shinichi Kako,[3] and Yoshiyuki Morishita[2]

[1]*Department of Clinical Engineering, Saitama Medical Center, Jichi Medical University, Saitama, Japan*
[2]*Division of Nephrology, First Department of Integrated Medicine, Saitama Medical Center, Jichi Medical University, Saitama, Japan*
[3]*Division of Hematology, First Department of Integrated Medicine, Saitama Medical Center, Jichi Medical University, Saitama, Japan*

Correspondence should be addressed to Susumu Ookawara; su-ooka@hb.tp1.jp

Academic Editor: Yoshihide Fujigaki

A 60-year-old woman with POEMS (polyneuropathy, organomegaly, endocrinopathy, monoclonal gammopathy, and skin changes) syndrome and intractable ascites presented with acute renal failure and received hemodialysis (HD) therapy. Due to frequent intradialytic hypotension, ultrafiltration with cell-free and concentrated ascites reinfusion therapy (CART) was performed to adequately manage the body fluid status and massive ascites. During HD with CART, her blood pressure was maintained compared with that during HD without CART, and an ultrafiltration volume of 3.7 L was achieved after HD with CART. In HD patients with intradialytic hypotension and massive ascites, the combination of CART and ultrafiltration during HD may be an effective therapeutic option for body-fluid management.

1. Introduction

Intradialytic hypotension (IDH) is a fatal and dangerous complication in hemodialysis (HD) patients [1]. Therapeutic strategies against IDH include setting an appropriate dry weight, evaluating cardiac function, and increasing serum protein by improving the nutritional status [2]. In addition, vasopressors or albumin may be administered to perform ultrafiltration during HD therapy.

Cell-free and concentrated ascites reinfusion therapy (CART) is employed for patients with massive ascites and has been implemented for more than 30 years in Japan [3]. CART is divided into three steps. First, there is aspiration of the massive ascites from the patient's abdominal cavity. Next, cells, such as red blood cells or white blood cells, are removed from the collected ascites, and ascites is concentrated by removing the excess fluid. Finally, cell-free and concentrated ascites is reinfused intravenously. The therapeutic effects of CART include amelioration of diuretic resistance, improvement in abdominal tension and quality of life, as well as an adjustment of body fluid status [4, 5]. Furthermore, CART may lead to a reduction in albumin administration, which is more economical (medically) [6].

Polyneuropathy, organomegaly, endocrinopathy, monoclonal gammopathy, and skin change (POEMS) syndrome is a rare refractory disease. POEMS is associated with various symptoms, including massive ascites caused by the overproduction of the vascular endothelial growth factor

(VEGF) [7] and has also been reported to lead to the deterioration of renal function and the development of acute renal failure [8]. In our case, HD was performed for the management of acute renal failure and body fluid excess, including massive ascites. However, IDH frequently occurred during HD with ultrafiltration. Therefore, to prevent the IDH occurrence in response to ultrafiltration, ultrafiltration with CART during HD was performed. Herein, we report a case of successfully managing body fluid excess and massive ascites without the development of IDH by combining CART with ultrafiltration during HD.

2. Case Description

A 60-year-old woman presented with repeated postmenopausal vaginal bleeding due to uterine myoma 3 months prior to admission. Her abdominal computed tomography (CT) was performed at her local hospital to evaluate the uterine myoma and coincidentally showed massive ascites with cirrhotic liver changes. Diuretics were administered in the management of her massive ascites. Thereafter, her renal function rapidly deteriorated, and she was admitted to our hospital. On admission, her height and body weight were 151 cm and 48.0 kg, respectively. Her vital signs were as follows: blood pressure (BP), 95/50 mm·Hg; pulse rate, 76 beats/minute; arterial oxygen saturation on pulse oximetry, 99%. Her physical examination revealed abdominal distension without jaundice or leg edema. Her laboratory findings are shown in Table 1, and the main data are as follows: white blood cell $4.56 \times 10^3/\mu L$, hemoglobin 12.3 g/dL, platelet $14.7 \times 10^4/\mu L$, total protein 6.4 g/dL, serum albumin 3.4 g/dL, serum potassium 7.7 mEq/L, blood urea nitrogen (BUN) 191 mg/dL, serum creatinine (Cr) 6.2 mg/dL, uric acid 18.2 mg/dL, C-reactive protein 4.7 mg/dL, and brain natriuretic peptide 61.6 pg/mL (Table 1). Chest *X*-ray on admission showed cardiac enlargement (cardiothoracic ratio, 57%), whilst computed tomography (CT) showed pleural effusion (Figure 1(a)), massive ascites (Figures 1(b), 1(c)), and multiple uterine myomas. After admission, HD was initiated for the treatment of acute renal failure with mineral and electrolyte disorders and was temporarily discontinued because of improvement in renal function. On day 31 of her hospitalization, her repeated laboratory findings confirmed the presence of serum VEGF >2000 pg/mL, IgG-lambda and kappa type M proteins in the immunoelectrophoretic study, and demyelinating polyneuropathy in the peripheral nerves, and she was diagnosed with POEMS syndrome. Although lenalidomide and dexamethasone therapy was initiated for the treatment of POEMS syndrome, her renal function gradually deteriorated (BUN 92 mg/dL, Cr 5.4 mg/dL) with massive ascites. HD was initiated again on day 63 of hospitalization. The details of her HD therapy were as follows: 3 h per session, 3 times per week; blood flow, 150 mL/min; dialysate flow, 500 mL/min; dialyzer, NV-13S® (Toray Medical, Japan); anticoagulant, nafamostat mesylate 30 mg/h. In addition to the progression of renal dysfunction, there was worsening of her body fluid excess, as she now had systemic edema and massive ascites. Ultrafiltration during HD was performed. However, body fluid excess could not be adequately removed because of the frequent IDH occurrence even with the use of vasopressors during HD on hospital day 80 (Figure 2(a)). To reduce the body fluid excess and prevent IDH occurrence, ultrafiltration with CART during HD was performed on hospital day 82 (Figure 2(b)). The procedure for ascites filtration and concentration was initiated using massive ascites (6.52 L) collected by intraperitoneal puncture. Aspiration of the massive ascites was performed slowly for more than 4 h to prevent the occurrence of hypotension; her systolic BP was maintained within 115 to 140 mm·Hg. Furthermore, the collected ascites was exudative ascites (serum albumin, 2.4 g/dL; ascites albumin, 1.7 g/dL; serum-ascites albumin gradient, 0.7 g/dL). The volume of the filtered concentrated ascites was 884 mL, which contained ascites albumin of 9.6 g/dL and ascites total protein of 16.2 g/dL. The concentrated ascites was stored in the refrigerator overnight and reinfused intravenously during the next HD therapy. The details of CART were as follows: filtration rate, 50 mL/min; processing time, 180 min/session; device name, ACH-Σ® (Asahi Kasei Medical Co., Japan); filter, AHF-MOW (Asahi Kasei Medical Co., Japan); concentrator, AHF-UP (Asahi Kasei Medical Co., Japan). During HD with CART, BP was maintained even under the faster ultrafiltration rate in comparison to what it is in HD without CART (Figure 2(b)). In this HD session with CART, the administrated albumin was consistent with around 85 g; therefore, her serum albumin concentration increased from 2.4 g/dL to 4.0 g/dL due to the albumin administration. In addition, the ultrafiltration volume reached 3.68 L. By removing massive ascites (6.52 L) and performing ultrafiltration (3.68 L) in this HD session with CART, more than 10 L of excessive body fluid was removed. Chemotherapy was continued for the treatment of POEMS syndrome, and her HD therapy was discontinued on hospital day 97 due to the improvement in renal dysfunction. Thereafter, autologous hematopoietic stem cell transplantation was performed, and the patient recovered fully after the bone marrow engraftment.

3. Discussion

In HD patients with massive ascites, IDH occurrence is associated with several factors, including a reduction in colloid osmotic pressure (COP), mismatch between ultrafiltration and plasma refilling in response to ultrafiltration during HD, and an increase in intraperitoneal pressure. COP reduction, which is mainly induced by hypoalbuminemia, leads to a decrease in body fluid movement from the interstitium into the intravascular space and was reportedly associated with the occurrence of IDH [1, 9]. Furthermore, the Kidney Disease Outcomes Quality Initiative guidelines recommend an ultrafiltration rate of less than 15 mL/kg/h to prevent IDH [10]; however, our patient developed IDH at an ultrafiltration rate of 8 mL/kg/h even with vasopressor use and excessive body fluid status in HD without CART. In addition, the increase in intraperitoneal pressure induced by massive ascites would be associated with a decrease in venous return to the central circulation, which leads to hemodynamic instability, including a reduction in cardiac

Table 1: Laboratory findings on admission.

Laboratory findings	
Total protein, g/dL	6.4
Albumin, g/dL	3.4
Total bilirubin, mg/dL	0.21
Aspartate transaminase, U/L	7
Alanine transaminase, U/L,	4
Lactate dehydrogenase, U/L	149
Alkaline phosphatase, U/L	260
Serum sodium, mEq/L	137
Serum potassium, mEq/L	7.7
Serum chloride, mEq/L	106
Serum corrected calcium, mg/dL	6.2
Serum phosphate, mg/dL	13.2
Serum magnesium, mg/dL	3.3
Blood urea nitrogen, mg/dL	191
Creatinine, mg/dL	6.2
Uric acid, mg/dL	18.2
White blood cells,/μL	4560
Neutrophil, %	85
Lymphocyte, %	5
Monocyte, %	9
Red blood cells, $\times 10^4/\mu$L	434
Hemoglobin, g/dL	12.3
Hematocrit, %	37.5
Platelet, $\times 10^4/\mu$L	14.7
C-reactive protein, mg/dL	4.7
Blood glucose, mg/dL,	75
Brain natriuretic peptide, pg/mL	61.6

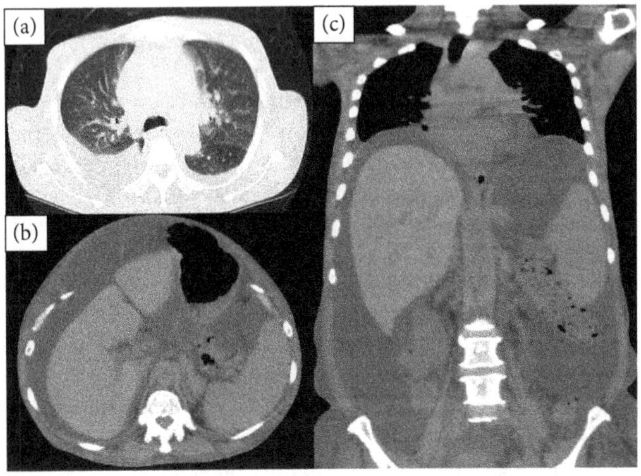

Figure 1: Computed tomography images, (a) lung image in transverse plane, (b) abdominal image in the transverse plane, and (c) thoracoabdominal image in the coronal plane.

output and a decrease in BP. Therefore, in HD patients with massive ascites, the increase in COP during HD and the decrease in intraperitoneal pressure would play an important role in preventing IDH. This would be due to the improvement in plasma refilling in response to ultrafiltration and the increase in venous return to the central circulation.

In this case, the patient's BP increased immediately and was maintained by combining CART and ultrafiltration during HD. Furthermore, the ultrafiltration rate gradually increased during reinfusion of the concentrated ascites, and the ultrafiltration volume reached approximately 3.7 L, which was approximately three times higher than that in HD without CART. Therefore, CART might cause an increase in plasma refilling from the interstitium into the blood vessels by increasing serum albumin concentration [11]. In this case, serum albumin concentration increased from 2.4 to 4.0 g/dL throughout HD with CART. This increase would be in favor of the increase in plasma refilling during HD. Instead of HD therapy with CART, combination therapy with simple ascites removal and albumin preparation might also be a therapeutic option. However, HD therapy with CART could be a better option when the collected ascites is exudative, rather than transudative. This is because the excess proteins, including albumin, could be reinfused in patients with exudative ascites because of the increase in protein concentration in ascites compared to the amount of ready-made albumin preparation. In recent reports, plasma proteins, including serum albumin, have been shown to form a crucial part of the endothelial surface layer [12, 13], which might prevent fluid leakage from blood vessels. It has also been suggested that the anti-inflammatory effects of albumin may contribute to the improvement of vascular permeability [14]. Therefore, concentrated albumin administration with CART might contribute to the promotion of water mobilization into the vascular space and prevention of water extravasation.

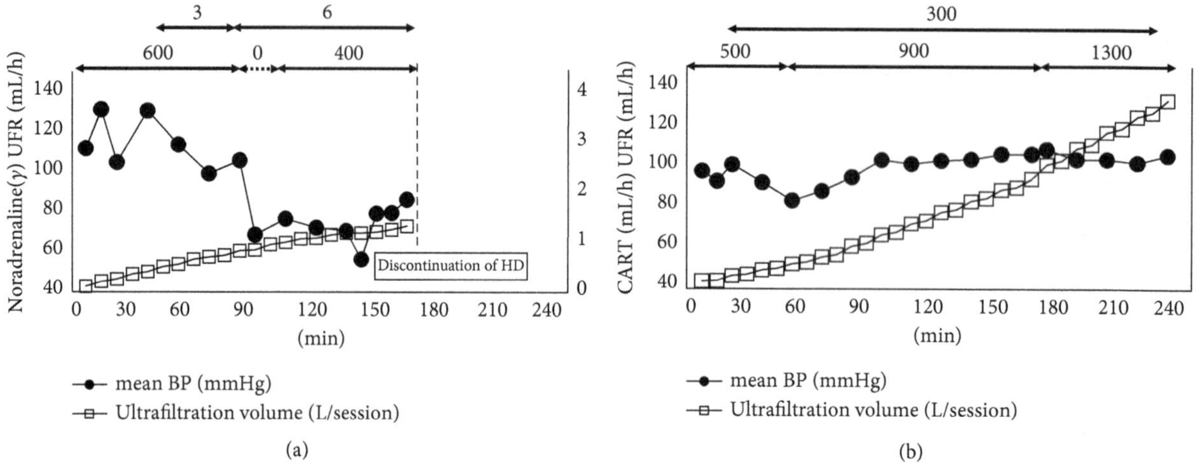

FIGURE 2: Differences in mean blood pressure and ultrafiltration volume during hemodialysis with or without CART. Abbreviations: BP, blood pressure; CART, cell-free and concentrated ascites reinfusion therapy; HD, hemodialysis; UFR, ultrafiltration rate. (a) HD without CART and (b) HD with CART.

Fever, an increase in BP, chest or abdominal pain, and dyspnea are known adverse effects of CART [15]. Particularly, in anuric HD patients, attention should be paid to the increase in BP, congestive heart failure, and pulmonary edema due to the increase in circulating blood volume induced by the increase in plasma refilling with CART, although this patient did not present with these symptoms. In addition, it is important to carefully preserve the filtered concentrated ascites derived from massive ascites. Previous reports have mentioned the possibility of refrigeration or frozen storage of the filtered concentrated ascites [16, 17]. Okamoto et al. reported that there was no change in endotoxin concentrations or properties even after storing ascites at 4°C for 24 h before treatment [16]. If filtered concentrated ascites is stored appropriately, its reinfusion might be considered permissible within 24 h.

In conclusion, we report a case of POEMS syndrome and acute renal failure in a patient who developed IDH and massive ascites. The combination of CART and ultrafiltration during HD could be an effective therapeutic option for body-fluid management in HD patients with massive ascites.

Authors' Contributions

Hideyuki Hayasaka and Kiyonori Ito contributed equally to this work.

Acknowledgments

The authors thank the dialysis staff at Saitama Medical Center, Jichi Medical University, Japan.

References

[1] T. Shoji, Y. Tsubakihara, M. Fujii, and E. Imai, "Hemodialysis-associated hypotension as an independent risk factor for two-year mortality in hemodialysis patients," *Kidney International*, vol. 66, no. 3, pp. 1212–1220, 2004.

[2] Y. Ohashi, K. Sakai, H. Hase, and N. Joki, "Dry weight targeting: the art and science of conventional hemodialysis," *Seminars in Dialysis*, vol. 31, no. 6, pp. 551–556, 2018.

[3] T. Utsugisawa, R. Kobayashi, A. Isoai et al., "Efficacy of cell-free and concentrated ascites for autologous albumin Products," *Japanese Journal of Transfusion and Cell Therapy*, vol. 64, no. 5, pp. 631–640, 2018, in Japanese.

[4] T. Ito, N. Hanafusa, S. Iwase et al., "Effects of cell-free and concentrated ascites reinfusion therapy (CART) on symptom relief of malignancy-related ascites," *International Journal of Clinical Oncology*, vol. 20, no. 3, pp. 623–628, 2015.

[5] H. Yamaguchi, J. Kitayama, S. Emoto et al., "Cell-free and concentrated ascites reinfusion therapy (CART) for management of massive malignant ascites in gastric cancer patients with peritoneal metastasis treated with intravenous and intraperitoneal paclitaxel with oral S-1," *European Journal of Surgical Oncology*, vol. 41, no. 7, pp. 875–880, 2015.

[6] K. Kozaki, M. Iinuma, T. Takagi et al., "Cell-free and concentrated ascites reinfusion therapy for decompensated liver cirrhosis," *Therapeutic Apheresis and Dialysis*, vol. 20, no. 4, pp. 376–382, 2016.

[7] A. Dispenzieri, "POEMS syndrome: 2019 update on diagnosis, risk-stratification, and management," *American Journal of Hematology*, vol. 94, no. 7, pp. 812–827, 2019.

[8] S. Sanada, S. Ookawara, H. Karube et al., "Marked recovery of severe renal lesions in POEMS syndrome with high-dose melphalan therapy supported by autologous blood stem cell transplantation," *American Journal of Kidney Diseases*, vol. 47, no. 4, pp. 672–679, 2006.

[9] H. Hirakata, K. Nitta, M. Inaba et al., "Japanese Society for Dialysis Therapy guidelines for management of cardiovascular diseases in patients on chronic hemodialysis," *Therapeutic Apheresis and Dialysis*, vol. 16, no. 5, pp. 387–435, 2012.

[10] K/DOQI Workgroup, "K/DOQI clinical practice guidelines for cardiovascular disease in dialysis patients," *American Journal of Kidney Diseases*, vol. 45, pp. S1–S153, 2005.

[11] K. L. Schroeder, J. E. Sallustio, and E. A. Ross, "Continuous haematocrit monitoring during intradialytic hypotension:

precipitous decline in plasma refill rates," *Nephrology Dialysis Transplantation*, vol. 19, no. 3, pp. 652–656, 2004.

[12] A. R. Pries, T. W. Secomb, and P. Gaehtgens, "The endothelial surface layer," *Pfluegers Archiv European Journal of Physiology*, vol. 440, no. 5, pp. 653–666, 2000.

[13] J. L. Vincent, J. A. Russell, M. Jacob et al., "Albumin administration in the acutely ill: what is new and where next," *Critical Care*, vol. 18, no. 6, p. 630, 2014.

[14] U. N. Das, "Albumin infusion for the critically ill--is it beneficial and, if so, why and how," *Critical Care*, vol. 19, no. 1, p. 156, 2015.

[15] N. Hanafusa, A. Isoai, T. Ishihara et al., "Safety and efficacy of cell-free and concentrated ascites reinfusion therapy (CART) in refractory ascites: post-marketing surveillance results," *PLoS One*, vol. 12, no. 5, Article ID e0177303, 2017.

[16] Y. Okamoto, Y. Nakahashi, M. Chino et al., "Towards the establishment of a safe cell-free and concentrated ascites reinfusion therapy," *Japanese Journal of Transfusion and Cell Therapy*, vol. 59, no. 3, pp. 470–475, 2013, in Japanese.

[17] S. Chiyoda, T. Morikawa, K. Matsuo, and S. Masuya, "Reinfusion of autogenous ascitic fluid concentrated by freezing in patients with intractable ascites," *Internal Medicine*, vol. 31, no. 3, pp. 325–332, 1992.

29

Bilateral Ureteral Stenosis with Hydronephrosis as First Manifestation of Granulomatosis with Polyangiitis (Wegener's Granulomatosis): A Case Report and Review of the Literature

Joelle Suillot,[1,2] Jürg Bollmann,[3] Samuel Rotman,[4] and Eric Descombes[1,2]

[1]*Service of Nephrology, HFR Cantonal Hospital Fribourg, Fribourg, Switzerland*
[2]*University of Fribourg, Fribourg, Switzerland*
[3]*Service of Urology, HFR Cantonal Hospital Fribourg, Fribourg, Switzerland*
[4]*Service of Clinical Pathology, Lausanne University Hospital, University of Lausanne, Lausanne, Switzerland*

Correspondence should be addressed to Eric Descombes; descombese@h-fr.ch

Academic Editor: Phuong Chi Pham

Ureteral stenosis is a rare manifestation of granulomatosis with polyangiitis (formerly known as Wegener's granulomatosis). We report the case of a 76-year-old woman with progressive renal failure in which bilateral hydronephrosis due to ureteral stenosis was the first manifestation of the disease. Our patient also had renal involvement with pauci-immune crescentic glomerulonephritis associated with high titers of anti-proteinase 3 c-ANCAs, but no involvement of the upper or lower respiratory tract. The hydronephrosis and renal function rapidly improved under immunosuppressive therapy with high-dose corticosteroids and intravenous pulse cyclophosphamide. We reviewed the literature and found only ten other reported cases of granulomatosis with polyangiitis/Wegener's granulomatosis and intrinsic ureteral stenosis: in two cases, the presenting clinical manifestation was unilateral hydronephrosis and in only two others was the hydronephrosis bilateral, but this complication developed during a relapse of the disease. This case emphasizes the importance of including ANCA-related vasculitis in the differential diagnosis of unusual cases of unilateral or bilateral ureteral stenosis.

1. Introduction

Granulomatosis with polyangiitis (GPA) (formerly known as Wegener's granulomatosis) is a necrotizing vasculitis of the small to medium vessels, according to the revised International Chapel Hill Consensus Conference Nomenclature of Vasculitides [1]. Its classic triad consists of necrotizing granulomatous vasculitis of the upper and lower respiratory tract in association with pauci-immune crescentic glomerulonephritis [2]. It is often associated with antineutrophilic cytoplasmic antibodies (ANCA) against proteinase 3 (anti-PR3), but occasionally also against myeloperoxidase (anti-MPO) [2]. GPA is an uncommon disease, with an annual incidence of about 10 cases per million inhabitants, a prevalence of 22–157 cases per million [3] and a peak incidence in the fourth and fifth decades of life [4]. Men and women are affected at a similar frequency. GPA was a fatal disease before the introduction of effective immunosuppressive treatments. The use of high-dose corticosteroids associated with cyclophosphamide has markedly improved survival as well as renal survival of patients with ANCA-associated vasculitis [3].

GPA can affect all organs of the body. Although rare, urogenital manifestation can occur during the course of the disease and may be asymptomatic [5]. Granulomatous inflammation of the prostate, bladder, penis, testes, seminal vesicles, ureters, urethra and epididymis have already been reported.

We are reporting on a case in which bilateral hydronephrosis due to bilateral ureteral stenosis was the first clinical manifestation of GPA. Ureteral stenosis is a rare complication of GPA: only 11 cases (including ours) have been reported in the literature to date and, to our knowledge, our case is the first one in which bilateral hydronephrosis was the presenting manifestation of the disease.

2. Case Report

A 76-year-old woman was transferred to our hospital after a 6-month history of progressive renal failure with bilateral hydronephrosis of unclear origin and normal cystoscopy.

At admission the patient complained of fatigue, bilateral leg oedema and a 10 kg weight loss. The patient denied any episode of macroscopic hematuria. Clinical examination found a patient in poor general condition with bilateral pitting edema of the legs. Temperature was 36.5°C, blood pressure 135/70 mmHg. The laboratory findings were as follows: serum creatinine was 601 μmol/l, urea 39.5 mmol/l, total protein 57.5 g/l, serum albumin 28 g/l, sodium 143 mmol/l, potassium 4.8 mmol/l. The sedimentation rate was 81 mm/h, C-reactive protein (CRP) 33 mg/l, hemoglobin 107 g/l, leukocyte count 7.2 G/l and platelets 333 G/l. Urinalysis showed microscopic hematuria with mild leukocyturia. Urine culture was sterile. Creatinine clearance was 4 ml/min. Proteinuria was present at 1.9 g/24 h, without paraproteins.

A native abdominal CT scan was performed showing bilateral hydro-uretero-nephrosis with massive dilatation of the upper ureters and of the renal pelvis (Figure 1(a)). The CT scan showed no signs of an obstructive abdomino-pelvic mass, of retroperitoneal fibrosis, urolithiasis or sloughed papillary necrosis. Bilateral ureteral catheterization using double J catheters was performed and the retrograde pyelography revealed that the bilateral hydronephrosis was due to a complete right ureteral stenosis and a partial stenosis on the left side (Figure 2). As bilateral malignancy was considered in the differential diagnosis a small periprocedural ureteral biopsy was performed showing only nonspecific inflammation without tumoral cells.

In the following days, despite an improvement of diuresis (≈2000 ml/day) with double J catheters, no improvement of renal function occurred. The diagnostic workup was therefore completed with immunological tests showing high c-ANCA titers (1 : 1280) with anti-PR3 positivity. Thereafter, a kidney biopsy detected pauci-immune crescentic glomerulonephritis (Figure 3). The ENT exam and a native pulmonary CT scan were normal.

Treatment with pulse methylprednisolone (4 × 1 gram) followed by oral prednisone in combination with monthly intravenous pulse cyclophosphamide (3 × 500 mg) was started. Renal function progressively improved in the following weeks and the creatinine stabilized at 140 μmol/l after 3 months, with negative c-ANCA. At the same time repeated ultrasounds showed a progressive regression of the hydro-uretero-nephrosis and the double J catheters were withdrawn. A follow-up CT scan at 3 months showed a complete regression of the hydronephrosis on the left side and a partial regression on the right side (Figure 1(b)). Of note this second CT scan, as the first one, showed no evidence of an obstructive abdomino-pelvic mass, of retroperitoneal fibrosis, urolithiasis or papillary necrosis.

3. Discussion

In adults, the most frequent causes of bilateral ureteral obstruction are retroperitoneal or pelvic neoplasms, calculi, or retroperitoneal fibrosis. However, the differential diagnosis also includes other rare etiologies. Table 1 summarizes the causes of bilateral, or potentially bilateral, ureteral obstruction according to the mechanism of obstruction and shows that different inflammatory or systemic diseases, including small and medium vessel vasculitis, can cause bilateral hydro-uretero-nephrosis. As we will discuss further below, sometimes, unilateral or bilateral ureteral stenosis with hydronephrosis may be due to ANCA-associated vasculitis. To our knowledge, we are reporting on the first patient with bilateral hydronephrosis as the presenting manifestation of ANCA-associated vasculitis.

Urogenital involvement is rare in GPA. Large series of GPA patients have reported between 1% and 10% of cases with urogenital involvement [6, 24]. Cases of asymptomatic urogenital involvement have also been reported in autopsy studies of patients with GPA, and urological manifestation may be underestimated because complete urological investigations are not routinely performed [5]. The main locations of the urogenital manifestations of GPA are summarized in Table 2. Prostatitis is the most common, followed by bladder involvement, orchitis, and penile ulcerations [5]. When urological involvement is present, it is usually observed as part of a generalized systemic disease associated with upper respiratory involvement in 90–100% of the cases, pulmonary lesions in 80%, and glomerulonephritis in 45–60% [5]. Isolated urological manifestations can precede GPA diagnosis in 12–18% of the cases having urological involvement [6, 24]. Intrinsic ureteral stenosis is a rare manifestation of GPA as only 11 cases (including ours) have been reported in the literature to date [6, 24–30]. Huong et al. [6] and Kamar et al. [27] each described two cases. One case was reported twice by the same author [6, 31]. Two other cases were published twice [26, 29, 32, 33] and another case three times [25, 34, 35]. It should be noted that cases of patients with GPA in which hydronephrosis was due to extrinsic ureteral obstruction caused by retroperitoneal inflammation, pseudotumors, or vascular compression as well as prostatic obstruction as a consequence of GPA-related inflammation have also been reported [36–44].

Table 3 summarizes the main clinical features of the 11 cases of ureteral stenosis reported in the literature. In most cases (8/11 = 73%), the ureteral involvement occurred during a relapse of GPA and in only two cases was the involvement bilateral [6, 26]. In the two remaining cases, the ureteral stenosis was, as in our patient, the initial manifestation of GPA, but in these two patients, the hydronephrosis was unilateral [27, 30]. Davenport et al. briefly described a case of initial manifestation of GPA with bilateral ureteral obstruction, but this was due to necrotic debris in the bladder and in the two ureters [43]. Interestingly, a case of ureteral stenosis has also been reported in a kidney transplant due to the recurrence of GPA after transplantation [28].

In 6 of these 11 cases, open ureteral surgery was performed as part of the diagnostic and/or therapeutic workup and granulomatous/vasculitic inflammation was found in all [24, 27–30]. In the other four cases that underwent only an endoscopic workup, no ureteral biopsy was performed [6, 25, 26]. Hence, our case is in fact the only one where a small

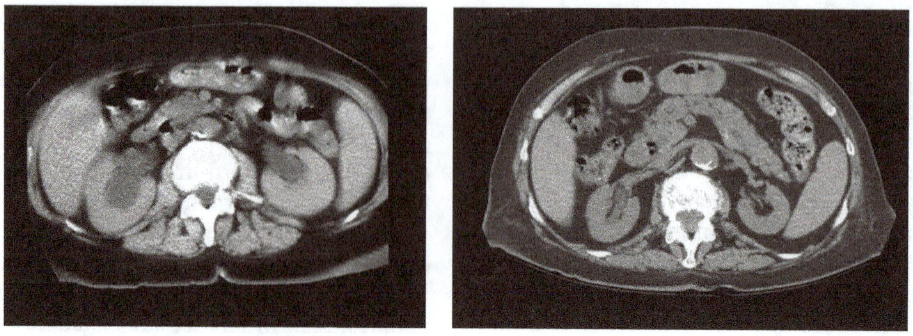

(a) (b)

Figure 1: Native CT scan (a) at admission showing massive bilateral hydronephrosis and (b) at 3 months showing a complete regression of the hydronephrosis on the left side and a partial regression on the right side.

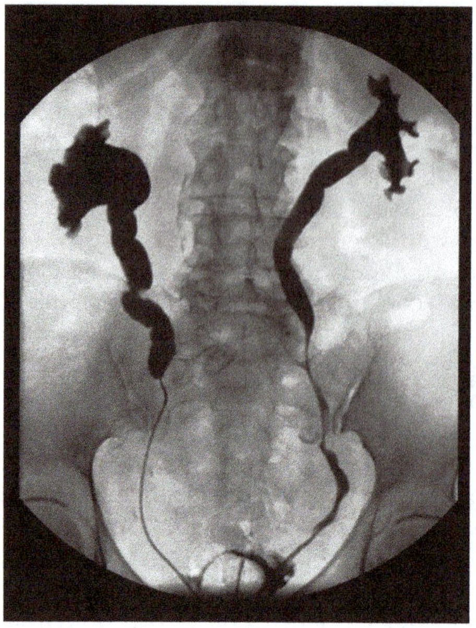

Figure 2: Retrograde pyelography showing bilateral hydro-uretero-nephrosis with a complete ureteral stenosis on the right and a partial ureteral stenosis on the left.

Table 1: Causes of bilateral or potentially bilateral ureteral obstruction*.

Urinary tract malformations	Several mainly congenital pediatric diseases
Urolithiasis and endoluminal obstruction	Calculi, papillary necrosis with sloughed papilla, blood clots, fungus balls
Intrinsic ureteral obstruction	Transitional cell carcinoma and other malignant neoplasms fibroepithelial polyps, ureteritis cystica
Extrinsic ureteral obstuction	Abdominopelvic tumors, lymphoma, retroperitoneal fibrosis endometriosis, sarcoidosis
Systemic and inflammatory diseases**	Small-vessel vasculitis, periarteritis nodosa, Churg–Strauss, Henoch–Schönlein purpura, eosinophilic ureteritis, RA
Ureteral localization of infections	Fungal (actinomycosis), tuberculosis, bacterial, viral (immunocompromised host)
Miscellaneous	Pregnancy, slowed peristalsis, obstructed stent, postoperative

*Adapted from references [6–23]. **Some can cause either intrinsic or extrinsic obstruction. RA = rheumatoid arthritis.

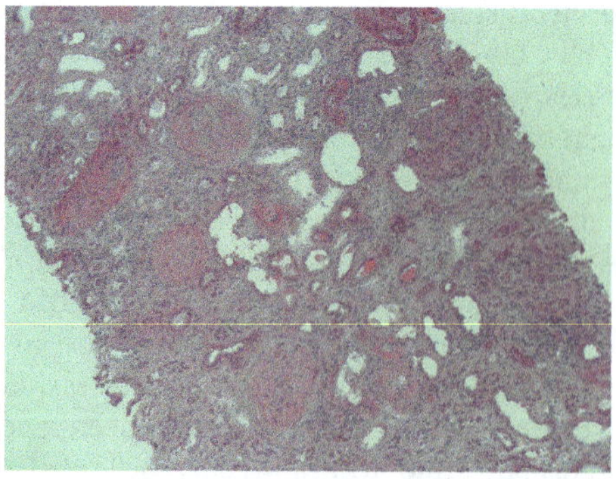

Figure 3: Renal biopsy showing extracapillary crescentic glomerulonephritis involving almost all glomeruli (HE, 100x).

Table 2: Relative frequency of the different urogenital manifestations of granulomatosis with polyangiitis.

Site	Clinical manifestations	Frequency
Prostate	Prostatitis, urinary retention, asymptomatic	+++++
Bladder	Cystitis, pseudotumor	++++
Penis	Ulcerations	+++
Testicles	Orchitis	+++
Kidneys	Pseudotumors, asymptomatic	+++
Urethra	Urethritis	++
Ureter	Stenosis, hydronephrosis	++
Epididymis	Epididymitis	+

Data adapted from Alba et al. [5].

endoscopic biopsy was performed in order to rule out malignancy. This biopsy showed only nonspecific inflammation, and we consider that our biopsy was too small and superficial to allow the detection of a granulomatous or vasculitic inflammation. However, one may question if the bilateral ureteric stenosis in our patient may eventually be unrelated to the ANCA-associated vasculitis. In this respect,

Table 3: Summary and characteristics of the reported cases of ureteral stenosis in GPA.

Reference	Year	Age	Sex	Ureteral stenosis		ANCA	Type	Treatment		Course
				Timing	Details			Urological	Medical	
27	2003	59	F	**Inaugural**	Left hydronephrosis with a 3 cm-long iliac ureteral stenosis	Negative		Double J stent, resection of the stenosis by open surgery	No	Remission at 12 months
30	2011	71	F	**Inaugural**	Right hydronephrosis related to a ureteral stenosis	Positive	PR3	Surgical exploration and resection of the stenosis	PRED + CYC	Remission at 6 months
Our case		76	F	**Inaugural**	**Bilateral** hydronephrosis related to ureteral stenosis	Positive	PR3	Bilateral ureteral double J stents	PRED + CYC	Remission at 3 months
6, 31*	1988	69	F	Relapse	**Bilateral** hydronephrosis related to pelvic bilateral ureteral stenosis	NA		Bilateral ureteral double J stents	PRED + CYC, and plasma exchanges	Died 3 yr later; no urologic relapse
26, 32*	2006	38	F	Relapse	**Bilateral** dilatation of both collecting systems with bilateral ureteral stenosis	Positive	MPO	Endoscopic dilatation and double J stent on the left side	PRED + CYC	Remission at 12 months
25, 34*, 35*	1977	60	F	Relapse	Left ureteral obstruction at the pelvic brim	NA		Transureter ureterostomy	PRED + CYC	Remission at 16 months
29, 33*	1982	50	M	Relapse	Moderate dilatation on the right urinary tract	NA		Ureteral resection	PRED + CYC	Remission at 10 yr
28	1994	25	F	Relapse	Hydronephrosis in a transplanted kidney by ureteral obstruction at the ureterovesical junction	Positive	NA	Ureteral resection	PRED + CYC + AZA	Remission at 15 yr
6	1995	55	M	Relapse	Right-sided ureteral stenosis	Positive	NA	None	PRED	Remission at 5 yr
27	2003	21	M	Relapse	Isolated right hydronephrosis with a 2 cm-long stenosis of the iliac ureter	Negative		Double J stent followed by open surgery excision	PRED + CYC	Remission at 6 months
24	2012	53	M	Relapse	Right-sided hydronephrosis with ureteral stenosis	Positive	PR3	Ureteral catheter	PRED and MTX	Died 3 yr later; no urologic relapse

*Cases reported two or three times. F: female, M: male, NA: not available, PRED: prednisone, CYC: cyclophosphamide, MTX: methotrexate, AZA: azathioprine, and yr: year.

we consider that the accurate initial diagnostic workup, the follow-up exams performed at 3 months, and the favourable response with the regression of the hydro-uretero-nephrosis under immunosuppressive therapy allow to reasonably rule out the alternative diagnosis listed in Table 1.

Concerning ANCAs, ANCA determinations were not performed on the oldest cases reported in the literature as this diagnostic test was not yet available at the time. Except for the two cases reported by Kamar et al., ANCA was positive in all other cases, with anti-PR3 positivity in three patients and anti-MPO positivity in one. The two ANCA-negative cases reported by Kamar et al. are unique since these two patients had isolated 2 and 3 cm long unilateral ureteral stenoses with granulomatous inflammation at surgical resection as the sole manifestation of the disease [27].

The treatment of GPA with a combination of glucocorticoids and immunosuppressants, mainly cyclophosphamide, has been well established. All but three of the reported patients received this treatment and responded well to it (Table 3). To the best of our knowledge, the recurrence of ureteral stenosis upon medical treatment has never been reported. Endoscopic placement of double J catheters was performed in our case, as well as in five others [6, 24, 26], followed by open surgery in two cases [27]. Open surgery was initially performed in four cases [28–30, 35]. The last case underwent no urological therapy as the patient responded rapidly to immunosuppression [6]. In general, surgical repair of the ureters is unnecessary because urological symptoms improve quickly on medical treatment. Consequently, all authors advocate that surgery should only be considered in patients who do not rapidly and effectively respond to the combination of corticoids and immunosuppressants.

In summary, the present review indicates that unilateral or bilateral ureteral stenosis can be the first clinical manifestation of GPA or may occur during a relapse of the disease. Since the clinical presentation may mimic cancer, the right diagnosis can avoid unnecessarily invasive procedures. Therefore, ANCA-related vasculitis should be considered in the differential diagnosis of unusual cases of unilateral or bilateral ureteral stenosis and ANCA testing should be performed in patients in whom a diagnosis is not readily apparent. The data from the reviewed literature suggest that ureteral stenosis responds well and rapidly to glucocorticoids and immunosuppressants.

References

[1] J. C. Jennette, "Overview of the 2012 revised international Chapel Hill Consensus conference nomenclature of Vasculitides," *Clinical and Experimental Nephrology*, vol. 17, no. 5, pp. 603–606, 2013.

[2] J. C. Jennette, R. J. Falk, K. Andrassy et al., "Nomenclature of systemic Vasculitides," *Arthritis & Rheumatism*, vol. 37, no. 2, pp. 187–192, 1994.

[3] C. Comarmond and P. Cacoub, "Granulomatosis with polyangiitis (Wegener): clinical aspects and treatment," *Autoimmunity Reviews*, vol. 13, no. 11, pp. 1121–1125, 2014.

[4] J. C. Jennette and P. H. Nachman, "ANCA glomerulonephritis and vasculitis," *Clinical Journal of the American Society of Nephrology*, vol. 12, no. 10, pp. 1680–1691, 2017.

[5] M. A. Alba, J. Moreno-Palacios, S. Beça, and M. C. Cid, "Urologic and male genital manifestations of granulomatosis with polyangiitis," *Autoimmunity Reviews*, vol. 14, no. 10, pp. 897–902, 2015.

[6] D. L. Huong, T. Papo, J. C. Piette et al., "Urogenital manifestations of Wegener's granulomatosis," *Medicine (Baltimore)*, vol. 74, no. 3, pp. 152–161, 1995.

[7] E. Yap, T. M. Salifu, A. A. Ahmad, M. Sanusi, A. Joseph, and M. Mallappallil, "Atypical causes of urinary tract obstruction," *Case Reports in Nephrology*, vol. 2019, Article ID 4903693, 5 pages, 2019.

[8] D. Bianchi, G. Vespasiani, and G. Bove, "Acute kidney injury due to bilateral ureteral obstruction in children," *World Journal of Nephrology*, vol. 3, no. 4, pp. 182–192, 2014.

[9] A. Dalpiaz, R. Schwamb, Y. Miao, J. Gonka, W. Walzter, and S. A. Khan, "Urological manifestations of henoch-schonlein purpura: a review," *Current Urology*, vol. 8, no. 2, pp. 66–73, 2015.

[10] C. Pfister, A. e. s. Liard-Zmuda, J.-N. Dacher, D. Dubois, P. Grise, and P. Mitrofanoff, "Total bilateral ureteral replacement for stenosing ureteritis in henoch-schönlein purpura," *European Urology*, vol. 38, no. 1, pp. 96–99, 2000.

[11] J. M. Powell, H. Ware, and G. Williams, "Recurrent ureteric obstruction in association with Henoch-Schonlein purpura," *Postgraduate Medical Journal*, vol. 63, no. 742, pp. 699–701, 1987.

[12] P. Cortellini, P. Manganelli, F. Poletti, P. Sacchini, U. Ambanelli, and E. Bezzi, "Ureteral involvement in the Churg-Strauss syndrome: a case report," *Journal of Urology*, vol. 140, no. 5 Part 1, pp. 1016–1018, 1988.

[13] B. Yoo, H. K. Kim, and H. B. Moon, "Case report: a case of polyarteritis nodosa with bilateral ureteral obstruction," *The Korean Journal of Internal Medicine*, vol. 11, no. 2, pp. 165–168, 1996.

[14] T. R. Hefty, P. Bonafede, and P. Stenzel, "Bilateral ureteral stricture from polyarteritis nodosa," *Journal of Urology*, vol. 141, no. 3 Part 1, pp. 600-601, 1989.

[15] J. P. Melin, P. Lemaire, P. Birembaut et al., "Polyarteritis nodosa with bilateral ureteric involvement," *Nephron*, vol. 32, no. 1, pp. 87–89, 1982.

[16] R.-X. Chen, S. "Stewart" Cao, L.-D. Zhao, and H.-X. Yang, "Obstructive uropathy associated with rheumatoid arthritis successfully treated with steroids and immunosuppressive therapy: a case report," *Medicine (Baltimore)*, vol. 98, no. 50, p. e18415, 2019.

[17] H. Bjorndalen and R. A. Hastings, "Ureteric obstruction secondary to retroperitoneal fibrosis leading to acute kidney injury," *BMJ Case Reports*, vol. 2013, 2013.

[18] J. V. Alonso, P. L. Cachinero, F. R. Ubeda, D. J. L. Ruiz, and A. Blanco, "Bilateral stones as a cause of acute renal failure in the emergency department," *World Journal of Emergency Medicine*, vol. 5, no. 1, pp. 67–71, 2014.

[19] P. Fraioli, L. Montemurro, L. Castrignano, and G. Rizzato, "Retroperitoneal involvement in sarcoidosis," *Sarcoidosis*, vol. 7, no. 2, pp. 101–105, 1990.

[20] E. Miyazaki, T. Tsuda, A. Mochizuki et al., "Sarcoidosis presenting as bilateral hydronephrosis," *Internal Medicine*, vol. 35, no. 7, pp. 579–582, 1996.

[21] W. Seidemann, "Hydronephrosis caused by enlarged retroperitoneal lymph nodes in sarcoidosis," *Deutsche Medizinische Wochenschrift*, vol. 112, no. 41, pp. 1583–1585, 1987.

[22] M. Grande, G. Lisi, D. Bianchi et al., "Bilateral ureteral obstruction in children after appendectomy," *Case Reports in Surgery*, vol. 2015, Article ID 740795, 3 pages, 2015.

[23] P. Jetty and G. G. Barber, "Aortitis and bilateral ureteral obstruction after endovascular repair of abdominal aortic aneurysm," *Journal of Vascular Surgery*, vol. 39, no. 6, pp. 1344–1347, 2004.

[24] J.-F. Dufour, T. Le Gallou, J.-F. Cordier et al., "Urogenital manifestations in wegener granulomatosis," *Medicine*, vol. 91, no. 2, pp. 67–74, 2012.

[25] T. W. Hensle, M. E. Mitchell, K. K. Crooks, and D. Robinson, "Urologic manifestations of Wegener granulomatosis," *Urology*, vol. 12, no. 5, pp. 553–556, 1978.

[26] I. Ben Ghorbel, W. Chebbi, M. Zouari, F. Hentati, M. Miled, and M. H. Houman, "Sténose urétérale au cours de la granulomatose de Wegener," *La Presse Médicale*, vol. 35, no. 11, pp. 1659–1663, 2006.

[27] N. Kamar, B. Malavaud, L. Alric et al., "Ureteral stenosis as the sole manifestation of Wegener's granulomatosis," *Urology*, vol. 62, no. 2, p. 352, 2003.

[28] L. M. Rich and W. F. Piering, "Ureteral stenosis due to recurrent Wegener's granulomatosis after kidney transplantation," *Journal of the American Society of Nephrology: JASN*, vol. 4, no. 8, pp. 1516–1521, 1994.

[29] P. Ronco, F. Mignon, Y. Lanoe, J. Roland, L. Morel-Maroger, and B. Gattegno, "Ureteral stenosis in Wegener's granulomatosis," *Nephron*, vol. 30, no. 3, pp. 201–204, 1982.

[30] J. Lillaz, S. Bernardini, M. P. Algros, H. Bittard, and

F. Kleinclauss, "Wegener's granulomatosis: a rare cause of hydronephrosis," *Case Reports in Medicine*, vol. 2011, Article ID 814794, 3 pages, 2011.

[31] D. Le Thi Huong, C. De Gennes, B. Wechsler, S. D. Etienne, and P. Godeau, "[Anuria caused by bilateral ureteral stenosis in Wegener's granulomatosis]," *La Presse Médicale*, vol. 17, no. 17, p. 870, 1988.

[32] S. Sataa, S. Ben Rhouma, M. Tanguour et al., "Ureteral stenosis due to Wegener's granulomatosis," *Tunisie Medicale*, vol. 89, no. 8-9, pp. 725-726, 2011.

[33] E. M. Plaisier, B. Mougenot, R. Khayat, B. Gattegno, F. Mignon, and P. M. Ronco, "Ureteral stenosis in Wegener's granulomatosis," *Nephrology Dialysis Transplantation*, vol. 12, no. 8, pp. 1759–1761, 1997.

[34] S. B. Baker and D. R. Robinson, "Unusual renal manifestations of Wegener's granulomatosis," *The American Journal of Medicine*, vol. 64, no. 5, pp. 883–889, 1978.

[35] "Case records of the Massachusetts general hospital, weekly clinicopathological exercises. Case 47-1977," *The New England Journal of Medicine*, vol. 297, no. 21, pp. 1164–1172, 1977.

[36] G. Middleton, D. Karp, E. Lee, and J. Cush, "Wegener's granulomatosis presenting as lower back pain with prostatitis and ureteral obstruction," *The Journal of Rheumatology*, vol. 21, no. 3, pp. 566–569, 1994.

[37] J. C. ter Maaten, C. F. Franssen, A. A. Daenekindt, and S. J. Hoorntje, "Triple Wegener's granulomatosis in the urogenital tract," *Nephron*, vol. 63, no. 3, pp. 358-359, 1993.

[38] A. P. V. B. Freitas, H. C. L. Filho, F. Gonzalez et al., "Ureteral stenosis secondary to granulomatous vasculitis," *JCR: Journal of Clinical Rheumatology*, vol. 11, no. 6, pp. 311–313, 2005.

[39] H. J. Metselaar, F. J. W. ten Kate, and W. Weimar, "Ureter obstruction as a complication of Wegener's granulomatosis," *European Urology*, vol. 11, no. 1, pp. 63-64, 1985.

[40] R. A. Adelizzi, F. K. Shockley, and J. R. Pietras, "Wegener's granulomatosis with ureteric obstruction," *The Journal of Rheumatology*, vol. 13, no. 2, pp. 448–451, 1986.

[41] L. Guillevin and M. Brauner, "Magnetic resonance imaging of ureter stenosis in Wegener's granulomatosis," *Annales de Medecine Interne*, vol. 149, no. 5, p. 287, 1998.

[42] J. Leche, C. Feuilhade, J. P. Ferroir, L. Moulonguet Doleris, and A. Guillard, "[Wegener's disease of urologic and neurologic onset]," *Ann Med Interne (Paris)*, vol. 136, no. 4, p. 353, 1985.

[43] A. Davenport, S. E. Downey, S. Goel, and A. G. Maciver, "Wegener's granulomatosis involving the urogenital tract," *BJU International*, vol. 78, no. 3, pp. 354–357, 1996.

[44] F. Farpour and A. Abrudescu, "A case of granulomatosis with polyangiitis causing hydroureter and hydronephrosis," *Case Reports in Rheumatology*, vol. 2014, Article ID 713957, 3 pages, 2014.

Liberation from Dialysis Dependence in a Patient with HIV-Associated Nephropathy (HIVAN) after Combined Antiretroviral Therapy (cART)

Virin Ramoutar[1] **Raafat Makary**[2] **Malleswari Ravi,**[3] **Leighton James,**[4] **and Charles Heilig**[5]

[1]*Nephrologist & Infectious Disease Specialist, Cumberland Kidney Specialists, Cookeville, TN, USA*
[2]*Pathology Department, University of Florida, Jacksonville, FL, USA*
[3]*Division of Infectious Disease, University of Florida, Jacksonville, FL, USA*
[4]*Division of Nephrology, Medical College of Georgia, Augusta University, Augusta, GA, USA*
[5]*Division of Nephrology, University of Florida, Jacksonville, FL, USA*

Correspondence should be addressed to Virin Ramoutar; virin.ramoutar@outlook.com

Academic Editor: Ze'ev Korzets

Prior to the advent of combined antiretroviral therapy (cART), human immunodeficiency virus-associated nephropathy (HIVAN) was inevitably associated with rapidly progressive renal failure and dialysis dependence. HIV-1 seropositive patients often met with untimely deaths due to complications of end-stage renal disease (ESRD), opportunistic infections, or other HIV-related end-organ failure. Although the association between cART and improved outcomes in HIVAN has been recognized for over 20 years, no randomized trials have specifically examined this effect to date. In terms of reversal of dialysis-dependent renal failure after cART initiation, only a handful of case reports exist. The authors report a case of a 44-year-old Latino male requiring thrice-weekly haemodialysis in the setting of biopsy-proven HIVAN who was able to stop dialysis in 7 months after being initiated on cART.

1. Introduction

HIVAN, the classic renal pathology associated with HIV infection, was first described in 1984 as a sequela of acquired immune deficiency syndrome (AIDS) [1, 2]. It is the most common cause of ESRD in HIV-1 seropositive patients [3] and manifests histologically as a collapsing form of focal segmental glomerulosclerosis (FSGS) accompanied by microcystic tubular dilatation and interstitial inflammation [4]. The prevalence ranges from 3.5% in clinical studies to 12% on postmortem evaluation [3], and it occurs more frequently in patients of African descent [5, 6]. Risk factors include CD4 cell count of less than 200 cells/mm^3 and a high viral load, but HIVAN has been seen in acute HIV infection [7, 8] as well as with undetectable viral loads [9]. The benefit of cART in HIVAN is based on observational data with isolated cases demonstrating remission within a few weeks [10, 11]. In terms of dialysis-dependent HIVAN, a literature search yielded only 3 prior published cases in which cART initiation improved renal function enough to reverse dependence on renal replacement therapy [12–14]. Two of these 3 cases were African-American males with no ethnicity reported by Winston et al. [13]. In this report, a 44-year-old Latino male with biopsy-proven HIVAN experienced reversal of dialysis dependence 7 months after cART initiation without the use of corticosteroids.

2. Case Presentation

A 44-year-old Latino male presented to the ER with complaints of generalized malaise, low grade fever, and watery stools for 1 to 2 weeks. He passed bowel movements

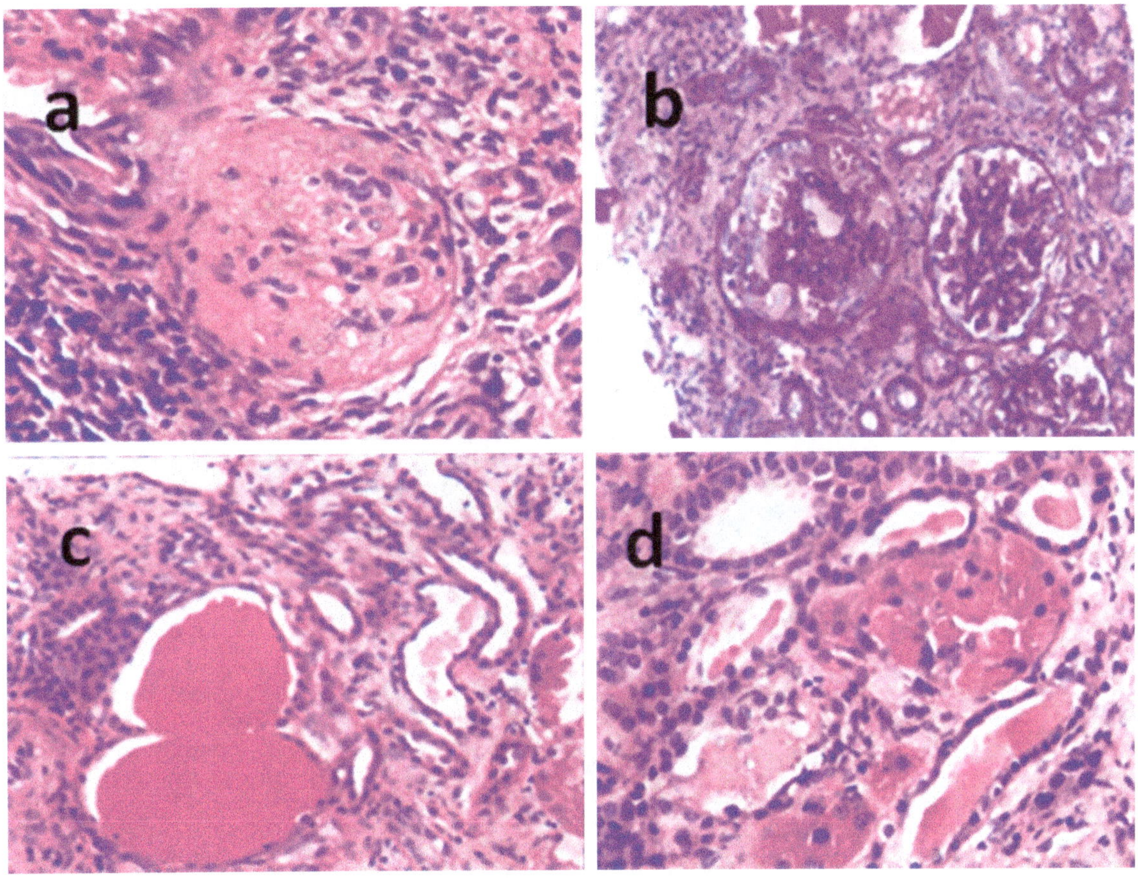

FIGURE 1: Haematoxylin and eosin stain (×20 magnification) showing (a) global to near global glomerulosclerosis, (b) collapsed glomerular tuft, (c) tubular microcystic dilatation, and (d) distended tubular epithelium from protein resorption droplets.

5 times per day without frank blood, melena, or mucus. He had a past medical history of chronic hypertension (HTN) and chronic kidney disease (CKD) with a baseline serum creatinine (sCr) in range 2.0 to 2.5 mg/dL. On presentation, his serum bicarbonate level was 9 mmol/L with blood urea nitrogen (BUN) 125 mg/dL and sCr 13.8 mg/dL. He had been initiated on lisinopril for HTN and to mitigate CKD progression 1 month prior to onset of symptoms. This was discontinued on presentation to the hospital and was his only prescribed medication. He denied any history of nonsteroidal anti-inflammatory drug (NSAID) use or intravenous drug abuse. Complete blood count revealed hemoglobin 7 g/dL, white cell count 4,800/mm^3, and mild thrombocytopenia 78,000/mm^3 (no abnormalities seen on peripheral smear). Urine microscopy revealed 2 normomorphic red blood cells, 9 white cells, and 3 hyaline casts per high power field. The spot urine protein to creatinine ratio was 10,417 mg/g, and urinalysis tested positive for protein at 2,000 mg/dL. He was volume expanded with an isotonic solution of sodium bicarbonate (150 mEq) in a litre of 5% dextrose solution. His serum bicarbonate normalized, but BUN remained elevated at 106 mg/dL with sCr 13.49 mg/dL. Urine culture was positive for pan-susceptible *Enterococcus faecalis*. He received a 10-day course of amoxicillin to sterilize the genitourinary tract in anticipation of a renal biopsy.

A renal ultrasound with Doppler sonography was performed to exclude obstructive uropathy and renal artery stenosis. There was no evidence of either condition, and both kidneys demonstrated increased echogenicity. The left kidney was measured at 10.3 cm and the right at 9.9 cm in the longitudinal axis. Serum complements were within normal range. Laboratory investigations returned negative for syphilis, hepatitis B and C, rheumatoid factor, antinuclear antibody (ANA), antineutrophil cytoplasmic antibody (ANCA), and monoclonal paraproteins in both urine and serum. Antistreptolysin O titres were within normal limits. HIV-1 Western blot returned positive with a viral load of 664,000 copies/ml and CD4 count of 40 cells/μL. Blood and stool samples did not yield any other infectious aetiology. His diarrhoea resolved within 36 hrs of hospital admission, but he exhibited continued anorexia and intermittent nausea in the setting of persistent azotaemia and oliguria (<800 cc urine/day). Haemodialysis was initiated via a tunnelled cuffed catheter.

A percutaneous renal biopsy was performed in light of proteinuria and HIV seropositivity. The biopsy revealed collapsing glomerulosclerosis, tubular dilatation (Figure 1), tubuloreticular inclusions, thickened glomerular basement membrane, foot process effacement, and absence of electron dense deposits (Figure 2). 20 glomeruli were sampled, and 5 (25%) were globally sclerotic. A variable degree of focal

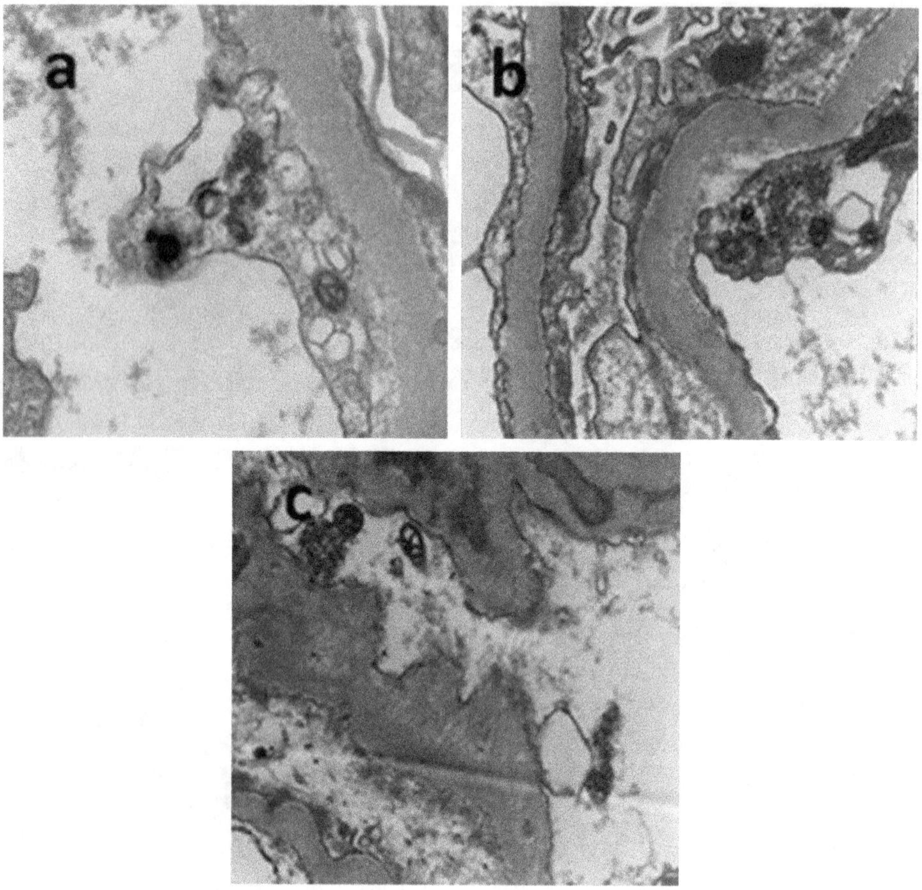

Figure 2: Electron microscopy (×35200–56200 magnification) showing (a) tubuloreticular inclusions (TRIs) in the endothelium of the glomerular capillaries, (b) thickened glomerular basement membrane with foot process effacement, and (c) absence of amorphous immune-type deposits (electron dense deposits).

segmental glomerulosclerosis (FSGS) with mesangial hypercellularity was present in the remaining glomeruli with collapsing features noted in 6 (30%) glomeruli. Immunofluorescence was negative, and there was no eosinophilic infiltrate. Additional findings included mild-to-moderate arteriosclerosis with moderate chronic interstitial inflammation comprising lymphocytes and plasma cells.

Human leukocyte antigen (HLA) B5701 testing returned negative, and the patient was initiated on cART with abacavir, lamivudine, atazanavir, and ritonavir prior to discharge. The patient was discharged with outpatient haemodialysis thrice weekly and followed up with infectious disease for HIV treatment. In 3 weeks, his viral load decreased to 17,000 copies/ml and then to 150 copies/ml in 2 months. Complete virologic suppression (undetectable viral load) was documented 11 months after cART initiation. His CD4 count improved to >200 cells/μL in 2 months. After 7 months on haemodialysis, it was noted that the patient was no longer oliguric and had no significant interdialytic change in BUN and sCr. Haemodialysis was discontinued, and the patient remained in stage 4 CKD range (as demonstrated in Figure 3).

3. Discussion

Classic HIVAN is identified by the following pathognomonic constellation of features: collapse of glomerular capillaries, visceral glomerular epitheliosis, podocyte hypertrophy and proliferation, mesangial prominence and hypercellularity, endothelial tubuloreticular inclusions (TRIs), and microcystic tubules [2,15]. It remains the most common renal histology finding in the HIV-infected [16], despite a decline in prevalence owing to the widespread use of cART. According to the US Renal Data System (USRDS), there has been 60% reduction in the risk of ESRD associated with HIVAN following the introduction of cART [17].

Three major groups of nephropathy are seen in HIV-positive patients: classic HIVAN, HIV-associated thrombotic microangiopathy, and HIV-associated immune-mediated glomerulonephritides [18]. The clinical presentation and pathological findings in this case were consistent with classic HIVAN. The duration of HIV infection for the patient was unknown, and although traditionally thought to occur later in the disease course, renal involvement may be seen as early as during acute seroconversion [13]. The exact pathogenesis of HIVAN and the mechanism by which cART improves renal function are unknown. Murine studies suggest that transgene expression is responsible for the histopathologic changes seen in HIVAN, and this process is mitigated by cART initiation [13, 19].

HIVAN is viewed as a disease that occurs as a direct effect of renal cellular HIV-1 infection and more so of HIV-1 gene products on the kidney. The effect of the HIV viral load

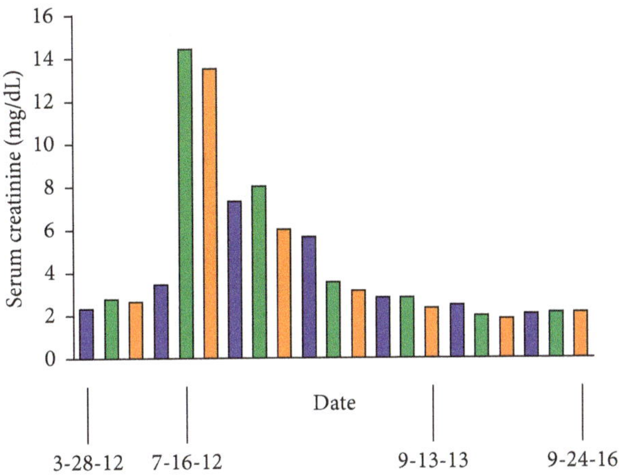

FIGURE 3: Demonstration of the change in serum creatinine over time showing return to stable baseline CKD 4 after cART initiation with sCr of approximately 2 mg/dL.

in the circulation on this process remains unclear. Reversal of dialysis dependence occurred in this case 4 months prior to complete virologic suppression. In the case by Vasquez et al., complete virologic suppression did not occur, not even 16 months after cessation of haemodialysis [14]. Wali et al. noted that after 13 weeks of cART and 12 weeks of haemodialysis, reversal of dialysis-dependence occurred with a detectable viral load (<500 copies/ml) [12]. Winston et al. noted that complete virologic suppression occurred within 6 weeks of cART, and in this case, haemodialysis was only required for 2-3 weeks [13].

In this case, only 5 (25%) of the sampled glomeruli were sclerotic without notable interstitial fibrosis or tubular atrophy (IFTA). Prior reports noted "patchy interstitial fibrosis" [13] and "mild periglomerular fibrosis" [12], while Vasquez et al. noted the presence of glomerular sclerosis but did not qualify its extent [14] (images of slides in this paper did not show significant IFTA). The initiation of cART before the onset of significant fibrosis appears to play a major role in recovery from and possibly progression to, dialysis dependence. However, there remains a paucity of data on this subject and despite use of cART many HIV patients progress to ESRD. Even in this subset, the survival of HIV-infected haemodialysis patients on cART is superior to those on suboptimal antiretroviral regimens or no treatment at all [20, 21].

In terms of treatment, ACE inhibitors and angiotensin II receptor blockade is recommended to slow disease progression in patients who have not shown significant improvement with cART alone. Renin-angiotensin blockade may help decrease proteinuria and slow progression of fibrosis, and this has been previously demonstrated in transgenic mice [22]. Glucocorticoids may provide benefit to cases with histologic evidence of dense tubulointerstitial inflammatory infiltrates. However, the evidence for this is limited, and their role remains controversial [23, 24]. Glucocorticoid therapy was neither employed in this case, nor the three prior referenced cases of HIVAN that recovered from dialysis dependence.

The Infectious Diseases Society of America (IDSA) recommends cART for all HIV-infected at time of diagnosis and referral to nephrology when there is albuminuria >300 mg per day, a clinically significant decline in glomerular filtration rate (GFR) or haematuria of renal origin [24]. Renal biopsy is encouraged as a definitive diagnosis may inform prognosis and treatment options. Further, the specificity and sensitivity of noninvasive testing is limited. The existing data have solidified the role of cART in the HIV-infected, regardless of whether renal disease is present or not. However, the interplay of host genetic factors and viral transgene expression that results in variable progression of nephropathy in those diagnosed with HIVAN remains largely unexplored.

4. Conclusion

The onset and progression of HIVAN remains variable, despite the widespread use of cART and an overall improved prognosis for the HIV-infected population. The authors describe the 4th case, as indexed in PubMed, of a patient with HIVAN who was liberated from dialysis dependence after the initiation of cART. There is a paucity of data on the subject and a lack of research into host genetic factors to account for the variable course of HIVAN in the era of cART. Further research is encouraged in this area since early cART initiation, prior to the onset of significant fibrosis in HIVAN, may prevent or reverse progression to ESRD.

References

[1] T. K. S. Rao, E. J. Filippone, A. D. Nicastri et al., "Associated focal and segmental glomerulosclerosis in the acquired immunodeficiency syndrome," *New England Journal of Medicine*, vol. 310, no. 11, pp. 669–673, 1984.

[2] V. Pardo, "Glomerular lesions in the acquired immunodeficiency syndrome," *Annals of Internal Medicine*, vol. 101, no. 4, pp. 429–434, 1984.

[3] J. Roling, H. Schmid, M. Fischereder, R. Draenert, and F. D. Goebel, "HIV-associated renal diseases and highly active antiretroviral therapy-induced nephropathy," *Clinical Infectious Diseases*, vol. 42, no. 10, pp. 1488–1495, 2006.

[4] A. Laurinavicius, S. Hurwitz, and H. G. Rennke, "Collapsing glomerulopathy in HIV and non-HIV patients: a clinico-pathological and follow-up study," *Kidney International*, vol. 56, no. 6, pp. 2203–2213, 1999.

[5] J. J. Bourgoignie, R. Meneses, C. Ortiz, D. Jaffe, and V. Pardo, "The clinical spectrum of renal disease associated with human immunodeficiency virus," *American Journal of Kidney Diseases*, vol. 12, no. 2, pp. 131–137, 1988.

[6] K. C. Abbott, I. Hypolite, P. G. Welch, and L. Y. Agodoa, "Human immunodeficiency virus/acquired immunodeficiency syndrome-associated nephropathy at end-stage renal disease in the United States: patient characteristics and survival in the pre highly active antiretroviral therapy era," *Journal of Nephrology*, vol. 14, pp. 377–383, 2001.

[7] A. H. Cohen and C. C. Nast, "HIV-associated nephropathy. A unique combined glomerular, tubular, and interstitial lesion," *Modern pathology*, vol. 1, pp. 87–97, 1988.

[8] P. Chander, A. Soni, A. Suri, R. Bhagwat, J. Yoo, and G. Treser, "Renal ultrastructural markers in AIDS-associated nephropathy," *The American Journal of Pathology*, vol. 126, no. 3, pp. 513–526, 1987.
[9] L. A. Szczech, S. K. Gupta, R. Habash et al., "The clinical epidemiology and course of the spectrum of renal diseases associated with HIV infection," *Kidney International*, vol. 66, no. 3, pp. 1145–1152, 2004.
[10] D. Scheurer, "Rapid reversal of renal failure after initiation of HAART: a case report," *The AIDS Reader*, vol. 14, no. 8, pp. 443–447, 2004.
[11] J. T. Kirchner, "Resolution of renal failure after initiation of HAART: 3 cases and a discussion of the literature," *The AIDS Reader*, vol. 12, no. 3, pp. 103–112, 2002.
[12] R. K. Wali, C. I. Drachenberg, J. C. Papadimitriou, S. Keay, and E. Ramos, "HIV-1-associated nephropathy and response to highly-active antiretroviral therapy," *The Lancet*, vol. 352, no. 9130, pp. 783-784, 1998.
[13] J. A. Winston, L. A. Bruggeman, M. D. Ross et al., "Nephropathy and establishment of a renal reservoir of HIV type 1 during primary infection," *New England Journal of Medicine*, vol. 344, no. 26, pp. 1979–1984, 2001.
[14] G. A. Vasquez, I. Brar, C. A. Abbud, and M. Faber, "Reversal of dialysis-dependent renal failure in a patient with HIV-associated nephropathy," *Infectious Diseases in Clinical Practice*, vol. 15, no. 6, pp. 415–418, 2007.
[15] M. H. Gardenswartz, C. W. Lerner, G. R. Seligson et al., "Renal disease in patients with AIDS: a clinicopathologic study," *Clinical Nephrology*, vol. 21, no. 21, pp. 197–204, 1984.
[16] A. Z. Rosenberg, S. Naicker, C. A. Winkler, and J. B. Kopp, "HIV-associated nephropathies: epidemiology, pathology, mechanisms and treatment," *Nature Reviews Nephrology*, vol. 11, no. 3, pp. 150–160, 2015.
[17] S. R. Chaudhary, B. T. Workeneh, M. E. Montez-Rath, A. R. Zolopa, P. E. Klotman, and W. C. Winkelmayer, "Trends in the outcomes of end-stage renal disease secondary to human immunodeficiency virus-associated nephropathy," *Nephrology Dialysis Transplantation*, vol. 30, pp. 1734–1740, 2015.
[18] S. D. Cohen, J. B. Kopp, and P. L. Kimmel, "Kidney diseases associated with human immunodeficiency virus infection," *New England Journal of Medicine*, vol. 377, no. 24, pp. 2363–2374, 2017.
[19] L. A. Bruggeman, S. Dikman, C. Meng, S. E. Quaggin, T. M. Coffman, and P. E. Klotman, "Nephropathy in human immunodeficiency virus-1 transgenic mice is due to renal transgene expression," *Journal of Clinical Investigation*, vol. 100, no. 1, pp. 84–92, 1997.
[20] T. S. Ahuja, J. Grady, and S. Khan, "Changing trends in the survival of dialysis patients with human immunodeficiency virus in the United States," *Journal of the American Society of Nephrology*, vol. 13, no. 7, pp. 1889–1893, 2002.
[21] T. S. Ahuja, M. Borucki, and J. Grady, "Highly active antiretroviral therapy improves survival of HIV-infected hemodialysis patients," *American Journal of Kidney Diseases*, vol. 36, no. 3, pp. 574–580, 2000.
[22] J. E. Bird, S. K. Durham, M. R. Giancarli et al., "Captopril prevents nephropathy in HIV-transgenic mice," *Journal of the American Society of Nephrology: JASN*, vol. 9, no. 9, pp. 1441–1447, 1998.
[23] J. A. Eustace, E. Nuermberger, M. Choi, P. J. Scheel, R. Moore, and W. A. Briggs, "Cohort study of the treatment of severe HIV-associated nephropathy with corticosteroids," *Kidney International*, vol. 58, no. 3, pp. 1253–1260, 2000.
[24] G. M. Lucas, M. J. Ross, P. G. Stock et al., "Clinical practice guideline for the management of chronic kidney disease in patients infected with HIV: 2014 update by the HIV medicine association of the infectious diseases society of America," *Clinical Infectious Diseases*, vol. 59, no. 9, pp. e96–e138, 2014.

Amlodipine-Induced Gingival Hyperplasia in a Young Male with Stage 5 Chronic Kidney Disease

Kevin John, Ajay Kumar Mishra, Karthik Gunasekaran, and Ramya Iyyadurai

Department of Medicine, Christian Medical College, Vellore, India

Correspondence should be addressed to Kevin John; kevinjohn619@gmail.com

Academic Editor: Ze'ev Korzets

Gingival hyperplasia is a rare finding in clinical practice. Nevertheless, when it occurs, it is a finding of great value as it can lead to definite clinical diagnosis. The present case is a 19-year-old male who was referred for further management of stage 5 chronic kidney disease. On evaluation, he was found to have gingival hyperplasia. He was evaluated for reversible causes of kidney disease, and since none were found, renal replacement therapy was advised. He had been taking amlodipine for blood pressure control. As this was presumed to be the cause of gingival hyperplasia, it was stopped and replaced by a combination of beta-blocker and prazosin. At six-month follow-up, he had complete resolution of gingival hyperplasia. Amlodipine as a cause of gingival hyperplasia is a rare occurrence. However, it is crucial to keep in mind such a possible side effect of this commonly prescribed antihypertensive drug.

1. Introduction

Gingival hyperplasia is a physical finding that is rarely encountered in clinical practice. However, once it is confirmed, it is an important sign as it can give a clue for the correct diagnosis of a patient. Over the years, various causes of gingival hyperplasia have been reported in the literature. The common causes of gingival hyperplasia are drugs, non-Hodgkin's lymphoma, acute monocytic leukemia, granulomatous diseases, and chronic periodontal infections [1]. This list can be further narrowed down with a focused history and physical examination. If a precise aetiology is established, it is often possible to avoid a biopsy, and treatment can be instituted by merely avoiding the etiological agent. In this context, it would be useful to know all the causes of gingival hyperplasia, both familiar and obscure. Here, we describe the rare case of a patient who presented with amlodipine-induced gingival hyperplasia in the background of stage 5 chronic kidney disease.

2. Case Presentation

A 19-year-old boy presented with nocturnal cough and bilateral lower limb swelling of 3 months duration. There were no complaints of frothy urine, decreased urine output, or hematuria. He was evaluated for these complaints at his hometown and diagnosed with hypertension and stage 5 chronic kidney disease. He did not have any addictions, allergies, or significant family history for kidney disease. He was started on 10 mg of amlodipine and referred to our hospital for further evaluation and management. After starting amlodipine, the patient noticed painless, gradually progressive, and irregular swelling of his gums with few episodes of bleeding while brushing his teeth. When he presented to us, he had been taking amlodipine for three months in total.

On presentation to the outpatient department, he had a blood pressure of 180/100 mmHg in both upper limbs. His heart rate was 84 beats/min, respiratory rate was 18 breaths/min, and arterial oxygen saturation on room air was 98%. He was afebrile. He was noted to have pitting pedal oedema of both lower limbs up to the midcalf. On intraoral examination massive, painless, gingival enlargement involving both the arches, encroaching buccal, palatal, and lingual vestibular spaces was found (Figure 1). The gingiva was pale pink, firm in consistency and not tender on palpation. There were no other positive findings on examination of the other systems.

He was evaluated for treatable causes of chronic kidney disease. Causes of gingival hyperplasia that were considered

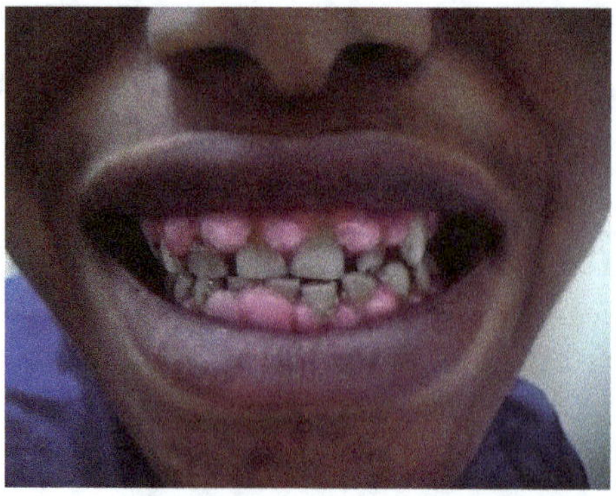

Figure 1: Photograph showing amlodipine-induced gingival hyperplasia.

included chronic periodontitis, drugs (calcium channel blockers such as amlodipine and nifedipine; cyclosporine and anticonvulsants such as phenytoin), acute monocytic leukemia, and non-Hodgkin's lymphoma.

The patient's initial blood investigations showed anaemia (Table 1). His creatinine was elevated, and an ultrasound scan showed bilateral shrunken kidneys with grade 3 renal parenchymal changes. The total duration of his kidney disease was not known. Kidney biopsy could not be performed given the small size and poor cortico-medullary differentiation. Hence, a complete evaluation of the cause of his kidney disease could not be conducted.

His blood leukocyte counts were normal, and this ruled out any blood dyscrasias. His blood picture did not show any blasts. He did not have lymphadenopathy. A diagnosis of stage 5 chronic kidney disease of unknown aetiology and secondary hypertension was made. A provisional diagnosis of amlodipine-induced gingival hyperplasia was made. Due to a clear temporal association, it was decided to assess response to the withdrawal of amlodipine before proceeding with further evaluation.

The patient was advised to take a low-salt renal diet. Amlodipine was stopped, and he was given a combination of atenolol and prazosin for blood pressure control. He was also started on febuxostat, torsemide, calcium and vitamin D supplements, phosphate binders, iron supplements, and erythropoietin. The need for renal replacement therapy was explained, and he was scheduled for the creation of an A-V(arteriovenous) fistula. The option of a renal transplant was also explained to him.

On follow-up after six months, the patient had complete resolution of gingival hyperplasia. A WHO-UMC causality assessment was performed, and the case fell into the "probable/likely" category. Proving "certain" causality would have required rechallenging the drug which would have been unethical. Therefore, it was considered to be sufficient evidence to attribute the cause of gingival hyperplasia to amlodipine. Chronic kidney disease was managed medically, and he was planned for an AV fistula creation for initiation of maintenance hemodialysis.

Table 1: Lab investigations.

Investigations	Result (normal range)
Haemoglobin (g/L)	90 (140–175)
Total count ($\times 10^9$/L)	6 (4.5–11.0)
Platelet count ($\times 10^9$/L)	154 (150–350)
HIV, HBV, HCV serology	Negative
Serum creatinine (μmol/L)	666.5 (62–106)
Erythrocyte sedimentation rate (ESR) (mm/hour)	22 (0–20)
Serum sodium (mmol/L)	138 (135–145)
Serum potassium (mmol/L)	5.2 (3.5–5)
Serum bicarbonate (mmol/L)	16 (22–29)
Serum uric acid (mg/dL)	5.8 (4–7)
Serum calcium (mg/dL)	7.81 (8.3–10.4)
Serum phosphorous (mg/dL)	5 (2.5–4.6)
Serum parathyroid hormone (pg/ml)	1305.3 (8–74)
c-ANCA(antineutrophilic cytoplasmic antibodies)	Negative
p-ANCA(antineutrophilic cytoplasmic antibodies)	Negative
Thyroid stimulating hormone (TSH) (μIU/ml)	2.6
Serum total complement	Normal
24-hour urine protein (g)	3.3 (50–150 mg)

3. Discussion

Amlodipine is a dihydropyridine calcium channel blocker that is commonly prescribed as an antihypertensive drug. The common side effects of amlodipine include headache, dizziness, and palpitations. Gingival hyperplasia is a rare side effect of this drug. The prevalence of gingival hyperplasia caused by amlodipine had been estimated by Jorgensen in 1997 as 3.3% for patients in the United States of America, while a study conducted in India in 2014 by Tejnaniet al. arrived at a similar number of 3.4% [2, 3]. This suggests that the prevalence of amlodipine induced gingival hyperplasia is similar across populations of different race and geography, and has remained stable over time. Other causes of gingival hyperplasia are drugs (other calcium channel blockers such as nifedipine; cyclosporine and anticonvulsants such as phenytoin), non-Hodgkin's lymphoma, acute monocytic leukemia, granulomatous diseases (sarcoidosis and Crohn's diseases), granulomatosis with polyangiitis, chronic periodontal infections, pyogenic granuloma, benign neoplasms such as fibroma or papilloma, malignant neoplasms such as carcinoma or malignant melanoma, syndromic causes (Rutherford syndrome, Cross syndrome, Ramon syndrome, and Laband syndrome), pregnancy, and idiopathic gingival hyperplasia [4].

It was known that calcium channel blockers such as nifedipine could cause gingival hyperplasia. When amlodipine was introduced into the market, there were similar reports of gingival hyperplasia with this drug also. This was first reported in 1993 by Ellis et al. [5]. Since then, there have been various reports of similar cases. It is seen to be three times more common in males than in females [6]. There is a reported case of amlodipine causing hyperplasia of the hard palate as well [7].

The exact mechanism of amlodipine-induced gingival hyperplasia is not known. Various mechanisms have been postulated. These include defective collagenase activity due to reduced folic acid uptake, increase in adrenocorticotrophic hormone (ACTH) due to block in aldosterone synthesis, increase in keratinocyte growth factor, inflammation due to the concentration of drug in the crevices and bacterial plaques, as well as upregulation of transforming growth factor-beta [8–10]. Other factors such as dental hygiene, nutritional deficiencies, comorbidities such as renal failure (as seen with our patient) and male sex may also contribute to the gingival hyperplasia [6]. This could also be a biased observation as a large proportion of patients with chronic kidney disease are on amlodipine therapy as an antihypertensive.

Substituting the drug amlodipine with another antihypertensive remains the basis of management. In our patient, gingival hyperplasia had resolved entirely within six months of stopping the drug. Regression within three months of stopping the drug has also been reported [11]. This suggests that amlodipine-induced gingival hyperplasia is reversible with cessation of the drug alone. However, some advocate surgical management for a better aesthetic outcome. Gingivectomy or periodontal flap surgery can be performed. Maintenance of good oral hygiene and regular brushing of teeth are also of paramount importance. In summary, amlodipine is a potentially reversible cause of gingival hyperplasia, and this needs to be considered while evaluating patients who present with gingival overgrowth.

Consent

Informed signed consent was obtained from the patient.

Acknowledgments

The authors would like to thank Prof. Varghese John for reviewing the manuscript.

References

[1] P. Holmstrup, J. Plemons, and J. Meyle, "Non-plaque-induced gingival diseases," *Journal of Periodontology*, vol. 89, no. S20, pp. S28–S45, 2018.

[2] M. G. Jorgensen, "Prevalence of amlodipine-related gingival hyperplasia," *Journal of Periodontology*, vol. 68, no. 7, pp. 676–678, 1997.

[3] A. Tejnani, A. Mani, N. Sodhi et al., "Incidence of amlodipine-induced gingival overgrowth in the rural population of Loni," *Journal of Indian Society of Periodontology*, vol. 18, no. 2, p. 226, 2014.

[4] F. Cekmez, O. Pirgon, and I. A. Tanju, "Idiopathic gingival hyperplasia," *International Journal of Biomedical Science: IJBS*, vol. 5, no. 5, pp. 198–200, 2009.

[5] J. Ellis, R. Seymour, J. M. Thomason, S. Monkman, and J. Idle, "Gingival sequestration of amlodipine and amlodipine-induced gingival overgrowth," *The Lancet*, vol. 341, no. 8852, pp. 1102-1103, 1993.

[6] S. Tavassoli, N. Yamalik, F. Çağlayan, G. Çağlayan, and K. Eratalay, "The clinical effects of nifedipine on periodontal status," *Journal of Periodontology*, vol. 69, no. 2, pp. 108–112, 1998.

[7] X. Wang, Q. Liu, G. Dong, and Q. Wang, "Reversible hard palate hyperplasia associated with amlodipine use: case report," *International Journal of Clinical Pharmacology and Therapeutics*, vol. 54, no. 9, pp. 712–715, 2016.

[8] A. Nyska, M. Shemesh, H. Tal, and D. Dayan, "Gingival hyperplasia induced by calcium channel blockers: mode of action," *Medical Hypotheses*, vol. 43, no. 2, pp. 115–118, 1994.

[9] S. J. Das and I. Olsen, "Keratinocyte growth factor is upregulated by the hyperplasia-inducing drug nifedipine," *Cytokine*, vol. 12, no. 10, pp. 1566–1569, 2000.

[10] W. A. Border and N. A. Noble, "Transforming growth factor beta in tissue fibrosis," *The New England Journal of Medicine*, vol. 331, no. 331, pp. 1286–1292, 1994.

[11] N. M. Aldemir, H. Begenik, H. Emre, F. M. Erdur, and Y. Soyoral, "Amlodipine-induced gingival hyperplasia in chronic renal failure: a case report," *African Health Sciences*, vol. 12, no. 12, pp. 576–578, 2012.

32

The Various Forms of Nephrotic Syndrome in a Patient with Systemic Lupus Erythematosus

Sophia Lionaki,[1] George Liapis,[2] Kalliope Vallianou,[1] Chrysovalantis Vergadis,[3] and Ioannis Boletis[1]

[1]*Nephrology Department and Transplantation Unit, Laiko Hospital, National & Kapodistrian University of Athens, Faculty of Medicine, Athens, Greece*
[2]*Pathology Department, Laiko Hospital, Athens, Greece*
[3]*Radiology Department, Laiko Hospital, Athens, Greece*

Correspondence should be addressed to Sophia Lionaki; sofia.lionaki@gmail.com

Academic Editor: Hernán Trimarchi

Kidney involvement is frequent in patients with systemic lupus erythematosus (SLE), although it may not be present from disease onset. Renal lupus itself is highly heterogenous with respect to the combination and/or severity of clinical and/or laboratory manifestations. This is a case of a 45-year-old Caucasian female with an established diagnosis of SLE, who presented four times with new onset of proteinuria during a follow-up time of ten years, since the diagnosis of SLE. Specifically, she experienced two episodes of lupus membranous nephropathy, and after she achieved remission, she developed twice overt nephrotic syndrome associated with new and biopsy proven lupus podocytopathy. All these episodes of nephrotic syndrome were combined with systemic symptoms, attributed to lupus itself, while serological activity of lupus was also noted. This case highlights the importance of performing a kidney biopsy in all patients with SLE who have new renal manifestations, including nephrotic proteinuria.

1. Introduction

Kidney involvement is very frequent in patients with systemic lupus erythematosus (SLE), although it may not be present from disease onset. Renal lupus itself is highly heterogenous with respect to the combination and/or severity of clinical and laboratory manifestations. The performance of each patient with kidney abnormalities is also variable but most importantly, different clinical settings and histopathological patterns may be found in the same patient over time. Nephrotic syndrome in patients with SLE is classically associated with proliferative glomerulonephritis or membranous nephropathy (WHO class III, IV, and V) [1, 2]. However, lupus podocytopathy associated with nephrotic proteinuria has been repeatedly reported in these patients [3], which is characterized by absent or scarce capillary wall immune complex deposition, or cellular proliferation, but diffuse effacement of the epithelial cell foot processes, identical to the histopathological pattern of minimal-change disease [4]. The diagnostic and classification criteria for lupus podocytopathy, which have been proposed by the American College of Rheumatology include the clinical diagnosis of full nephrotic syndrome combined with histopathology showing normal glomeruli by light microscopy, i.e., minimal-change disease (MCD), or focal segmental glomerulosclerosis (FSGS) with or without mesangial proliferation but with no endocapillary proliferation, necrosis, and/or crescents by immunofluorescence microscopy without deposits confined to the mesangium, and by electron microscopy diffuse and severe (typically >70%) foot process effacement [1]. It is considered to be rather pertinent than a simple coincidence [3], given the statistical unlikelihood of concurrent active lupus and idiopathic minimal change glomerulopathy. Accumulated evidence from clinical experience and epidemiologic observations indicate that lupus podocytopathy is related to the disease itself and is not random. Herein, we describe a case of a lupus patient, who developed overt nephrotic syndrome associated with new and biopsy proven lupus podocytopathy, following therapy and remission of previously diagnosed lupus membranous nephropathy. Furthermore, mesangial proliferation is the most common presentation (56%) followed by MCD (26%) and FSGS (18%). Undoubtedly, patients with FSGS have worse outcomes, higher rates of hypertension, and acute kidney injury on clinical presentation, with more severe tubulointerstitial involvement on kidney biopsy compared to patients with MCD and mesangial proliferative lesions.

2. Case Description

This is a case of a 45-year-old Caucasian female with an established diagnosis of SLE, who presented four times with new onset of proteinuria during a follow-up time of ten years since the diagnosis of SLE. The first time, 2 years after the diagnosis of lupus, she presented with proteinuria (mean value 3.3 grams), glomerular hematuria, and normal serum creatinine, combined with musculoskeletal symptoms, leukopenia, rash, positive antinuclear antibodies (ANA) >1: 640, and low serum complements. The kidney biopsy clearly revealed lupus membranous nephropathy (WHO class V), i.e., subepithelial deposits and a full house pattern by immunofluorescence. She was started on therapy with oral methylprednisolone, cyclosporine, and hydroxychloroquine with complete remission of proteinuria and hematuria within 4 months (Table 1). However, 11 months later, she relapsed on therapy with new onset of proteinuria (14 grams per day), inactive urine sediment, normal renal function, fatigue, lymphadenopathy, generalized skin rash, and increased anti-dsDNA antibodies. A new kidney biopsy was performed, showing again lupus membranous nephropathy, with numerous, well-defined subepithelial, dense deposits by electron microscopy (EM). Mycophenolate mofetil was initiated in combination with glucocorticoids, and cyclosporine was withdrawn. She achieved complete remission again within a few months. Two years later, while on mycophenolate mofetil and low-dose prednisolone, she presented with new onset of nephrotic syndrome, i.e., edema anasarca and proteinuria (3.6 grams per day), combined with microscopic hematuria, skin rash, anemia, arthralgias, myalgias, high titers of antinuclear and anti-dsDNA antibodies, and low serum complement levels. The third kidney biopsy showed glomeruli of normal size, mild hyper cellularity, and normal thickness of the basement membrane. Immunofluorescence was negative, and EM revealed diffuse effacement of the podocyte foot processes >70%, consistent with lupus podocytopathy with the morphologic type of MCD and mild mesangial hyper cellularity. Mycophenolate mofetil was discontinued, and the patient was treated with high-dose glucocorticoids, i.e., 1 mg/kg body weight (BW) prednisolone daily, leading to remission within two months. However, tapering of glucocorticoids resulted in proteinuria increase, and thus, oral cyclophosphamide (2 mg/kg BW) was initiated for a total of three months with achievement of complete remission. The patient was maintained on 4 mg of methylprednisolone but unfortunately, six months later, she experienced again full-blown nephrotic syndrome. Of note, arterial pressure was well controlled with low dose of fosinopril. At this point, we performed a fourth biopsy, which was diagnostic again for lupus podocytopathy. She was treated with cyclosporine (3 mg/kg BW) and glucocorticoids (0.25 mg/kg BW) with a remarkable improvement of 24-hour urinary protein excretion, which returned to normal values within two months. Glucocorticoids were gradually reduced to 4 mg per day, while cyclosporine was tapered slowly until discontinuation. To date, she remains on hydroxychloroquine, with normal renal function and 24-hour urinary protein excretion, without extrarenal manifestations.

3. Discussion

Nephrotic syndrome or nephrotic range proteinuria in the context of SLE is often associated with identification of immune deposits in the glomerular capillary wall, with or without endocapillary proliferation and/or necrosis. However, there are reports of lupus patients who developed nephrotic syndrome in the absence of capillary wall immune deposits or cellular proliferation [3–10]. The lupus patient, who is described here, presented with nephrotic proteinuria with or without symptoms of nephrotic syndrome in four separate circumstances. In two occasions, histopathology revealed lupus membranous nephropathy (WHO class V) [1, 2] and in the other two, lupus podocytopathy, manifested as minimal-change disease. The probability of lupus podocytopathy, manifested as idiopathic minimal-change disease or idiopathic focal segmental glomerulosclerosis, has been estimated by Hertig et al. to be in <1 in 10,000 [3]. Yet, the observed prevalence of lupus podocytopathy was far higher than expected by chance, i.e., 2 per 132 patients with lupus involvement, in that study. Kraft et al. [4] reported 8 cases, derived from a pool of 470 renal biopsies performed in patients with SLE and abnormal renal indexes. Another series of seven lupus patients with diffuse podocyte effacement on renal biopsy manifested with nephrotic syndrome was presented by Dube et al. [5].

In our patient, like in most other cases, onset of nephrotic syndrome was observed in combination with clinical systemic symptoms of SLE and/or serological findings indicative of active disease and the discovery of lupus podocytopathy by histopathology. This is supportive of the notion that lupus podocytopathy is the result of active disease, more likely than the coexistence of two separate clinical entities who run concurrently [4]. More recently, Hu et al. studied fifty patients with lupus podocytopathy, counting for the 1.3% of all biopsies performed in lupus patients in their registry during the period 2000–2013 [11]. All had nephrotic syndrome and more than 70% foot process effacement [11]. Besides, a

Table 1: Laboratory indexes and serological parameters at the time of kidney biopsy.

	24 h proteinuria (grams)	Glomerular hematuria	Serum creatinine (mg/dl)	Serum albumin (g/dl)	C3 (>80 mg/dl)	C4 (>10 mg/dl)	Antinuclear antibodies (<7 IU)
Biopsy #1	3.5	Yes	0.6	3.7	57	7	1/640
Biopsy #2	3.0	Yes	0.6	3.2	124	23	1/640
Biopsy #3	3.6	Yes	0.7	2.9	68	9	1/640
Biopsy #4	3.7	No	0.9	3.3	79	9.8	1/640

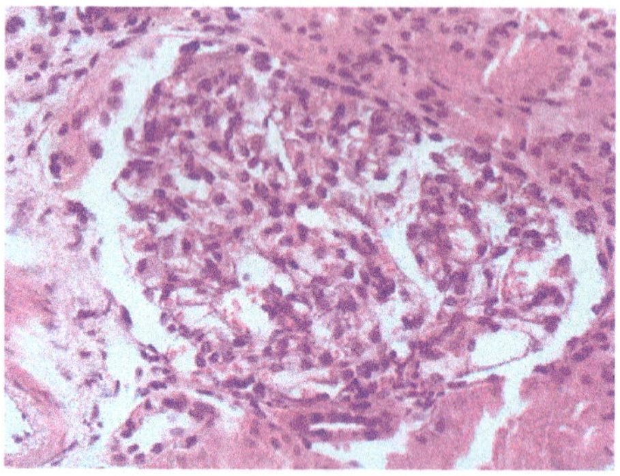

Figure 1: Glomerulus with no essential abnormalities; segmental and mild mesangial expansion at the time of lupus podocytopathy diagnosis (H&E, 400X).

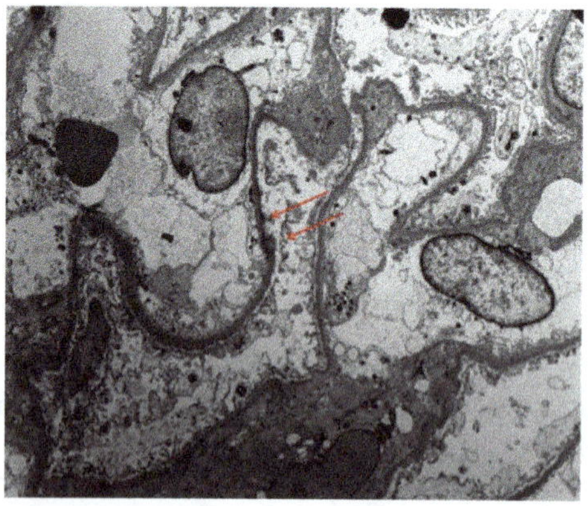

Figure 2: Diffuse foot process effacement (>70%) with scarce subepithelial deposits (red arrows), which represent residual scar from previous episodes of membranous nephropathy (uranyl acetate and lead citrate, 2800X).

pathological transition can occur after renal relapse. In the study of Hu et al. [11], six patients changed from lupus podocytopathy to lupus nephritis class IV ($n = 3$) and class V ($n = 3$) while in our case transition occurred form class V to lupus podocytopathy. Based on their findings, Hu et al. proposed certain criteria for the diagnosis of lupus podocytopathy using clinical and pathological parameters. In this regard, and considering this entity as a distinct one, we need to establish a more specific connection between its pathogenesis and the activity of SLE [12] than the observation that these two occur concurrently. Furthermore, addition of this disease in the new revised classification of lupus nephritis is another requirement.

The patient received therapy guided by the histopathological findings in each of these instances and finally achieved sustained remission. The treatment of lupus podocytopathy is based on observational and retrospective studies as the disease is quite rare. It generally follows the concept of therapy of MCD (glucocorticoids alone) or FSGS (combined with another immunosuppressive agent, i.e., calcineurin inhibitors, cyclophosphamide, or rituximab) considering that FSGS has a low rate of complete remission (22%) and a higher relapse rate (30–60%). Most patients with FSGS have a partial remission (55%) or do not respond to therapy (22%), with a longer median time to achieve remission (Figures 1 and 2).

Overall, the proposed criteria for the diagnosis of lupus podocytopathy in Oliva-Damaso and Chen [1, 13] are similar. In addition, Oliva-Damaso and co-authors proposed criteria for the clinical classification and also the inclusion of lupus podocytopathy in the classification of lupus nephritis, in between class II and Class III lupus nephritis. These authors proposed to include lupus podocytopathy in the International Society of Nephrology/Renal Pathology Society classification of lupus nephritis, as it is becoming clear now, that lupus podocytopathy is not a coexisting histological lesion but an independent type of renal involvement in SLE.

4. Conclusion

Lupus podocytopathy, which is characterized by diffuse foot process effacement without peripheral capillary wall immune deposits or glomerular proliferation, has been repeatably described in lupus patients with nephrotic syndrome and is becoming clear that it represents an independent type of renal involvement in patients with SLE. A kidney biopsy is mandatory in any new episode of renal involvement in lupus patients. Therapy should always be guided by histopathology, because renal indexes alone cannot precisely predict the type of the renal lesion.

Acknowledgments

The authors thank Dr. George Baltatzis for technical support in EM.

References

[1] N. Oliva-Damaso, J. Payan, E. Oliva-Damaso, T. Pereda, and A. S. Bomback, "Lupus podocytopathy: an overview," *Advances in Chronic Kidney Disease*, vol. 26, no. 5, pp. 369–375, 2019.

[2] J. J. Weening, V. D. D'agati, M. M. Schwartz et al., "The classification of glomerulonephritis in systemic lupus eryth-

ematosus revisited," *Kidney International*, vol. 65, no. 2, pp. 521–530, 2004.

[3] A. Hertig, D. Droz, P. Lesavre, J.-P. Grünfeld, and P. Rieu, "SLE and idiopathic nephrotic syndrome: coincidence or not?," *American Journal of Kidney Diseases*, vol. 40, no. 6, pp. 1179–1184, 2002.

[4] S. W. Kraft, M. M. Schwartz, S. M. Korbet, and E. J. Lewis, "Glomerular podocytopathy in patients with systemic lupus erythematosus," *Journal of the American Society of Nephrology*, vol. 16, no. 1, pp. 175–179, 2005.

[5] G. K. Dube, G. S. Markowitz, J. Radhakrishnan, G. B. Appel, and V. D. D'Agati, "Minimal change disease in systemic lupus erythematosus," *Clinical Nephrology*, vol. 57, no. 2, pp. 120–126, 2002.

[6] N. Stankeviciute, W. Jao, A. Bakir, and J. P. Lash, "Mesangial lupus nephritis with associated nephrotic syndrome," *Journal of the American Society of Nephrology: JASN*, vol. 8, no. 7, pp. 1199–1204, 1997.

[7] G. Nishihara, M. Nakamoto, C. Yasunaga et al., "Systemic lupus erythema- tosus in a patient with remitting minimal change nephrotic syndrome," *Clinical Nephrology*, vol. 48, no. 5, pp. 327–330, 1997.

[8] C. Perakis, A. Arvanitis, F. Sotsiou, and D. S. Emmanouel, "Nephrotic syndrome caused by minimal-change disease in a patient with focal proliferative SLE nephritis (WHO III) in remission," *Nephrology Dialysis Transplantation*, vol. 13, no. 2, pp. 467–470, 1998.

[9] T. E. Hunley, A. Yared, A. Fogo, and R. C. MacDonell, "Nephrotic syndrome in an adolescent: the cry of the wolf," *American Journal of Kidney Diseases: The Official Journal of the National Kidney Foundation*, vol. 31, no. 1, pp. 155–160, 1998.

[10] H. Makino, T. Haramoto, K. Shikata, T. Ogura, and Z. Ota, "Minimal-change nephrotic syndrome associated with systemic lupus erythematosus," *American Journal of Nephrology*, vol. 15, no. 5, pp. 439–441, 1995.

[11] W. Hu, Y. Chen, S. Wang et al., "Clinical-morphological features and outcomes of lupus podocytopathy," *Clinical Journal of the American Society of Nephrology*, vol. 11, no. 4, pp. 585–592, 2016.

[12] A. S. Bomback and G. S. Markowitz, "Lupus podocytopathy: a distinct entity," *Clinical Journal of the American Society of Nephrology*, vol. 11, no. 4, pp. 547-548, 2016.

[13] D. Chen and W. Hu, "Lupus podocytopathy: a distinct entity of lupus nephritis," *Journal of Nephrology*, vol. 31, no. 5, pp. 629–634, 2018.

ANCA-Negative Vasculitis in Eosinophilic Granulomatosis with Polyangiitis Complicated with Membranous Nephropathy: A Case Report and Brief Literature Review

Eri Kasama,[1] Jun Ino,[1] Fumika Iemura,[1] Saeko Kumon,[1] Mio Kodama,[1] Keitaro Sato,[1] Hitoshi Eizumi,[1] Kosaku Nitta,[2] and Junichi Hoshino[2]

[1]*Department of Nephrology, Kidney Center, Toda Central General Hospital, 1-19-3 Hon-cho, Toda City, Saitama 335-0023, Japan*
[2]*Department of Nephrology, Tokyo Women's Medical University, 8-1 Kawada-cho, Shinjyuku-ku, Tokyo 162-0054, Japan*

Correspondence should be addressed to Jun Ino; pikkun46@hotmail.com

Academic Editor: Kouichi Hirayama

Renal involvement in eosinophilic granulomatosis with polyangiitis (EGPA) typically occurs in anti-neutrophil cytoplasmic autoantibody (ANCA)-positive cases presenting with rapidly progressive renal insufficiency and urinary abnormalities induced by primarily necrotizing crescentic glomerulonephritis (NCGN). Recently, ANCA-negative EGPA has also been reported to manifest with renal involvement, such as NCGN or non-NCGN, including membranous nephropathy (MN). Herein, we report a 70-year-old female who presented with purpura on the lower legs, upper limb numbness, renal dysfunction (eGFR, 20.5 ml/min/1.73 m^2), and eosinophilia (eosinophils, 37,570/μl). MPO-and PR3-ANCA were negative, and urinalysis revealed urine protein (0.63 g/day) but without red blood cells in the urine sediment. Thus, she was diagnosed with ANCA-negative EGPA with rapidly progressive renal dysfunction. A renal biopsy revealed vasculitis in the interlobular arteries without NCGN, with the vasculitis being complicated by MN. Micrograph findings on fluorescence immunostaining contained both primary and secondary characteristics of MN (dominance of IgG subclass 4 more than subclass 1 vs. negativity of PLA2R and THSD7A). After treatment with prednisolone, her eosinophil counts normalized, and renal dysfunction improved. Furthermore, urine protein did not increase above 1.0 g/day during the clinical course. This is a rare case of ANCA-negative EGPA presenting with acute renal dysfunction without NCGN and subclinical MN with unknown etiology. It is important to recognize that EGPA pathology varies widely throughout the disease course, and the clinical course of subclinical MN should be carefully assessed in further follow-ups.

1. Introduction

Eosinophilic granulomatosis with polyangiitis (EGPA) is a systemic vasculitis that is involved in anti-neutrophil cytoplasmic autoantibody (ANCA)-associated vasculitis (AAV). Although EGPA shares some common pathologies with AAV, microscopic polyangiitis, and granulomatosis with polyangiitis, EGPA has distinct clinical findings of severe asthma and eosinophilic sinusitis. Specifically, there is a significant increase in peripheral blood eosinophils that occurs several years before eosinophilic inflammation and vasculitis become apparent. ANCA occurs in approximately 40–60% of patients with EGPA [1]; however, the exact mechanism of the prevalence of EGPA and the role of ANCA in EGPA, particularly the association between ANCA and eosinophilic inflammation, remain unclear [2]. Moreover, ANCA-positive patients present with a greater frequency of renal insufficiency, sinusitis, and peripheral neuropathy than that in ANCA-negative patients [2].

Meanwhile, a typical renal histological finding in patients with EGPA is necrotizing crescentic glomerulonephritis (NCGN) that leads to rapid progressive renal deficiency. However, it was recently reported that 10% of EGPA was complicated with non-NCGN, such as membranous nephropathy (MN), of which most were ANCA negative [3]. Furthermore, MN complicated in EGPA has been previously reported for both ANCA-positive [4–6] and -negative [7, 8] cases. Although ANCA is recognized as a useful marker to differentiate the heterogeneous clinical spectrum of EGPA [9], it is difficult to clarify all clinical findings from ANCA results given the aforementioned exceptions.

We experienced a rare case of ANCA-negative EGPA, wherein rapid progressive renal insufficiency was caused by small vasculitis in the interlobular arteries rather than NCGN and was complicated with MN without nephrotic syndrome. We present herein the clinical course of this rare case, assessing the relationships among ANCA-negative EGPA, renal damage, and MN.

2. Case Presentation

A 70-year-old Japanese female, who was previously diagnosed with asthma 10 years ago and received steroid inhalation therapy from her primary doctor, developed general fatigue, appetite loss, numbness in the upper limb, and a red rash on the lower legs. Examination revealed a rapid decrease in renal function (creatinine [Cr], 1.78 mg/dL and estimated glomerular filtration rate [eGFR], 22.5 mL/min/1.73 m^2 vs. Cr, 0.73 mg/dL and eGFR, 60.1 mL/min/1.73 m^2 4 months prior), so the patient was referred to our hospital. Blood examination on the day of admission revealed the following: peripheral eosinophilia (eosinophils, 37,570/μL), upregulated inflammatory markers (white blood cells, 47,560/μL; C-reactive protein, 1.0 mg/dL), renal dysfunction (Cr, 1.94 mg/dL; eGFR, 20.5 mL/min/1.73 m^2), and negative PR3-ANCA and MPO-ANCA. Additionally, there were no prescriptions that could cause drug-induced eosinophilia. Urinalysis revealed urine protein (0.63 g/day) but without red blood cells in urine sediment. Although chest and brain computed tomography (CT) revealed no abnormal findings, CT of the sinuses demonstrated not only poor air-containing and hyper-absorptive areas predominantly in the left ethmoid sinus, which indicated rhinosinusitis, but also scattered polyps in the bilateral maxillary sinuses. The red rash on the lower legs and numbness in the upper limb were diagnosed as purpura by a dermatologist and as mononeuropathy by a neurologist, respectively. The patient met the new classification criteria for EGPA, recently published by the American College of Rheumatology/European Alliance of Association for Rheumatology (a minimum score of 6 points is required for the classification of EGPA) [10]. The patient scored 11 points: (1) bronchial asthma as an obstructive airway disease; +3 points, (2) Nasal polyps; +3 points, and (3) blood eosinophil count $\geq 1 \times 10^9$/liter; +5 points.

After administration of prednisolone (PSL) 50 mg/day (1.0 mg/kg/day), the patient's general condition improved, eosinophils disappeared, and renal function showed slight recovery (Cr, 1.30 mg/dl; eGFR, 28.2 mL/min/1.73 m^2). Percutaneous renal biopsy was performed 8 days after PSL administration, wherein light microscopy findings (Figures 1(a)–1(d)) showed 41 glomeruli without crescentic formation or apparent membrane changes. There was also moderate-to-severe infiltration of inflammatory cells into the interstitial lesion but without eosinophil infiltration and granuloma formation. Additionally, we observed inflammatory cell infiltration into the lumen in some interlobular arteries, fibrin deposition, necrotizing lesions on the vascular wall, and rupture of elastic fibers. Fluorescence immunostaining (Figure 1(e)) further showed dominant granular to linear glomerular capillary deposits in IgG4; however, PLA2R and THSD7A were negative. Electron microscopy (Figure 1(f)) showed subepithelial electron-dense deposits (EDDs) and a thickened basement membrane with spike formation. The EDDs were limited to the subepithelium and were relatively uniform in size and distribution. Considering these findings, two major histological diagnoses were made: (1) fibrinoid necrotizing vasculitis in microvessels and (2) early-stage MN.

After PSL was reduced to 40 mg/day, the patient was discharged and followed up at our outpatient clinic. She is currently well, and her renal function has recovered to almost equivalent to age-appropriate levels (Cr, 0.89 mg/dl; eGFR, 47.5 mL/min/1.73 m^2). No abnormality in proteinuria was found 4 months prior (0.07 g/day) and at the latest visit in December 2021 (0.10 g/day). Symptoms including numbness and purpura improved after the administration of steroids, and no recurrence of these symptoms have been observed since. However, continuous inhalation therapy was necessary to stabilize asthma.

3. Discussion

We encountered a rare case of ANCA-negative EGPA that caused rapid progressive renal insufficiency and was complicated with MN without nephrotic syndrome. Histological findings revealed necrotizing vasculitis in the interlobular arteries and moderate-to-severe infiltration of inflammatory cells (not eosinophils) into the interstitial lesion as the EGPA pathology. Meanwhile, MN pathology was characterized by subepithelial EDDs and a thickened basement membrane with spike formations in the glomerular capillaries, as observed on electron microscopy.

The difference in the clinical findings of EGPA is reported to be related to two types of tissue damage linked to the diversity of ANCA: ANCA-mediated small vessel inflammation in ANCA-positive cases or eosinophilic inflammation in ANCA-negative cases [2]. In particular, the kidney is recognized as a representative target organ in ANCA-positive EGPA, with 80% of EGPA patients with renal involvement being ANCA positive [11]. A previous multicenter study also reported that rapid progressive renal insufficiency (52%) and isolated urinary tract abnormalities (48%) were two major renal clinical findings and that, as an important histological sign supporting renal insufficiency, NCGN presented in ANCA-positive EGPA patients [12]. Therefore, the rare feature of our case is acute renal impairment in ANCA-negative EGPA, which was likely caused by necrotizing vasculitis of the interlobular arteries rather than the typical NCGN. Other reports of ANCA-negative EGPA with renal involvement

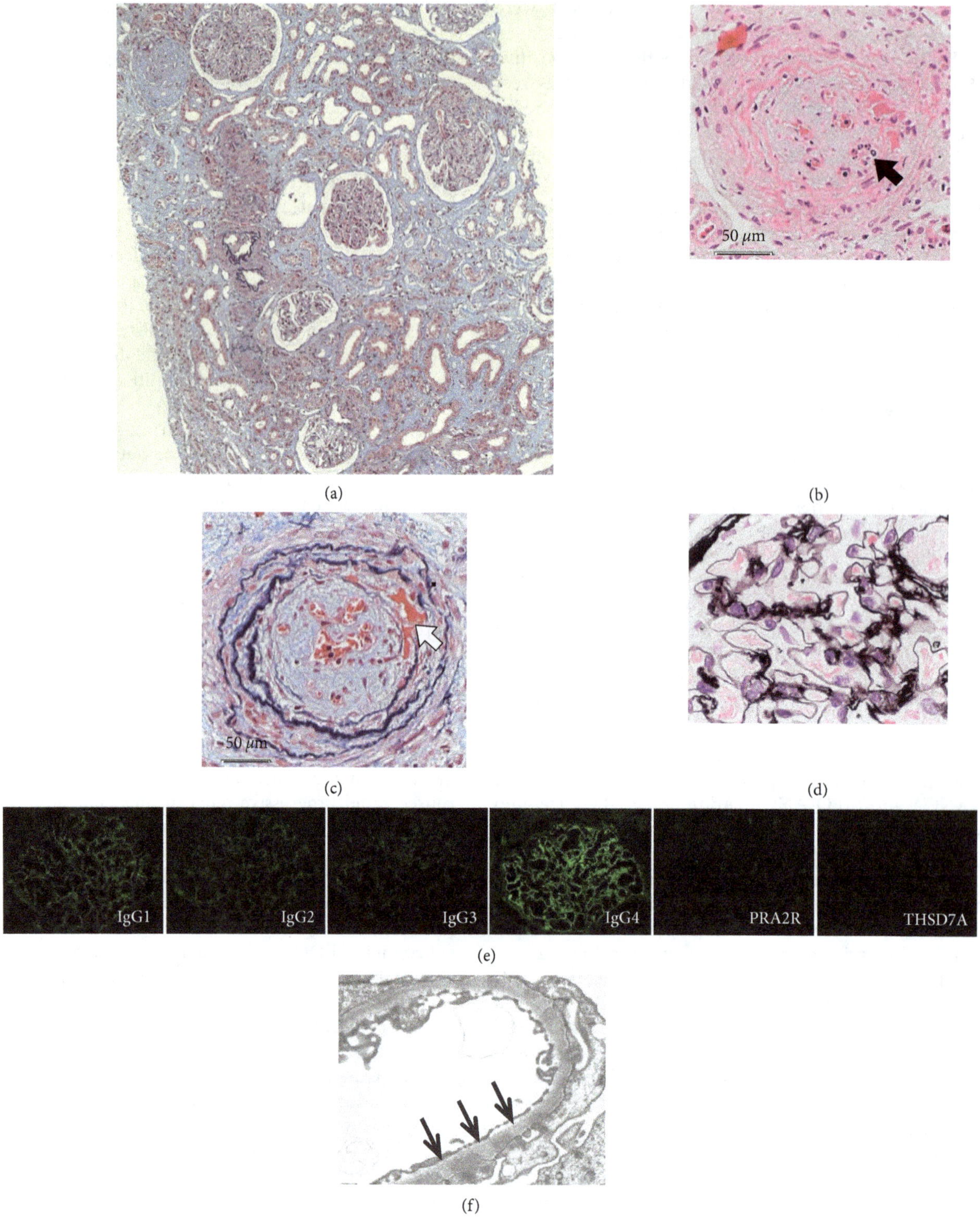

FIGURE 1: Histological findings of the renal specimen. Light microscopy image showing infiltration of inflammatory cells in the interstitial area and a severe degree of interstitial fibrosis and tubular atrophy (about 60%) but without granulomas ((a): PAS staining, original magnification ×100). Among the interlobular arteries, some show inflammatory cell infiltration in the lumen ((b): black arrow, hematoxylin and eosin staining, original magnification ×400), fibrin deposition in the vascular wall, and rupture of the elastic fibers ((c): white arrow, PAS staining, original magnification ×400). There are no significant abnormal findings in the glomerulus, including membrane changes ((d): periodic acid-methenamine silver staining, original magnification ×400). As shown in the micrograph of fluorescence immunostaining ((e): original magnification ×400), glomerular capillary deposits are dominant in IgG4. PLA2R and THSD7A are negative, suspicious of a secondary pathology. Electron microscopy image ((f): original magnification ×3000) showing subepithelial electron-dense deposits (EDDs) and a thickened basement membrane with spike formation (arrow). EDDs are limited to the subepithelium and are relatively uniform in size and distribution, which is not a finding of a secondary pathology.

that were evaluated with renal biopsy also showed a heterogeneous clinical picture of vasculitis. Notably, one case reported pauci-immune crescentic glomerulonephritis and pulmonary hemorrhage [13], and another case reported isolated proteinuria with glomerular angionecrosis and eosinophil infiltration complicated by intracardiac thrombus [14].

Clinical diversity in patients with ANCA-negative EGPA might be associated with the pathological diversity that could occur over the long-term process of EGPA development. Originally, EGPA development involves three common phases [15]: prodromal localized inflammation by an unknown antigen with a genetic component, eosinophilic inflammation triggered by Th2-related cytokines [16], and ANCA-induced vasculitis [17]. Considering the transition of these phases, EGPA does not always show a consistent clinical picture within each phase. Therefore, we speculated that ANCA-negative vasculitis could occur as a clinical picture that is different from the completed picture of phase 3. This means that ANCA in tissues could cause vasculitis even if the circulating ANCA is not yet at an identifiable level. Although the precise mechanisms leading to the occurrence of ANCA-negative vasculitis remain unclear, ANCA-negative pauci-immune NCGN appears to be a part of a systemic vasculitis disease process [18]. Therefore, depending on the timing of the examination and diagnosis in the long-term course, EGPA could present with varying pathophysiological findings, including the extent of ANCA involvement.

On the other hand, a recent report of 63 renal biopsy-proven EGPA cases revealed that eosinophilic infiltration could contribute to renal involvement in EGPA [3]. In the present case, there was no significant infiltration of eosinophils into the interstitial tissues, which made it difficult to determine the connection between renal dysfunction and eosinophilic inflammation. However, the absence of eosinophilic inflammation in the renal tissue in our case could be explained by the patient's good response to steroids for EGPA, thereby resolving eosinophil infiltration after steroid treatment [9]. Hence, rapid progressive renal insufficiency without NCGN in the present case was deemed to have occurred due to necrotizing vasculitis in the interlobular arteries and, possibly, eosinophil infiltration.

The unique features of MN in this case included the absence of nephrotic syndrome, which is reported to occur in 70–80% of MN patients [19], and histological findings of both primary and secondary characteristics. If the present case was primary MN that was accidentally identified in subclinical nephrotic syndrome, old age would be the most likely trigger, and further examinations and treatments for proteinuria should be considered in the future. Whereas, in a case of secondary MN complicated with EGPA, a relationship beyond accidental coexistence is most likely, based on the following reports: MN could occur secondary to systemic diseases, such as autoimmune diseases [20]; 10% of EGPA was identified to be complicated with MN, of which most were ANCA-negative [3]; both conditions may share a genetic background of a common HLA allele; and both pathological conditions are similarly mediated by Th2 inflammatory response [21]. However, if the present case was a secondary MN related to EGPA, it makes sense to clinically and pathologically recognize large amounts of urinary protein and more advanced MN findings, respectively, in line with the timing of EGPA onset due to its increased activity. Similarly, although the dominance of IgG4 staining, which is characteristic of primary MN [22], could occur in advanced-stage secondary MN [23], the fact that our case was in the early stage without spike formation prompted us to consider primary MN. Additionally, although recent studies have revealed the distinct genetic predisposition of primary MN patients [24] and the involvement of self-antigens PLA2R and THSD7A in the development of primary MN [25, 26], primary MN with negative results for both self-antigens is not uncommon, with an incidence of up to 40% in Japan [27]. A previous study also reported that self-antigens other than PLA2R and THSD7A were possibly involved in MN [23], further supporting that MN was likely to be primary in our case. Furthermore, the localization pattern of EDDs to the subepithelium was also suggestive of primary MN [28].

We compared the clinicopathological features described in the six previous case reports of EGPA complicated with MN, including both ANCA-positive [4–6] and negative cases [7, 8], with our case (Table 1). We found that those with rapidly progressing renal deficiency demonstrated NCGN histologically, except for our case, and that renal function was recovered in almost all cases. Contrarily, those without renal dysfunction had no NCGN. Although eosinophilic infiltration was 50%, the close association between eosinophilic infiltration and MN, as previously reported [3], remained unclear, owing to scarce information on histological findings. All cases also demonstrated nephrotic syndrome, except for our case, and showed good responsiveness to therapies, reaching complete or partial remission. Moreover, all clinicopathological and prognostic factors appeared to be independent of ANCA positivity. A notable difference we found was that the present patient was older than the six previous ones. Thus, it was considered that the accidental finding of age-related MN complication and age-related effects on immune response were responsible for the different clinical findings.

In the present case, we determined that active treatment was not required for subclinical MN. Although our EGPA case presented with renal impairment, for which immunosuppressive agents are recommended based on FFS scoring [29], the consent for these therapies was not obtained by the family due to the patient's age. Furthermore, 2 weeks after azathioprine was induced for maintaining remission, cytopenia, which was thought to be due to azathioprine-induced myelosuppression, occurred. As a result, steroid monotherapy for EGPA was conducted, and the patient's clinical course was uneventful and improved without any particular symptoms in our outpatient management.

Table 1: Cases of EGPA complicated with MN.

Author (year)	Age/sex	Before treatment renal function (Cre mg/dL) Proteinuria	Other organ comorbidities	ANCA	NCGN/EOS	IF	Treatments	After treatments Cre (mg/dL)/proteinuria Other organ comorbidities
Ayuzawa (2012)	65/F	Decreased (Cre 0.9) 9.9 g/gCre	Purpura, neuropathy, pneumonia	Negative	+/+	IgG1 > 4	mPSL 1 g × 3 days PSL 40 mg (initial dose)	Cre 0.6/CR Improved
Ram (2014)	37/M	Decreased (Cre 2.3) 8.7 g/day	Respiratory syndromes, subcutaneous nodules, arthritis	Positive	+/ND	IgG	mPSL 15 mg/kg/day × 3 days PSL 0.5 mg/kg/day (initial dose) IVCY × 9 times, AZA 2 mg/kg/day	Cre 1.2/CR ND
Mahmood (2019)	63/F	Preserved (Cre ND) 8.0 g/gCre	Purpura, neuropathy, pneumonia	Positive	−/ND	IgG	Rituximab (regimen unknown)	ND/PR Improved
Kondo (2020)	50/F	Preserved (Cre 0.54) 8.4 g/gCre	IgG4-related disease, neuropathy	Negative	−/−	IgG4 > 1	PSL 0.8 mg/kg/day (initial dose) CsA 1.5 mg/kg/day (initial dose) MZB 3.0 mg/kg/day, IVIg × 3 times	ND/CR Neuropathy did not improve
Zhu (2019)	50/M	Preserved (Cre 0.87) 6.4 g/gCre	Purpura, pneumonia	Positive	−/+	IgG4, PLA2R	PSL 60 mg IVCY × 9 times	ND/CR ND
Our case	70/F	Decreased (Cre 1.94) 0.63 g/gCre	Purpura, neuropathy,	Negative	−/−	IgG4 > 1	mPSL 0.5 g × 3 days PSL 40 mg (initial dose)	Cre 0.86/CR Improved

ANCA, anti-neutrophil cytoplasmic antigen; AZA, azathioprine; Cre, creatinine; CsA, cyclosporine; CR, complete remission; EOS, eosinophilic infiltration; IF, immunofluorescence staining; IVCY, intravenous cyclophosphamide; IVIg, intravenous immunoglobulin; mPSL, methylprednisolone; MZB, mizoribine; ND, no data; NCGN, necrotizing crescentic glomerulonephritis; PR, partial remission; PSL, prednisolone.

4. Conclusions

In EGPA, ANCA positivity, clinical, and histological findings may not appear consistently with each other as these could depend on the timing of diagnosis during the long-term process of EGPA development. It also remains unclear whether the etiology of the present MN was primary or secondary. Therefore, it is important to pay close attention to the critical pathologies of MN and the possibility of reactivation of EGPA in the future.

Consent

Informed consent was obtained from the patient and her family.

Acknowledgments

This research did not receive specific funding but was performed as part of the employment of the authors. The authors' employers were Toda Central General Hospital and Tokyo Women's Medical University.

References

[1] R. A. Sinico, L. Di Toma, U. Maggiore et al., "Prevalence and clinical significance of antineutrophil cytoplasmic antibodies in Churg-Strauss syndrome," *Arthritis & Rheumatism*, vol. 52, no. 9, pp. 2926–2935, 2005.

[2] S. Furuta, T. Iwamoto, and H. Nakajima, "Update on eosinophilic granulomatosis with polyangiitis," *Allergology International*, vol. 68, no. 4, pp. 430–436, 2019.

[3] C.-A. Durel, R. A. Sinico, V. Teixeira et al., "Renal involvement in eosinophilic granulomatosis with polyangiitis (EGPA): a multicentric retrospective study of 63 biopsy-proven cases," *Rheumatology*, vol. 60, no. 1, pp. 359–365, 2021.

[4] R. Ram, C. S. Rao, G. Swarnalatha et al., "Membranous nephropathy superimposed on Churg-Strauss syndrome," *Indian Journal of Nephrology*, vol. 24, no. 1, pp. 57–59, 2014.

[5] S. Mahmood, H. Ahmad, J. Wu, D. Haselby, M. LeClaire, and R. Nasr, "Anti-neutrophil cytoplasmic antibody-positive eosinophilic granulomatosis with polyangiitis: can it cause membranous nephropathy?" *Scandinavian Journal of Rheumatology*, vol. 48, no. 3, pp. 256-257, 2019.

[6] Y. Zhu, Q. Chang, X. Cao et al., "Co-occurrence of PLA2R-positive membranous nephropathy without crescents, and PR3-positive eosinophilic granulomatosis with polyangiitis," *Clinical Nephrology*, vol. 92, no. 4, pp. 208–215, 2019.

[7] N. Ayuzawa, Y. Ubara, S. Keiichi et al., "Churg-Strauss syndrome with a clinical condition similar to igg4-related kidney disease: a case report," *Internal Medicine*, vol. 51, no. 10, pp. 1233–1238, 2012.

[8] I. Kondo, Y. Arai, E. Sakamoto, D. Katagiri, and F. Hinoshita, "The First Case of Eosinophilic Granulomatosis with Polyangiitis simultaneously demonstrating various clinical manifestations with retroperitoneal fibrosis and membranous nephropathy," *Internal Medicine*, vol. 60, no. 12, pp. 1963–1969, 2021.

[9] A. Vaglio, I. Casazza, C. Grasselli, D. Corradi, R. A. Sinico, and C. Buzio, "Churg-Strauss syndrome," *Kidney International*, vol. 76, no. 9, pp. 1006–1011, 2009.

[10] P. C. Grayson, C. Ponte, R. Suppiah et al., "2022 American College of Rheumatology/European Alliance of Associations for Rheumatology classification criteria for eosinophilic granulomatosis with polyangiitis," *Annals of the Rheumatic Diseases*, vol. 81, no. 3, pp. 309–314, 2022.

[11] C. Comarmond, C. Pagnoux, M. Khellaf et al., "Eosinophilic granulomatosis with polyangiitis (Churg-Strauss): clinical characteristics and long-term followup of the 383 patients enrolled in the French vasculitis study group cohort," *Arthritis & Rheumatism*, vol. 65, no. 1, pp. 270–281, 2013.

[12] R. A. Sinico, L. D. Toma, U. Maggiore et al., "Renal involvement in Churg-Strauss syndrome," *American Journal of Kidney Diseases*, vol. 47, no. 5, pp. 770–779, 2006.

[13] B. D. Munshi, S. Sengupta, A. Sharan et al., "Anti-neutrophil cytoplasmic antibody (ANCA)-negative small vessel vasculitis: a rare cause of pulmonary renal syndrome," *Internal Medicine*, vol. 54, no. 21, pp. 2759–2763, 2015.

[14] Y. Saito, S. Okada, N. Funabashi, and Y. Kobayashi, "ANCA-negative eosinophilic granulomatosis with polyangitis (EGPA) manifesting as a large intracardiac thrombus and glomerulonephritis with angionecrosis," *BMJ Case Reports*, vol. 2016, Article ID bcr2016216520, 2016.

[15] J. G. Lanham, K. B. Elkon, C. D. Pusey, and G. R. Hughes, "Systemic vasculitis with asthma and eosinophilia: a clinical approach to the Churg-Strauss syndrome," *Medicine*, vol. 63, no. 2, pp. 65–81, 1984.

[16] E. Clutterbuck, E. Hirst, and C. Sanderson, "Human interleukin-5 (IL-5) regulates the production of eosinophils in human bone marrow cultures: comparison and interaction with IL-1, IL-3, IL-6, and GMCSF," *Blood*, vol. 73, no. 6, pp. 1504–1512, 1989.

[17] A. Radice, L. Bianchi, and R. A. Sinico, "Anti-neutrophil cytoplasmic autoantibodies: methodological aspects and clinical significance in systemic vasculitis," *Autoimmunity Reviews*, vol. 12, no. 4, pp. 487–495, 2013.

[18] U. Eisenberger, F. Fakhouri, P. Vanhille et al., "ANCA-negative pauci-immune renal vasculitis: histology and outcome," *Nephrology Dialysis Transplantation*, vol. 20, no. 7, pp. 1392–1399, 2005.

[19] H. Shiiki, T. Saito, T. Saito et al., "Prognosis and risk factors for idiopathic membranous nephropathy with nephrotic syndrome in Japan," *Kidney International*, vol. 65, no. 4, pp. 1400–1407, 2004.

[20] P. Ronco and H. Debiec, "Molecular pathomechanisms of membranous nephropathy: from Heymann nephritis to alloimmunization," *Journal of the American Society of Nephrology*, vol. 16, no. 5, pp. 1205–1213, 2005.

[21] A. Kronbichler and E. L. Bettac, "Kidney disease in eosinophilic granulomatosis with polyangiitis: expect the unexpected," *Rheumatology*, vol. 60, no. 1, pp. 1-2, 2021.

[22] D. B. Oliveira, "Membranous nephropathy: an IgG4-mediated disease," *The Lancet*, vol. 351, no. 9103, pp. 670-671, 1998.

[23] C. C. Huang, A. Lehman, A. Albawardi et al., "IgG subclass staining in renal biopsies with membranous glomerulonephritis indicates subclass switch during disease progression," *Modern Pathology*, vol. 26, no. 6, pp. 799–805, 2013.

[24] H. C. Stanescu, M. Arcos-Burgos, A. Medlar et al., "Risk HLA-DQA1 and PLA(2)R1 alleles in idiopathic membranous nephropathy," *New England Journal of Medicine*, vol. 364, no. 7, pp. 616–626, 2011.

[25] L. H. Beck, R. G. B. Bonegio, G. Lambeau et al., "M-type phospholipase A2 receptor as target antigen in idiopathic membranous nephropathy," *New England Journal of Medicine*, vol. 361, no. 1, pp. 11–21, 2009.

[26] N. M. Tomas, L. H. Beck, C. Meyer-Schwesinger et al., "Thrombospondin type-1 domain-containing 7A in idiopathic membranous nephropathy," *New England Journal of Medicine*, vol. 371, no. 24, pp. 2277–2287, 2014.

[27] T. Iwakura, N. Ohashi, A. Kato, S. Baba, and H. Yasuda, "Prevalence of enhanced granular expression of thrombospondin type-1 domain containing 7A in the glomeruli of Japanese patients with idiopathic membranous nephropathy," *PLoS One*, vol. 10, no. 9, Article ID e0138841, 2015.

[28] K. Nagahama, H. Matsushita, M. Hara, Y. Ubara, S. Hara, and A. Yamada, "Bucillamine induces membranous glomerulonephritis," *American Journal of Kidney Diseases*, vol. 39, no. 4, pp. 706–712, 2002.

[29] M. Groh, C. Pagnoux, C. Baldini et al., "Eosinophilic granlomatosis with polyangiitis (Churg-Strauss) (EGPA) Consensus task force recommendations for evaluation and management," *European Journal of Internal Medicine*, vol. 26, no. 7, pp. 545–553, 2015.

34

Acute Kidney Injury Caused by Superior Mesenteric Artery Syndrome

Nur Ezzaty Mohammad Kazmin,[1] Lydia Kamaruzaman,[2] Zhiqin Wong,[3] Voon Ken Fong,[2] Rozita Mohd,[2] and Ruslinda Mustafar[2]

[1]*Medical Department, National University of Malaysia Medical Centre, Kuala Lumpur, Malaysia*
[2]*Nephrology Unit, Medical Department, National University of Malaysia Medical Centre, Kuala Lumpur, Malaysia*
[3]*Gastroenterology Unit, Medical Department, National University of Malaysia Medical Centre, Kuala Lumpur, Malaysia*

Correspondence should be addressed to Ruslinda Mustafar; ruslinda.m@gmail.com

Academic Editor: Yoshihide Fujigaki

Background. Superior mesenteric artery (SMA) syndrome is a rare cause of upper gastrointestinal obstruction leading to acute kidney injury (AKI). *Methods.* We report a case of 23-year-old army personnel who presented with persistent vomiting leading to severe hypokalaemia, metabolic alkalosis, and acute kidney injury resulting in cardiorespiratory arrest. *Results.* After successful resuscitation, he was supported with haemodialysis and aggressive electrolytes correction. He was repeatedly not able to tolerate nasogastric (NG) tube feeding and computerised tomography of abdomen was performed, and the diagnosis of SMA syndrome was made. Gastroscopy examination revealed duodenal ulcer at D1, pinhole D1-D2 junction, but there was no evidence of intraluminal mass or lesions leading to upper gastrointestinal obstruction. A nasojejunal tube was inserted to bypass the narrow segment of the duodenum, and he was put on nutritional support. He was subsequently weaned off dialysis support as his renal function gradually improved and later on normalised. He remains symptoms free, and he gained five kilograms in four months after discharge. *Conclusions.* SMA syndrome is a rare cause of upper gastrointestinal obstruction but should be considered as a differential diagnosis in a patient who presented with recurrent vomiting and AKI with metabolic alkalosis.

1. Introduction

Superior mesenteric artery (SMA) syndrome is one of the rare causes of upper gastrointestinal (GI) obstruction with reported a very low prevalence of 0.013–0.3% [1, 2]. It was first described following autopsy findings by Carl Freiherr von Rokitansky in 1842. SMA syndrome is characterised by extraluminal vascular compression of the third segment of the duodenum (D) between SMA and aorta, leading to complete or partial duodenal obstruction. Patients could present with symptoms varying from chronic abdominal discomfort lasting for months to recurrent vomiting and acute upper intestinal ileus [3]. Diagnosis is usually challenging and requires a high index of suspicion due to the nonspecific presentations and its rarity, while radiological imaging with computerised tomography (CT) is considered a gold standard for diagnosis. To date, limited cases had described the association of metabolic alkalosis in a patient with significant renal impairment [4–6]. Management includes supportive measures by nutrition supplementation to help weight gain and build retroperitoneal fat tissue, although the majority of patients will require surgical intervention to relieve the obstruction [7].

2. Case Report

A 23-year-old man who was previously fit army personnel presented to our emergency department (ED) with a history of intermittent postprandial vomiting and leg cramps for one month which had worsened two days before his presentation where he vomited for ten times a day. He also had no loin pain or haematuria. Clinically, he was alert, not pale, neither jaundice nor cachexic, and without any abnormality on physical examination. On arrival, his blood pressure (BP) was 130/73 mmHg, pulse rate of 92 beats per minute, and oxygen saturation of 98% under room air.

The initial blood investigations in ED showed severe metabolic alkalosis with hypokalaemia, hypocalcaemia, and renal impairment. Blood urea was 9.1 mmol/L, serum creatinine of 218.3 μmol/L (eGFR 35.5 ml/min/1.73 m^2), potassium of 1.6 mmol/L, and sodium of 126 mmol/L. Venous blood gas showed metabolic alkalosis with pH of 7.56, bicarbonate of 62 mmol/L, pCO_2 of 73.3, mm Hg, pO_2 of 29.1, and SO_2 of 52.2%. Corrected serum calcium was 2.04 mmol/L while serum phosphate was 1.0 mmol/L. Full blood count showed haemoglobin of 12.2 g/L, total white blood cell count of 10.2×10^9/L, and platelet of 302×10^9/L. Meanwhile, C-reactive protein was 0.28 mg/dL. There were no baseline investigations for comparison and also no arterial blood gas results.

Shortly after reviewing him, he developed generalised tonic seizure followed by cardiac arrest with pulseless electrical activity. The blood pressure was not recordable; hence, cardiopulmonary resuscitation was carried out for a total of 70 minutes, with 14 direct current shocks delivered for ventricular tachycardia and fibrillation before he regained full and sustained recirculation. He was intubated and required inotropic support for persistent hypotension despite adequate volume resuscitation. He had 300 ml of urine following urinary bladder catheterisation after the resuscitation, which was most likely reflective of residual urine prior to the collapsed, but later he became anuric and was initiated on renal replacement therapy.

Placement of nasogastric tube (NG) postintubation drained almost 2 L gastric content, and even after emptying, he was unable to tolerate feeding via the tube. He required multiple corrections for hypokalaemia and hypocalcaemia with intravenous potassium chloride and calcium gluconate infusion, respectively. CT thorax, abdomen, and pelvis was done and showed distended elongated stomach with air contrast level (Figure 1). There was no enhancing lesion or compression at the pylorus and antrum of the stomach. However, the D3 segment of the duodenum was significantly smaller in calibre at the precaval and preaortic region with lack of mesenteric fat. There was a reduced aortomesenteric angle measuring 21 degrees (normal: 25–60 degree) with reduced distance measuring 8 mm (normal: 10–28 mm). The contrast was seen opacifying the duodenum, jejunum and ileal loops.

He required intermittent haemodialysis and extubated after four days and could give more detailed histories which help to exclude the possibility of congenital related disorders or drug abuse which were not present. He was well before but gave a history of progressive weight loss with intermittent vomiting, which goes back to almost a year. Although it was not initially alarming, for the past two months, he lost 2 kilograms, despite normal appetite and no associated diarrhoea or vomiting. His body mass index on admission was 17.8 kg/m^2 only with a weight of 48 kg and height of 1.64 m.

He had a full neurological recovery but remained intolerance to NG feeding. Gastroscopy examination showed Forrest 3 ulcer at D1, pinhole D1-D2 junction, which was dilated during the scope, and the nasojejunal (NJ) tube was inserted to facilitate oral feeding. He was given parenteral nutritional support throughout the hospital stay together with oral erythromycin ethylsuccinate as a prokinetic agent until he tolerates the tube feeding very well. He was then successfully discharged without the feeding tube after one month of admission. His renal function was also gradually recovered (Figure 2). He was taken off dialysis support after three months. With proper dietary advice, he gained five kilograms in a span of four months.

3. Discussion

SMA syndrome, apart from being very rare, can present with a broad spectrum of clinical manifestations and cause confusion with other causes of intestinal obstruction or motility disorders. The syndrome mostly affects female between the age 10 and 39 years [3] and those with low BMI < 18 kg/m^2 or weight percentile for the height of <5% [8].

Its underlying pathophysiology involves narrowing of the aortomesenteric angle to 6 to 8 mm or reduction of its distance to 16 to 22 mm which results in extraluminal compression of the third part of the duodenum between the aorta and SMA. The predisposing factors can be divided into congenital or acquired. Some patients were born with shortened ligaments of Treitz causing the duodenum to be suspended nearer to the origin or SMA, thus prone for compression. More commonly, this condition is acquired as a result of retroperitoneal and mesenteric fat tissue loss in patients with chronic illness, dietary disorders, or severe malnutrition. Local pathology such as tumours or anatomical changes following injury, intra-abdominal surgical repair of aortic aneurysm, or spinal instrumentation has also been reported as predisposing factors [3].

So far, this condition has been described in patients with rapid weight loss with comorbidities or following surgery [9], but uncommon in a healthy individual. In this case, the patient did not have typical risk factors for the disease as he was previously fit army personnel with no known medical illness. Apart from the loss of retroperitoneal fat tissue due to progressive weight loss for past one year that probably attributed to his vigorous physical training, thus resultant to intermittent vomiting, CT scan, and gastroscopy examination with biopsy ruled out any local cause such as tumours that could contribute to the narrowing of the aortomesenteric angle.

Due to low suspicion index and delay in diagnosis of SMA syndrome, most of the patients present late with a long-standing history of upper abdominal discomfort, intermittent vomiting, and weight loss which could last up to 8 to 28 months [3, 9, 10]. Rarely, as in this case, the patient could present acutely with gastric dilation and upper intestinal ileus [3, 11–13] mimicking more common causes of acute vomiting such as gastroenteritis, pancreatitis, peptic ulcer disease, cholecystitis, mesenteric ischemia, and medication-related side effects [14, 15]. Mortality has also been

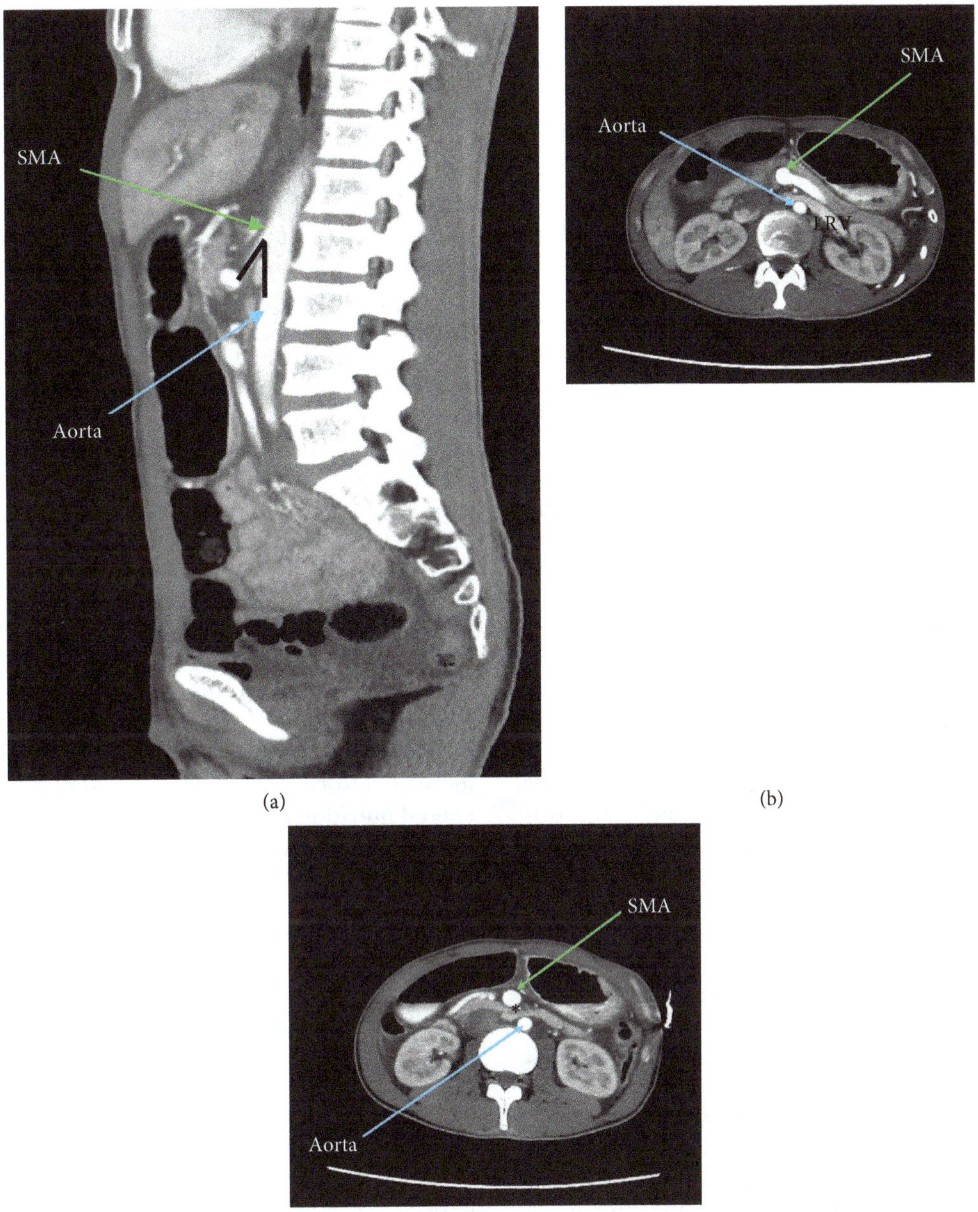

FIGURE 1: Contrasted CT abdomen image in (a) showing the narrow-angle created by the SMA anteriorly and descending aorta posteriorly. (b) and (c) showing dilated left renal vein (LRV) and third D3 (marked by*), respectively, which are compressed by descending aorta posteriorly and SMA anteriorly.

reported due to gastric necrosis and perforation as a complication of the condition [11, 13].

AKI is a common presentation to medical attention and can be categorised by prerenal, renal, and postrenal causes. In general, most of the causes of AKI were apparent from histories such as volume loss following bleeding, burns, severe gastrointestinal (GI) loss, hypotension, sepsis, use of nephrotoxic drugs, or obstructive uropathy. Intrinsic renal causes of AKI such as glomerulonephritis and infiltrative disease are more difficult to diagnose and need a renal biopsy for confirmation.

On the other hand, AKI as a primary presenting feature of SMA syndrome remains uncommon, and only a few cases had reported AKI in association with the condition [12, 16, 17]. In severe GI obstruction with a massively distended stomach, AKI could occur as a result of increased abdominal compartment pressure, resulting in decreased renal artery perfusion as well as impaired venous drainage. Clinically, the patient presents with massively distended abdomen accompanied by tenderness and rigidity, as well as metabolic acidosis due to bowel hypoperfusion and ischemia [16]. Rarely, a patient can present with AKI due to simultaneous renal vein compression by superior mesenteric artery [8], a condition called nutcracker syndrome [18].

Nutcracker syndrome is also another possibility; however, apart from the incidental finding of left renal vein

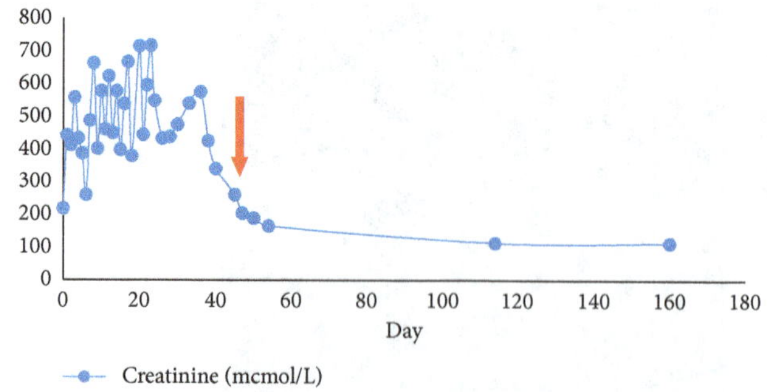

FIGURE 2: Showed serum creatinine trend over time, with a red arrow indicating the point when the patient was taken off haemodialysis support.

compression on the CT imaging which would suggest this phenomenon, the patient did not complain of any loin pain or haematuria prior to the presentation. Unfortunately, there was no urine sample sent on admission to check for the presence of any microscopic haematuria or sediment of red blood cells. Due to these limitations, the diagnosis of SMA syndrome is very clear based on the clinical findings; however, coexistence of nutcracker syndrome remains speculative in this case.

Recurrent vomiting in this case could lead to volume depletion and prerenal AKI, as well as metabolic alkalosis due to loss of hydrogen ion from the gastric juice. Apart from the initial prerenal insult due to hypovolemia from excessive vomiting and third space loss, this patient developed worsening AKI and subsequent oligoanuria likely due to hypotensive acute tubular necrosis (ATN) secondary to prolonged cardiorespiratory collapse and hypotension requiring renal replacement therapy.

Nevertheless, it was unusual for severe metabolic alkalosis to occur in a patient with significant renal impairment, as the latter is commonly associated with metabolic acidosis. Despite only two days history of excessive vomiting, this patient presented with life-threatening metabolic alkalosis causing neuromuscular irritability, seizure, and cardiac arrest likely due to a combination of low serum calcium, hypokalaemia, and hypoventilation induced cerebral hypoxemia. Raised venous pCO_2 concentration on arrival suggests that somewhere following arrival and onset of the seizure, hypoxemia likely had occurred due to secondary hypoventilation in response to severe metabolic alkalosis [4].

Mechanism of severe metabolic alkalosis, in this case, is postulated to be initiated by hypergastrinemia following cholinergic stimulation due to acute gastric distention. This results in an increased volume of gastric juice produced, as well as hydrogen ion secreted, which was subsequently lost [4]. In a healthy patient, bicarbonate ion (HCO_3) generated from hydrogen ion (H+) secreted from the parietal cell will be buffered by pancreatic HCO_3 loss into the small intestine. However, in this case, there was a net HCO_3 gained as gastric acid produced in the stomach failed to enter the small intestine to stimulate pancreatic secretion of HCO_3. This HCO_3 gain is maintained as the kidney is unable to excrete the excess HCO_3 due to impaired glomerular filtration. At the same time, intravascular volume depletion secondary to excessive vomiting and third space loss causes secondary hyperaldosteronism which increases HCO_3 reabsorption, causing worsening of metabolic alkalosis as well as renal potassium K+ ion loss [6]. Some cases had used low bicarbonate dialysate for the treatment of severe metabolic alkalosis [19]. However, here, haemodialysis using normal dialysate had successfully decreased serum bicarbonate concentration and brought down blood pH to normal.

In patients considered at risk for SMA syndrome, a high index of suspicion is needed to minimised delay in the diagnosis. Contrasted CT has been considered the gold-standard imaging to visualise aortomesenteric angle and distance accurately for diagnosis of SMA syndrome. CT will also be able to pick up local pathologies such as neoplasm or aneurysm that could be the cause of anatomical change and compression. On the other hand, upper endoscopic examination is usually required to exclude intraluminal causes of obstruction, including ulcers which could mimic the syndrome or develop as a complication secondary to reflux of gastric acids [3]. Rarely, an experienced endoscopist will be able to demonstrate pulsatile extrinsic compression which supports the diagnosis during the examination [2].

Management of SMA syndrome varies from medical to surgical procedures aiming to promote weight gain and to increase retroperitoneal fat tissue. Medical management via enteral nutrition given through a feeding tube bypassing the obstruction or a parenteral nutrition with or without prokinetic agents are the preferred strategies and has been proven to be successful in certain cases [20, 21]. Knee-chest or side-lying positional change after a meal had been tried to provide partial obstruction relief by widening the aortomesenteric angle [22, 23]. Surgical management, on the other hand, is usually reserved for patients not responding to medical management, and these include procedures such as gastrojejunostomy, open or laparoscopic duodeno-jejunostomy, and Strong procedure [8, 24].

The severities of complications reported are mainly related to delay in diagnosis, and these include electrolyte imbalances, dehydration, peptic ulcer, stomach perforation, aspiration pneumonia, pancreatitis, and even death [3, 24]. A patient whose diagnosis was picked up early during illness without significant complication usually has a good prognosis. In this case, although the patient was fortunate to be revived following cardiac arrest, he developed AKI and was temporarily dependent on haemodialysis support for seven weeks.

4. Conclusion

SMA syndrome is rare but should be considered as a differential diagnosis when a patient presents with recurrent vomiting and AKI with metabolic alkalosis. CT contrast is the gold-standard imaging for diagnosis together with an endoscopic examination to identify potential secondary causes for the narrowing of aortomesenteric angle causing D3 compression. Conservative medical management with nutritional support should be attempted in most patients, whereas surgical procedures are reserved for those not responding or came with complications that warrant immediate surgery. Generally, the prognosis of SMA syndrome, in this case, is good given that the condition is identified and intervenes early.

Disclosure

The abstract of this case was presented as a poster presentation at the Malaysian Society of Nephrology Congress 2019.

References

[1] T. Welsch, M. W. Büchler, and P. Kienle, "Recalling superior mesenteric artery syndrome," *Digestive Surgery*, vol. 24, no. 3, pp. 149–156, 2007.

[2] E. Sinagra, D. Raimondo, D. Albano et al., "Superior mesenteric artery syndrome: clinical, endoscopic, and radiological findings," *Gastroenterology Research and Practice*, vol. 2018, Article ID 1937416, 7 pages, 2018.

[3] M. T. Mandarry, L. Zhao, C. Zhang, and Z. Q. Wei, "A comprehensive review of superior mesenteric artery syndrome," *European Surgery*, vol. 42, no. 5, pp. 229–236, 2010.

[4] L. Huber and F. J. Gennari, "Severe metabolic alkalosis in a hemodialysis patient," *American Journal of Kidney Diseases*, vol. 58, no. 1, pp. 144–149, 2011.

[5] J. Jacobi, S. Schnellhardt, M. Opgenoorth et al., "Severe metabolic alkalosis and recurrent acute on chronic kidney injury in a patient with Crohn's disease," *BMC Nephrology*, vol. 11, no. 1, p. 6, 2010.

[6] M. E. Ostermann, "Metabolic alkalosis in patients with renal failure," *Nephrology Dialysis Transplantation*, vol. 18, no. 11, pp. 2442–2448, 2003.

[7] N. Van Horne and J. P. Jackson, *Superior Mesenteric Artery Syndrome*, StatPearls, Treasure Island, FL, USA, 2018.

[8] F. J. Bohanon, O. N. Lopez, B. M. Graham, L. W. Griffin, and R. Radhakrishnan, "A case series of laparoscopic duodenojejunostomy for the treatment of pediatric superior mesenteric artery syndrome," *International Journal of Surgery and Research*, vol. 2016, no. 1, pp. 1–5, 2016.

[9] G. Cicero, T. D'Angelo, A. Bottari et al., "Superior mesenteric artery syndrome in patients with crohn's disease: a description of 2 cases studied with a novel magnetic resonance enterography (MRE) procedure," *American Journal of Case Reports*, vol. 19, pp. 431–437, 2018.

[10] N. D. Merrett, R. B. Wilson, P. Cosman, and A. V. Biankin, "Superior mesenteric artery syndrome: diagnosis and treatment strategies," *Journal of Gastrointestinal Surgery*, vol. 13, no. 2, pp. 287–292, 2009.

[11] M. K. Demir and T. Cevher, "A rare cause and complication of acute gastric dilatation: superior mesenteric artery syndrome and perforation," *The Eurasian Journal of Medicine*, vol. 50, no. 1, pp. 60-61, 2018.

[12] Z. A. Zhang, "Superior mesenteric artery syndrome: a vicious cycle," *BMJ Case Reports*, vol. 2018, 2018.

[13] Y. M. Feng, D. Wan, and R. Guo, "Case report of gastric distension due to superior mesenteric artery syndrome mimicking hollow viscus perforation: considerations in critical care ultrasound," *Medicine*, vol. 97, no. 20, Article ID e10757, 2018.

[14] R. Jain, "Superior mesenteric artery syndrome," *Current Treatment Options in Gastroenterology*, vol. 10, no. 1, pp. 24–27, 2007.

[15] W. D. Anderson and S. M. Strayer, "Evaluation of nausea and vomiting: a case-based approach," *American Family Physician*, vol. 88, no. 6, pp. 371–379, 2013.

[16] K. Reece, R. Day, and J. Welch, "Superior mesenteric artery syndrome with abdominal compartment syndrome," *Case Reports in Emergency Medicine*, vol. 2016, Article ID 7809281, 4 pages, 2016.

[17] M. Inal, B. Unal Daphan, and M. Y. Karadeniz Bilgili, "Superior mesenteric artery syndrome accompanying with nutcracker syndrome: a case report," *Iranian Red Crescent Medical Journal*, vol. 16, no. 10, Article ID e14755, 2014.

[18] M. Polguj, M. Topol, and A. Majos, "An unusual case of left venous renal entrapment syndrome: a new type of nutcracker phenomenon?" *Surgical and Radiologic Anatomy*, vol. 35, no. 3, pp. 263–267, 2013.

[19] S. Tripathy, "Extreme metabolic alkalosis in intensive care," *Indian Journal of Critical Care Medicine*, vol. 13, no. 4, pp. 217–220, 2009.

[20] K. Takehara, K. Sakamoto, R. Takahashi et al., "Superior mesenteric artery syndrome improved by enteral nutritional therapy according to the controlling nutritional status score," *Case Reports in Gastroenterology*, vol. 11, no. 3, pp. 729–735, 2017.

[21] D. K. Chan, K. S. Mak, and Y. L. Cheah, "Successful nutritional therapy for superior mesenteric artery syndrome," *Singapore Medical Journal*, vol. 53, no. 53, pp. e233–e236, 2012.

[22] E. A. Milner, W. G. Cioffi, W. F. McManus, and B. A. Pruitt Jr., "Superior mesenteric artery syndrome in a burn patient," *Nutrition in Clinical Practice*, vol. 8, no. 6, pp. 264–266, 1993.

[23] S. W. Munns, R. T. Morrissy, E. S. Golladay, and C. N. McKenzie, "Hyperalimentation for superior mesenteric-artery (cast) syndrome following correction of spinal deformity," *The Journal of Bone & Joint Surgery*, vol. 66, no. 8, pp. 1175–1177, 1984.

[24] N. Mathenge, S. Osiro, I. I. Rodriguez, C. Salib, R. S. Tubbs, and M. Loukas, "Superior mesenteric artery syndrome and its associated gastrointestinal implications," *Clinical Anatomy*, vol. 27, no. 8, pp. 1244–1252, 2014.

35

Severe Hyponatremia Precipitated by Acute Urinary Retention in a Patient with Psychogenic Polydipsia

C. M. H. Hilton,[1,2] L. Boesby,[1] and K. E. Nelveg-Kristensen[1]

[1]*Department of Cardiology, Nephrology and Endocrinology, Nordsjællands Hospital-Hillerød, 3400 Hillerød, Denmark*
[2]*Department of Otorhinolaryngology, Nordsjællands Hospital-Hillerød, 3400 Hillerød, Denmark*

Correspondence should be addressed to C. M. H. Hilton; carro_hilton@hotmail.com

Academic Editor: Mahzuz Karim

A woman in her late sixties presented with severe hyponatremia and acute kidney injury (AKI) as consequence of psychogenic polydipsia and acute urinary retention due to urinary tract infection. Urinary catheterization promptly drained 5.5 L of urine with resulting polyuria, leading to an initial swift raise in plasma (P) sodium concentration, disregarding the course of fluid resuscitation. After the polyuric phase, normal range P-sodium levels were reestablished by oral water restriction. Treatment with psychoactive drugs, e.g., zuclopentixol, may have contributed to the severity of the condition. There are few published reports regarding water intoxication and urinary retention, but none reflecting severe hyponatremia precipitated by acute urinary retention in a patient with polydipsia. By this report, we illustrate the detrimental consequences on water and electrolyte homeostasis of urinary retention and polydipsia resulting in acute water intoxication. The purpose of presenting this case is firstly to draw attention to the potentially fatal combination of polydipsia and postrenal acute kidney injury, where the kidneys are unable to correct the enormous excess water, then to focus on the difficulty in correcting hypervolemic hyponatraemia in the context of polyuria after relief of urinary retention, and finally, to point out that patients in treatment with antipsychotics may have further worsening of electrolyte derangement.

1. Introduction

Hyponatremia is a frequently encountered electrolyte abnormality [1]. Of all hospitalized patients, 14–38% develop hyponatremia during hospital stay, [2, 3] and approximately 15% of all patients acutely admitted to hospital have a P-sodium < 135 mmol/L [4]. Hyponatremia is associated with a marked increase in mortality and morbidity resulting from, e.g., cerebral oedema and central pontine myelinolysis. Even mild cases are independently associated with a higher risk of in-hospital and long-term mortality [5, 6]. Psychogenic water intoxication is a well-known cause of hyponatremia and, hence, plasma hypo-osmolality [7]. People with normal kidney function are protected from developing severe electrolyte derangements by effective renal compensation. Impaired renal function, as a consequence to postrenal obstruction, potentiates the harmful effects of excessive water intake.

Hyponatremia in acutely admitted medical patients is often multifactorial. Causes are Syndrome of Inappropriate Antidiuretic Hormone Secretion (SIADH) (22%), heart-, liver- or kidney-insufficiency (23%), thiazides (20%), correction of fluid losses with hypotonic solutions (17%), loop-diuretics (8%), and others (10%) [8]. In-hospital acquired hyponatremia is primarily caused by hypotonic fluid therapy. Hypo-, hyper-, and normovolemic hyponatremia should be treated differently.

2. Case Presentation

A woman in her late sixties with schizoaffective disorder, managed with zuclopenthixol and oxazepam, was transferred from the psychiatric department to the acute care facility with polydipsia, urinary retention, and hyponatremia. She had no history of hyponatremia, polydipsia, or urinary retention and was not treated with diuretics. The laboratory charts showed P-sodium within the normal range of 136–142 mmol/l and a normal kidney function (P-creatinine 55–70 μmol/l).

The patient was initially admitted to the psychiatric ward in a psychotic condition with a Glasgow Coma Scale (GCS) of 14-15 and polydipsia, suspected of not having taken her antipsychotic medication. The excessive water intake was handled by fluid restriction, which was not fully followed. P-sodium was not initially measured. Four days after admission, the P-sodium was 122 mmol/L (137–145 mmol/L), and at day six, after several episodes of vomiting, the P-sodium concentration had decreased to 98 mmol/L (Figure 1). The patient was transferred to the acute care facility, presenting with GCS 10 and diffuse abdominal soreness. A urinary catheter was placed, and 5.5 L of red coloured urine was emptied immediately. Fluid therapy with 0.9% saline at an infusion rate of 50 ml/hour (h), daily weighing, fluid input/output registration, blood samples every 3-4 hours, and a 24-h urine sample were initiated. During the next nine hours, the patient became increasingly polyuric with a total diuresis of 5.5 L. Simultaneously, after an additional decrease to 90 mmol/L, P-sodium rose to 112 mmol/L, after which the saline infusion was removed. Antibiotics were given empirically due to leucocytosis, elevated C-reactive protein, and signs of urinary tract infection. After these initial days of fluctuation, the P-sodium slowly rose, primarily due to water restriction.

3. Investigations

Blood samples obtained in the acute care facility showed a P-osmolality of 216 mosmol/kg (280–290 mosmol/kg), P-creatinine 333 μmol/L (45–90 μmol/L), and P-potassium 6.0 mmol/L (3.5–4.4 mmol/L). Urine- (U-) osmolality was 235 mosmol/kg (>560 mosmol/kg), and U-sodium was 83 mmol/L (20–40 mmol/L).

Nine hours from admission, the P-sodium had risen to 112 mmol/L, and after another four hours, it further rose to 131 mmol/L (Figure 1). P-sodium returned to the normal range after eight days. Hyperkalemia was corrected as the renal function returned to normal 12–15 hours after urinary catheterization.

An abdominal computed tomography (CT) imaging described a flaccid, slightly thickened urinary bladder and a uterus fibroma, discreet free abdominal fluid, slight hydroureteres bilaterally, discreet unilateral hydronephrosis, and discreet pleural effusion, predominantly on the right side.

4. Outcome and Follow-Up

One week after admission to the acute care facility the patient had two general tonic clonic seizures lasting more than two minutes. There was no lateralization upon neurological examination. The patient was treated with diazepam, fentanyl, propofol, a loading dose of fosphenytoin and was intubated. Thereafter, she was treated with tinzaparin, lamotrigine, and valproate. The patient had no history of epilepsy, seizures, or any other neurologic disease. A cerebral CT scan and magnetic resonance imaging (MRI) showed no focal cerebral damage, specifically no pontine signal changes, and it was concluded that the seizures should be explained by vast electrolyte fluctuation and treatment with zuclopenthixol, which lowers the convulsive threshold.

5. Discussion

By the present case report on a patient with psychogenic water intoxication, we demonstrate the detrimental consequences of acute urinary retention and AKI, resulting in impaired renal fluid and electrolyte regulation. This was indeed emphasized by the abrupt fall in P-sodium, which initially was forced by the inability of free-water clearance as the urinary tract was obstructed. Furthermore, after urinary catheterization, the relatively high U-osmolality to P-osmolality of 1.09, which under normal renal conditions should have been much lower in the setting of acute water intoxication [9], is most reasonably explained by renal tubule damage as a consequence to severe urinary retention, resulting in an inability of adequate sodium reabsorption [10]. This was further stressed by a relatively long resuscitation period, before normal-range P-sodium was achieved. Water intoxication with resulting hyponatremia and hypoosmolality is a well-known challenge among patients with psychiatric disorders [7, 8]. In addition to the massive water overload, hyponatremia itself, in patients with psychiatric diseases, has been associated with resetting of the hypothalamic osmoreceptors, resulting in secretion of ADH (Anti Diuretic Hormone) at a lower P-osmolality [11]. Effective fluid restriction was not carried out prior to acute care facility admission, as indicated by a drop in the P-sodium from 122 to 98 mmol/l.

A timely differentiation between acutely and chronically developed hyponatremia of 48 hours has been widely accepted. Nevertheless contemporary international guidelines recommend that severe symptomatic hyponatremia should be treated promptly with 100 ml 3% saline administered intravenously over 10 minutes and that this procedure may be repeated up to three times, since the risk of acute cerebral oedema far exceeds the risk of osmotic demyelination [12]. Subsequent correction of the condition should proceed with the administration of 0.9% saline intravenously (IV) at an infusion rate of 50 ml/h. Furthermore, guidelines recommend a maximal change in the P-sodium of 8 mmol/L over 24 hours and no more than 1 mmol/L/h in acute hyponatremia and 0.5 mmol/L/h in chronic conditions. If correction has proceeded more rapidly than desired, the risk of osmotic demyelination may be reduced by IV administration of 5% glucose, 0.45% NaCl, or desmopressin. In the current case report, our patient was initially treated with 50 ml 0.9% saline/h; however, one can argue that a bolus of 3% saline should have been initiated as she presented with a GCS of 10 and other neurologic symptoms. Interpretation of the neurologic evaluation was hampered by her psychotic condition. Moreover, as the patient became polyuric, putatively with a rapid rise in free-water clearance, administration of hypertonic saline could cause a fatal increase in

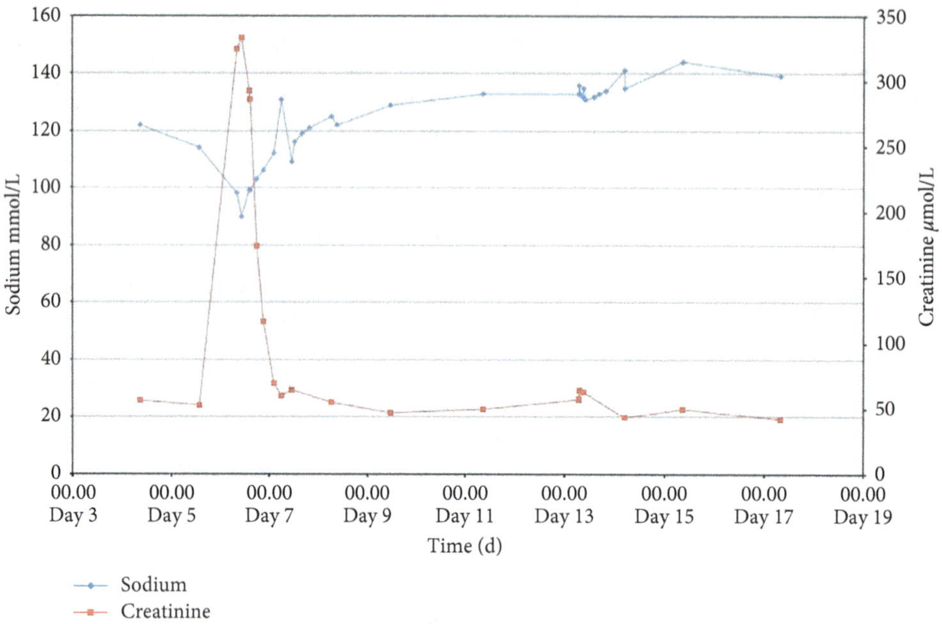

FIGURE 1: Blood samples reflecting P-sodium (mmol/L) and P-creatinine (μmol/L) levels over days.

P-sodium concentration. It is difficult to predict the tubular function in a patient with AKI; however, in this case, where the hyponatremia was induced by severe fluid overload, expanding the ECV with IV isotonic saline did not increase p-sodium. The subsequent fall in s-sodium could be explained by, e.g., residual water absorption from the gut or excessive tubular sodium excretion coincided by fluid retention due to an increased ADH response, which would be in keeping with the initial high U-sodium concentration [13].

The kidneys possess counteracting mechanisms that allow for urinary concentration and dilution. With normal renal function, the total solute concentration of body fluids remains constant, despite fluctuations in solute and water intake. During excessive water intake, the renal free-water clearance may produce up to 25 L of urine per day; however, in cases of severe water deprivation, the daily urine production can be reduced to less than 0.5 L [12]. In incidents of impaired kidney function, as in the current case with postobstructive AKI, the harmful effects of polydipsia increase.

Although our patient was unable to adequately dilute her urine, the subsequent polyuric phase may have contributed to the fast initial rise in P-sodium (Figure 1). We interpret the outlying blood sample with a P-sodium of 131 mmol/L as a measurement error, as P-sodium before and after this measurement, with a four-hour margin between each blood sample, was 112 mmol/L and 109 mmol/L, respectively. Fluctuations in the P-sodium of 18–21 mmol/L within four hours in the current case are most unlikely to have occurred.

Urinary tract obstruction per se can lead to hyponatremia. A patient undergoing urea diuresis after relief of urinary tract obstruction will lose sodium and water leading to hypovolemia and hyponatremia [12]. This patient's drastic rise and fall in P-creatinine, before and after urinary catheterization, respectively, suggests acute urinary obstruction as a contributing factor to AKI, although there probably pre-existed some level of chronic urinary retention. In this regard, a previous report showed that correction of chronic urinary obstruction reduced the incidence of hyponatremia in a polydipsic patient, [14], and urinary retention and polyuria are both registered as common (1–10%) side effects to zuclopenthixol, with which this patient was treated upon admission. Nonetheless, these considerations taken into account, we believe that urinary tract infection was the primary cause of acute total obstruction in the current case [15].

Collectively, the combination of polydipsia, urinary retention, and postobstructive AKI holds a serious risk of severe hyponatremia and hypoosmolality, with subsequent increased morbidity and risk of fatal outcomes. Furthermore, in the setting of acute water intoxication, postobstructive polyuria and sodium loss due to postobstructive tubular damage may contribute to a less predictable and prolonged resuscitation period [16]. Physicians should be aware of these mechanisms, especially among patients with psychogenic polydipsia treated with psychoactive drugs.

6. Learning Points/Take-Home Messages

(i) Be aware of urinary retention in patients with water intoxication

(ii) Follow sodium levels more frequently after relieving urinary retention in a patient with hyponatremia

(iii) Patients with urinary retention are not able to adequately regulate sodium levels

(iv) Possibly, urinary retention can cause a picture similar to SIADH

(v) Possibly, urinary retention should be relieved more gently

Consent

Informed consent was obtained from the patient.

Acknowledgments

The authors would like to thank Ulrik Pedersen-Bjergaard for his contribution with insight, expertise, and valuable comments, which greatly improved the manuscript.

References

[1] E. A. Holm, S. W. Brorson, J. S. Kruse, J. O. Faber, and B. Jespersen, "Hyponatremia in acutely admitted medical patients--occurrence and causes," *Ugeskr Laeger*, vol. 166, no. 45, pp. 4033–4037, 2004.

[2] H.-M. Chung, R. Kluge, R. W. Schrier, and R. J. Anderson, "Clinical assessment of extracellular fluid volume in hyponatremia," *The American Journal of Medicine*, vol. 83, no. 5, pp. 905–908, 1987.

[3] W. Fenske, S. K. G. Maier, A. Blechschmidt, B. Allolio, and S. Störk, "Utility and limitations of the traditional diagnostic approach to hyponatremia: a diagnostic study," *The American Journal of Medicine*, vol. 123, no. 7, pp. 652–657, 2010.

[4] L. Holland-Bill, C. F. Christiansen, U. Heide-Jorgensen et al., "Hyponatremia and mortality risk: a Danish cohort study of 279508 acutely hospitalized patients," *European Journal of Endocrinology*, vol. 173, no. 1, pp. 71–81, 2015.

[5] S. S. Waikar, D. B. Mount, and G. C. Curhan, "Mortality after hospitalization with mild, moderate, and severe hyponatremia," *The American Journal of Medicine*, vol. 122, no. 9, pp. 857–865, 2009.

[6] C. Giuliani and A. Peri, "Effects of hyponatremia on the brain," *Journal of Clinical Medicine*, vol. 3, no. 4, pp. 1163–1177, 2014.

[7] F. Gebel, H. Meng, F. Michot, and B. Truniger, "Psychogenic water intoxication," *Schweiz Med Wochenschr*, vol. 119, no. 6, pp. 169–177, 1989.

[8] T. Berl and R. W. Schrier, "Disorders of water metabolism," in *Renal and Electrolyte Disorders*, R. W. Schrier, Ed., pp. 1–44, Lippincott Williams & Wilkins, Philadelphia, PA, USA, 6th edition, 2010.

[9] L. E. Armstrong, E. C. Johnson, C. X. Munoz et al., "Evaluation of Uosm:Posm ratio as a hydration biomarker in free-living, healthy young women," *European Journal of Clinical Nutrition*, vol. 67, no. 9, pp. 934–938, 2013.

[10] S. Klahr, K. Harris, and M. L. Purkerson, "Effects of obstruction on renal functions," *Pediatric Nephrology*, vol. 2, no. 1, pp. 34–42, 1988.

[11] M. B. Goldman, G. L. Robertson, D. J. Luchins, D. Hedeker, and G. N. Pandey, "Psychotic exacerbations and enhanced vasopressin secretion in schizophrenic patients with hyponatremia and polydipsia," *Archives of General Psychiatry*, vol. 54, no. 5, pp. 443–449, 1997.

[12] C. Parikh and T. Berl, "Disorders of water metabolism," *Comprehensive Clinical Nephrology*, pp. 100–17, Elsevier, Amsterdam, Netherlands, 2010.

[13] A. Steele, M. Gowrishankar, S. Abrahamson, C. D. Mazer, R. D. Feldman, and M. L. Halperin, "Postoperative hyponatremia despite near-isotonic saline infusion: a phenomenon of desalination," *Annals of Internal Medicine*, vol. 126, no. 1, p. 20, 1997.

[14] N. Itoh, S. Fuwano, N. Matsui, and R. Takagi, "Reduction of hyponatremia in a schizophrenic with polydipsia-hyponatremia syndrome by surgical intervention," *Psychiatry Research*, vol. 70, no. 2, pp. 125–129, 1997.

[15] B. A. Selius and R. Subedi, "Urinary retention in adults: diagnosis and initial management," *American Family Physician*, vol. 77, no. 5, pp. 643–650, 2008.

[16] C. Halbgewachs and T. Domes, "Postobstructive diuresis: pay close attention to urinary retention," *Canadian Family Physician*, vol. 61, no. 2, pp. 137–142, 2015.

The Use of Pleural Fluid to Serum Glucose Ratio in Establishing the Diagnosis of a Not So Sweet PD-Related Hydrothorax: Case Report and Literature Review

Nidrit Bohra,[1] Abigayle Sullivan,[1] Haseeb Chaudhary,[1] and Trudy Demko[2]

[1]Internal Medicine Department, Reading Hospital, West Reading, PA, USA
[2]Nephrology Department, Reading Hospital, West Reading, PA, USA

Correspondence should be addressed to Nidrit Bohra; nidrit.bohra@towerhealth.org

Academic Editor: Rumeyza Kazancioglu

Hydrothorax is a well-known but rare complication of peritoneal dialysis (PD), with an average incidence of 2% mainly in cases of continuous ambulatory peritoneal dialysis (CAPD). In more than 80% of these cases, the hydrothorax is attributed to an abnormal pleuroperitoneal communication. It commonly manifests as unilateral effusion, predominantly on the right. A thoracentesis to determine pleural glucose has been a diagnostic aid well relied on, as the dextrose rich dialysate raises the pleural fluid glucose. A pleural fluid glucose to serum glucose gradient greater than 50 mg/dL is suggestive of a leak with a specificity of 100% according to some studies; however, its sensitivity is variable. Our case illustrates a diagnostic dilemma due to a relatively low pleural fluid to serum glucose gradient of 21 mg/dL that caused a delay in diagnosis. A pleural fluid to serum glucose ratio >1.0 was used as a diagnostic marker that pointed toward a peritoneal leak. For confirmation, a peritoneal scintigraphy with nuclear technetium 99 scan was performed that revealed a pleuroperitoneal fistula as the source of the recurring hydrothorax in the setting of automated peritoneal dialysis (APD). The hydrothorax completely resolved with termination of APD on follow-up as the patient was transitioned to intermittent hemodialysis (HD).

1. Background

Given its safety and convenience as a renal replacement therapy, peritoneal dialysis (PD) is preferred at many centers around the world. Noninfective complications related to PD that are commonly seen include outflow failure, pericatheter leak, abdominal wall herniation, catheter cuff extrusion, and intestinal perforation. PD-related hydrothorax is a rare complication mainly in cases of continuous ambulatory peritoneal dialysis (CAPD) with an incidence of 1.6% according to a study [1] in 328 patients that underwent PD where 6 developed pleuroperitoneal leak.

The pleural fluid glucose, which is a representative of glucose in the dialysate, to serum glucose gradient greater than 50 mg/dL is suggestive of a peritoneal leak causing hydrothorax with a specificity of 100% according to some studies [2]; however, its sensitivity is variable [3]. We describe a case of PD-related hydrothorax with a low pleural fluid to serum (PF-S) glucose gradient but a PF-S glucose ratio >1.0 that led to the final diagnosis.

2. Case Presentation

We describe a case of a 63-year-old gentleman with history of heart failure with reduced ejection fraction (HFrEF) due to ischemic cardiomyopathy, bioprosthetic aortic valve, and end-stage renal disease (ESRD) on automated peritoneal dialysis (APD) for 3 months who presented with dyspnea secondary to recurrent right-sided hydrothorax. The patient reported worsening dyspnea that correlated with the initiation of peritoneal dialysis; however, pleural fluid studies performed at prior admission had revealed a transudative effusion. The low pleural fluid to serum glucose gradient was not suggestive of a peritoneal source. The patient was not in overt heart failure and was being treated with recurrent therapeutic thoracentesis, and nightly continuous cyclic

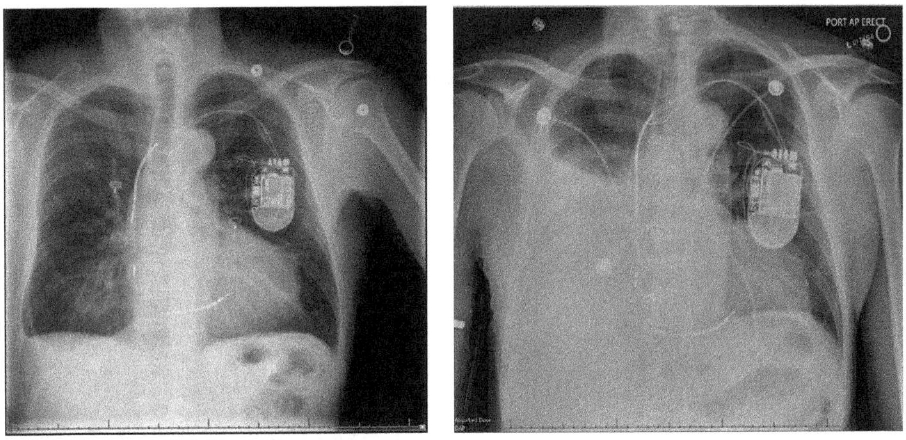

(a) (b)

FIGURE 1: Chest radiograph illustrating worsening right pleural effusion (b) after thoracentesis (9 days prior) (a).

TABLE 1

	Pleural fluid	Serum	PF-S gradient	PF-S ratio
Glucose (mg/dl)	104	83	21	1.2530

peritoneal dialysis (CCPD) for 3 hours with 4.25% dialysate in a semirecumbent position was performed.

He presented this time with worsening dyspnea. His vitals were within normal limits. Pertinent physical exam included right-sided dull percussion note with near-absent breath sounds. The patient appeared euvolemic otherwise. Chest radiograph (CXR) showed worsening large volume right-sided hydrothorax despite a paracentesis a week prior to presentation (Figure 1). The B-type natriuretic peptide level was 172 pg/mL (0–100), and troponin I was 0.07 ng/mL (<0.06). Basic metabolic panel was significant for elevated serum creatinine (Se-Cr) 7.46 mg/dL (0.6–1.30). He initially required oxygen and had another ultrasound-guided large-volume thoracentesis, owing to his symptoms and drained 2.5 liters of clear, straw-colored fluid.

Repeat pleural fluid analysis was sent which revealed a transudative fluid with normal lactate dehydrogenase (76 IU/L) and protein (<3.0 g/dL) with a glucose level of 104 mg/dl (Table 1). Pleural fluid to serum glucose gradient was 21 mg/dL. Due to the high clinical index of suspicion of a peritoneal source for recurrent hydrothorax, a PF-S glucose ratio was also evaluated which was >1.0 mg/dL. In order to confirm the source, a technetium 99 peritoneal scintigraphy was performed with continuous images over a 5-hour period (Figure 2). The scan showed traversing of the isotope from the peritoneal dialysate into the pleural cavity, thus confirming the abnormal pleuroperitoneal communication.

Peritoneal dialysis was discontinued permanently with removal of the Tenckhoff catheter, and the patient was started on hemodialysis (HD). He was deemed a poor candidate for video-assisted thoracoscopic surgery (VATS) given his comorbidities and continued HD with complete resolution of the hydrothorax within 2 weeks.

3. Discussion

Peritoneal dialysis can be complicated by development of a hydrothorax and is most commonly seen with CAPD. Hydrothorax development is often attributed to a pleuroperitoneal fistula, an abnormal communication created between the pleural and peritoneal space that can be congenital or acquired. Acquired communication results from an abnormal increase in pressure gradient between the two spaces from an increase in intraperitoneal pressure due to the volume of dialysate [4]. Intra-abdominal pressures are higher when in a vertical, rather than supine position, and therefore predispose patients to complications including dialysate leaks. CCPD, an automated peritoneal dialysis, was developed to allow for a nightly process with larger solute and fluid removal in the supine position [5], and thus it is recommended in those at risk of complications related to increased intra-abdominal pressure gradient [4].

Initial diagnosis can be supported by increased PF-S glucose gradient, indicating presence of dialysate, but in our case, this did not prove to be a reliable indicator. There are several factors that can affect the glucose concentration in the pleural fluid coming from a peritoneal leak. It depends on the diameter of the defect causing the leakage, the rate of absorption of glucose from the pleural surface, glucose concentration of the dialysate, and a delay between the dialysate exchange and pleural fluid sample collection [6]. Literature suggests that the pleural effusion is unlikely to be due to a pleuroperitoneal communication with a low PF-S glucose gradient of <50 mg/dL [7, 8]. However, there is also limited evidence that argues in favor of pleuroperitoneal communication in a PD patient as the only cause for a pleural glucose to be higher than the serum, i.e., a PF-S glucose ratio >1.0 in cases where gradient was lower than 50 mg/dl [3, 9, 10]. The PF-S glucose >1.0 in our case also supports the higher sensitivity of this approach. Pleural fluid analysis for lactate D-isomer that is only found in the dialysate is an alternate method to identify the peritoneal source [11] which was not utilized in our case.

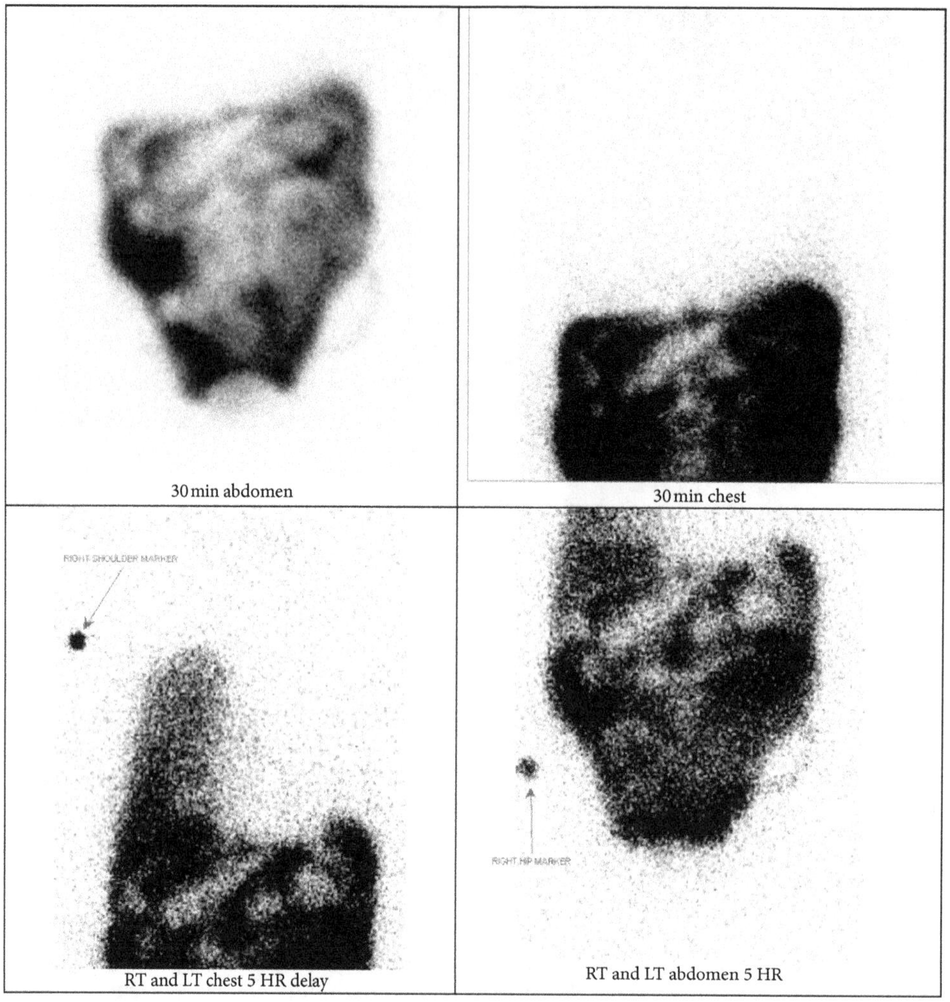

FIGURE 2: Right pleural-peritoneal fistula demonstrated on peritoneal scintigraphy after 5th hour.

The confirmatory tests to diagnose a peritoneal leak mainly include instillation of methylene blue, CT peritoneography, or a technetium scan, followed by serial imaging which can visualize the rate and amount of dye seepage and assess the location and size of the defect which helps in guiding management [12]. A technetium scan also has the additional advantage of being able to assess if a fistula repair has been successful, although this is often limited by cost.

First-line treatment is usually temporary halt of the PD for 2–6 weeks or switching to HD [13]. In cases where this is not attainable, conventional treatment methods involve the instillation of pleural irritants via the intercostal catheter into pleural space, such as tetracycline or talc, for pleurodesis. Surgical correction with VATS with direct pleurodesis or surgical diaphragmatic repair is more definitive with no reported recurrence but is often limited due to its invasive nature. In our case, a surgical repair was deemed high risk because of our patient's poor cardiopulmonary reserve, and he was transitioned to HD with a further plan for pleurodesis and follow-up by cardiothoracic surgery. The pleural effusion resolved with HD on follow-up.

4. Conclusion

PD irrespective of duration with either CAPD or APD can be complicated by a pleuroperitoneal leak. A high index of suspicion is warranted in PD patients presenting with new-onset unilateral hydrothorax when common causes are ruled out. As depicted in our case, the PF-S ratio may have higher sensitivity than PF-S gradient.

Authors' Contributions

NB was involved in manuscript writing and literature review, SA was responsible for manuscript editing and literature review, HC contributed in identification of the case, manuscript writing, literature review, and final manuscript review and approval, and TD approved the final manuscript.

References

[1] R. Diaz Mancebo, G. Del Peso Gilsanz, M. Rodriguez et al., "Pleuroperitoneal communication in patients on peritoneal

dialysis one hospital's experience and a review of the literature," *Nefrologia*, vol. 31, no. 2, pp. 213–217, 2011.

[2] M. Mohamad Alahmad and R. Kasmani, "Sweet hydrothorax: a common presentation of a rare condition," *Avicenna Journal of Medicine*, vol. 9, no. 3, pp. 111–114, 2019.

[3] S. Tang, W. H. Chui, A. W. C. Tang et al., "Video-assisted thoracoscopic talc pleurodesis is effective for maintenance of peritoneal dialysis in acute hydrothorax complicating peritoneal dialysis," *Nephrology Dialysis Transplantation*, vol. 18, no. 4, p. 804, 2003.

[4] S. Q. Lew, "Hydrothorax: pleural effusion associated with peritoneal dialysis," *Peritoneal Dialysis International: Journal of the International Society for Peritoneal Dialysis*, vol. 30, no. 1, pp. 13–18, 2010.

[5] Z. J. Twardowski, R. Khanna, K. D. Nolph et al., "Intra-abdominal pressures during natural activities in patients treated with continuous ambulatory peritoneal dialysis," *Nephron*, vol. 44, no. 2, pp. 129–135, 1986.

[6] N. Momenin, P. M. Colletti, and E. M. Kaptein, "Low pleural fluid-to-serum glucose gradient indicates pleuroperitoneal communication in peritoneal dialysis patients: presentation of two cases and a review of the literature," *Nephrology Dialysis Transplantation*, vol. 27, no. 3, pp. 1212–1219, 2012.

[7] K. M. Chow, C. C. Szeto, WongTY et al., "Hydrothorax complicating peritoneal dialysis: diagnostic value of glucose concentration in pleural fluid aspirate," *Peritoneal Dialysis International*, vol. 22, 2002.

[8] C. C. Szeto and K. M. Chow, "Pathogenesis and management of hydrothorax complicating peritoneal dialysis," *Current Opinion in Pulmonary Medicine*, vol. 10, no. 4, pp. 315–319, 2004.

[9] P. Mangana, D. Arvanitis, and D. Vlassopoulos, "Acute hydrothorax in peritoneal dialysis patients: diagnosis and treatment options," *Nephrol Dial Transplant*, vol. 18, p. 2451, 2003.

[10] L. Ortiz, D. Hazley, and M. G. Seikaly, "Thoracocentesis helps diagnose diaphragmatic defects in peritoneal dialysis patients," *Pediatric Nephrology*, vol. 16, no. 2, pp. 105-106, 2001.

[11] K. N. Ramakrishna, D. Lowe, and U. K. Murthy, "Hunt for the shunt: an unusual case of late-onset hydrothorax in a patient on peritoneal dialysis," *Cureus*, vol. 11, no. 1, Article ID e3839, 2019.

[12] M. Nishina, M. Iwazaki, M Koizumi et al., "Case of peritoneal dialysis-related acute hydrothorax, which was successfully treated by thoracoscopic surgery, using collagen fleece," *The Tokai Journal of Experimental and Clinical Medicine*, vol. 36, no. 4, pp. 91–94, 2011.

[13] V. Puri, F. A. Orellana, G. G. Singer, and M. S. Wald, "Diaphragmatic defect complicating peritoneal dialysis," *The Annals of Thoracic Surgery*, vol. 92, no. 4, p. 1527, 2011.

Acute Kidney Injury in a Case Series of Patients with Confirmed COVID-19 (Coronavirus Disease 2019): Role of Angiotensin-Converting Enzyme 2 and Renin-Angiotensin System Blockade

Avantika Chenna,[1] Venu Madhav Konala,[2] Subhasish Bose,[3] Sasmit Roy,[3] Bhaskar Reddy Madhira,[4] Vijay Gayam,[5] Srikanth Naramala,[6] and Sreedhar Adapa[7]

[1]*Department of Internal Medicine, Division of Nephrology, Phobe Putney Memorial Hospital, Medical College of Georgia, 417 W 3rd Avenue, Albany 31701, GA, USA*
[2]*Department of Internal Medicine, Division of Medical Oncology, Ashland Bellefonte Cancer Center, 122 St Christopher Dr, Ashland 41169, KY, USA*
[3]*Lynchburg Nephrology Physicians, Lynchburg, VA, USA*
[4]*Fellow in Hematology and Oncology, Sunny Upstate Medical University, Syracuse, NY, USA*
[5]*Department of Medicine, Interfaith Medical Center, Brooklyn, NY, USA*
[6]*Department of Internal Medicine, Division of Rheumatology, Adventist Medical Center, Hanford 93230, CA, USA*
[7]*Department of Internal Medicine, Division of Nephrology, Adventist Medical Center, Hanford 93230, CA, USA*

Correspondence should be addressed to Sreedhar Adapa; sreedharadapa@gmail.com

Academic Editor: Rumeyza Kazancioglu

The renin-angiotensin system plays a very critical role in hypertension, diabetes, and kidney and heart diseases. The blockade of the renin-angiotensin system results in the prevention of progression of renal and cardiac damage. There have been controversial hypotheses raised regarding the safety of angiotensin-converting enzyme inhibitors and angiotensin receptor blockers in COVID-19 (coronavirus disease 2019). We present the case series of four patients (2 men and 2 women; 1 Caucasian and 3 African Americans; two survived and two died) with confirmed COVID-19, presenting with respiratory symptoms and acute kidney injury, who have been on angiotensin-converting enzyme inhibitors or angiotensin receptor blockers. Membrane-bound angiotensin-converting enzyme 2 (ACE2) has been implicated as the gateway for viral entry into the human cell in causing the infection. The factors contributing to acute kidney injury are diuretics, iodinated contrast administration, hemodynamic instability apart from ACE inhibitors, and angiotensin receptor blockers. The ACE inhibitors and ARBs were stopped in these patients due to acute kidney injury. We also discussed the role of ACE2 and the renin-angiotensin system (RAS) blockade in patients with COVID-19 infection along with pathogenesis.

1. Introduction

The severe acute respiratory syndrome by coronavirus 2 (SARS-CoV-2) has resulted in mortality worldwide and has been declared a global pandemic. The United States has the highest number of positively tested cases in the world, and the virus has been spreading relentlessly. The lung is the main organ affected by COVID-19 resulting in respiratory failure, but there is also the involvement of other organs like the heart, kidney, and gastrointestinal tract. The patients who tend to have severe disease or need intensive care unit (ICU) admission have multiorgan involvement. Membrane-bound angiotensin-converting enzyme 2 (ACE 2) has been implicated as the gateway for viral entry into the human cell in causing the infection [1, 2].

The renin-angiotensin system (RAS) plays a very critical role in hypertension, diabetes, and kidney and heart diseases. The blockade of RAS results in the prevention of progression of renal and cardiac damage. The role of angiotensin-converting enzyme inhibitors (ACEIs) and angiotensin receptor blockers (ARBs) needs to be elucidated in COVID-19. There have been controversial hypotheses raised regarding the safety of ACEIs/ARBs in COVID-19 [1]. Here, we describe the case series of four patients with confirmed COVID-19 who developed AKI. We also discuss the role of ACE2 in pathogenesis and in AKI and the perspectives of ACEIs/ARBs in COVID-19.

1.1. First Case. A 49-year-old male presented to the emergency room with complaints of cough and shortness of breath started getting worse for one week. Associated symptoms included fever, chills, and generalized body aches. The patient was found to be hypoxic in the emergency room, requiring oxygen via a nasal cannula. Past medical history was significant for type 2 diabetes mellitus, hypertension, dyslipidemia, depression, and gastroesophageal reflux disease. The patient had a 28-pack-year smoking history and quit smoking four years ago. The patient denied any chest pain, orthopnea, paroxysmal nocturnal dyspnea, or swelling of his extremities. The patient denied any recent travel history. His home medications included metformin 1000 mg by mouth twice a day, hydrochlorothiazide 25 mg by mouth daily, amlodipine 10 mg by mouth daily, duloxetine 60 mg by mouth daily, atorvastatin 40 mg by mouth daily, lisinopril 40 mg by mouth daily, and aspirin 81 mg by mouth daily. The patient had no significant family history.

Initial vital signs showed a blood pressure of 132/89 mmHg, heart rate of 88 beats per minute (bpm), oxygen saturation of 80% on room air, which improved to 89% on a 5 L nasal cannula, respiratory rate of 30 breaths/min, and temperature of 99.1°F. Physical examination revealed an unkempt obese male with mild tachypnea and coarse breath sounds bilaterally. The rest of the physical examination was within normal limits.

Laboratory data revealed normal hemoglobin at 13.9 g/dL and platelet count of 220K/mm^3. Liver function tests were within normal limits. Lactic acid was slightly elevated at 1.7 mmol/L. The rest of the laboratory data are summarized in Table 1. His influenza A and B testing was negative. Chest X-ray PA and lateral view revealed bibasilar infiltrate consistent with bilateral pneumonia. The patient had a CT of the chest with IV contrast showing bilateral ground-glass opacities. The patient's nasopharyngeal swab was sent for COVID-19 testing, and he was placed in isolation.

The patient's clinical course was complicated by transferring to the intensive care unit due to worsening hypoxic respiratory failure requiring high flow oxygen. He was subsequently intubated. The patient was started on treatment for possible community-acquired pneumonia with ceftriaxone 1 g intravenously daily and azithromycin 500 mg once followed by 250 mg by mouth daily. The patient was also started on lopinavir and ritonavir as per protocol at that time.

His clinical course was also complicated by worsening renal function with the increased blood urea nitrogen to 21 mg/dL and serum creatinine to 2.2 mg/dL. The patient's lisinopril and hydrochlorothiazide were held, and he was started on 0.9% normal saline intravenously. His urine analysis was significant for 2+ protein and no RBC casts. The patient complement levels were within normal limits. Testing for hepatitis B, hepatitis C, and HIV screen was all negative. Serum protein electrophoresis did not reveal any monoclonal protein. His COVID-19 testing returned positive. The patient's urine output subsequently continued to drop, and hence he was started on dialysis due to volume overload and hyperkalemia in the setting of acute respiratory distress syndrome type. The patient is currently receiving dialysis three times a week, and his antibiotic coverage was expanded to pulse-dose vancomycin and cefepime. The patient remains intubated and ventilated in the intensive care unit.

1.2. Second Case. A 48-year-old female was admitted with worsening shortness of breath for two days after attending a funeral where some people have tested positive for COVID-19. The patient complained of dry cough but denied any chest pain, orthopnea, or paroxysmal nocturnal dyspnea. The patient denied any nausea, vomiting, or diarrhea. Her past medical history was significant for hypertension, dyslipidemia, and hypothyroidism. Her surgical history was positive for thyroidectomy in 2001. The patient denied any history of smoking or illicit drug use. Her home medications included rosuvastatin 20 mg by mouth daily, hydrochlorothiazide/losartan 25–100 mg by mouth daily, amlodipine 10 mg by mouth daily, levothyroxine 150 mcg by mouth daily, and aspirin 81 mg by mouth daily.

Initial vital signs were a blood pressure of 132/56 mmHg, heart rate of 109 bpm, respiratory rate of 22 breaths/min, oxygen saturation of 80% on room air, which improved to 90% on 5 L of oxygen via a nasal cannula, and temperature of 101°F. Her physical examination was significant for morbidly obese female in mild acute distress with decreased breath sounds and positive rales bilaterally. The rest of the physical examination was unremarkable.

Laboratory testing: CBC was significant for hemoglobin of 12 g/dL and platelet count of 160K/mm^3. Liver function testing was within normal limits. The rest of the laboratory data are summarized in Table 1. Initial arterial blood gas showed a pH of 7.3, PO_2 of 58 mmHg, PCO_2 of 63 mmHg, and oxygen saturation of 83% on a high flow nasal cannula at 40 liters. Influenza A and B testing was negative. Chest X-ray PA and lateral showed cardiomegaly and pulmonary edema. The patient's nasopharyngeal swab was sent for COVID-19 testing, and she was placed in appropriate isolation.

The patient was initially admitted to the medical floor, and subsequently, her oxygen requirements escalated to high flow oxygen and venti mask and she was subsequently transferred to the intensive care unit for worsening hypercapnic hypoxic respiratory failure requiring

Table 1: Laboratory data for all the patients on admission.

Patient	Sodium (mmol/l)	Potassium (mmol/l)	Bicarbonate (mmol/dl)	Blood urea nitrogen (mg/dl)	Serum creatinine (mg/dl)	CPK (units/L)	White cell count (K/mm^3)	Lymphocyte count (K/mm^3)	Urine analysis	Urine protein creatinine ratio (mg/g)
1	130	4.4	22	14	0.96	233	5.3	0.8	2+ protein and no RBC casts	Not available
2	130	4.0	34	22	0.87	458	6.9	0.6	No protein and no RBC casts	Not available
3	143	3.5	17	26	1.1	287	8.8	0.7	No protein and no RBC casts	524
4	154	3.2	23	25	1.8	278	10.6	0.3	3+ protein and no RBC casts (RBC—30/HPF)	270

intubation and ventilation. The patient was started on intravenous Lasix 80 mg every 8 hours and was also started on hydroxychloroquine 200 mg twice a day and azithromycin 500 mg once followed by 250 mg daily for five days as per protocol. The patient's creatinine continued to increase to 3.65 mg/dL, and blood urea nitrogen increased to 92 mg/dL over three days. Lisinopril and hydrochlorothiazide were held since admission, and later Lasix was also held. Her urine analysis was negative for any protein or RBC casts. The patient is currently being monitored without any requirement for dialysis at present.

1.3. Third Case. A 64-year-old female was admitted with complaints of cough and shortness of breath getting worse over one week. She also had fever, nausea, vomiting, and diarrhea. The patient also complained of decreased appetite. Her cough was productive with greenish sputum. The patient denied any chest pain, orthopnea, paroxysmal nocturnal dyspnea, or pedal edema. The patient denied any history of recent travel. The patient's past medical history was significant for type 2 diabetes mellitus, hypertension, dyslipidemia, and seasonal allergies. The patient denied any history of smoking or illicit drug use. The patient's home medications included metformin 750 mg by mouth twice a day, spironolactone 25 mg by mouth daily, amlodipine 10 mg by mouth daily, and azilsartan 80 mg by mouth daily.

Initial vital signs showed a blood pressure of 132/89 mmHg, heart rate of 88 bpm, respiratory rate of 30 breaths/min, temperature of 100.1°F, and oxygen saturation of 82% on room air, which improved to 89% on 5 L of oxygen via a nasal cannula. Her physical examination revealed an obese female with mild respiratory distress. Her respiratory examination revealed coarse breath sounds bilaterally. The rest of her physical examination was unremarkable.

Laboratory testing: the patient's initial CBC revealed anemia with hemoglobin 9.5 g/dL and platelet count 121K/mm^3. Liver function tests were within normal limits. The rest of the laboratory data are summarized in Table 1. Patient's influenza A and B testing was negative. Chest X-ray PA and lateral view suggested multifocal pneumonia. The patient had a CT angiogram of the chest with PE protocol showing bilateral ground-glass opacities concerning COVID-19. The patient's nasopharyngeal swab was sent for COVID-19 testing, and she was placed in appropriate isolation.

The patient was admitted to the medical floor initially but later transferred to the intensive care unit due to hypoxic respiratory failure requiring high flow oxygen. The patient was also started on lopinavir and ritonavir per protocol at that time. The patient's clinical course continued to get worse with continued worsening of renal function with an increase in creatinine from 1.1 mg/dL to 1.7 mg/dL and then to 6.9 mg/dL for the next 3-4 days. The patient was treated with IV fluids and intravenous bicarbonate. Her medications, azilsartan and spironolactone, were discontinued because of hypotension and worsening renal function. Urine analysis was negative for protein or RBC casts. Testing for hepatitis B and C and HIV screening were negative. Testing for antinuclear antibody, anti-neutrophilic cytoplasmic antibody, and anti-glomerular basement membrane antibodies was either negative or within normal limits. Complement levels, including C3 and C4, were 65 mg/dL and 8 mg/dL, respectively, which were low. Serum protein electrophoresis revealed no M spike.

The patient's COVID-19 testing came back as positive. Her urine output dropped to 5–10 milliliters/hour. The patient developed acute respiratory distress syndrome with fluid overload and was started on Lasix 80 mg IV every 8 hours and was also placed in a prone position. The patient failed medical management and was started on dialysis due to oliguric renal failure. Despite the above efforts, the patient's clinical condition continued to deteriorate with hypoxia and hypotension, which persisted despite being maximized on four vasopressors. The family decided to opt for comfort measures only, and the patient, unfortunately, died 11 days after the presentation.

1.4. Fourth Case. A 77-year-old African American male presented with a chief complaint of dry cough, shortness of breath, and fever for one week. The patient was encephalopathic on presentation and went into cardiac arrest, received 1 round of cardiopulmonary resuscitation, and was able to achieve the return of spontaneous circulation. He was then placed on the hypothermic protocol. The patient was also hypotensive, requiring norepinephrine. The patient's past medical history was significant for type 2 diabetes mellitus, hypertension, dyslipidemia, and hypothyroidism. The patient has no travel history, but the wife reported a concern that he might have encountered a person who was sick. The patient has no history of smoking or illicit drug use. His home medications were pioglitazone 30 mg by mouth daily, olmesartan 40 mg by mouth daily, levothyroxine 100 mcg by mouth daily, glimepiride 4 mg by mouth daily, fenofibrate 160 mg by mouth daily, aspirin 81 mg by mouth daily, and sitagliptin 100 mg by mouth daily. His vital signs were a blood pressure of 102/66 mmHg, heart rate of 92 bpm, respiratory rate of 26 breaths per minute, oxygen saturation of 89% on 100% FiO_2, and temperature of 95.8°F. Physical examination revealed an obese patient who was intubated and sedated. Respiratory examination revealed coarse breath sounds bilaterally.

His laboratory examination was significant for hemoglobin 14.1 g/dL and platelet count 306K/mm^3. The rest of the laboratory data are summarized in Table 1. Liver function tests were significant for AST elevated at 125 U/L. Lactic acid was elevated at 14 mmol/L. The patient's influenza A and B testing was negative. The patient's nasopharyngeal swab was sent for COVID-19 testing, and he was placed in isolation, with the result being positive couple of days later. A portable chest X-ray revealed bilateral pulmonary infiltrates concerning COVID-19.

All antihypertensives and hypoglycemics were held, including olmesartan. The patient was treated with aggressive IV fluid resuscitation along with IV bicarbonate. The patient was administered insulin therapy for hyperglycemia.

The patient's vasopressor requirement continued to increase due to hypotension. His renal failure continued to get worse. Dialysis was considered but was not done due to hemodynamic instability, and the patient was able to urinate. Due to persistent hypotension despite the use of vasopressors and continued hypoxia despite intubation and ventilation, after discussion with the family, the family chose to opt for do not resuscitate (DNR) and comfort care only. The patient died immediately after extubation.

2. Discussion

We presented the case series of four patients who were on angiotensin-converting enzyme inhibitors (ACE inhibitors) or angiotensin receptor blockers (ARBs) with COVID-19 infection and acute renal failure. We summarize the findings, including patient characteristics, comorbidities, presenting symptoms, types of ACE inhibitors, or ARB use, including diuretic use at home as well as in the hospital, whether the patient had a computed tomography with IV contrast, dialysis initiation in hospital, and outcome of the patients in Table 2. In our case series, there were two men and two women: 1 Caucasian and 3 African Americans. All of them developed acute kidney injury and mortality was 50%. We summarized creatinine trends during hospital stay in Table 3.

SARS-CoV-2 utilizes ACE2 and type 2 transmembrane serine proteases (TMPRSS 2) to enter the human cell [2]. The spike (S) protein of the virus binds to the catalytic domain of the ACE2 with high affinity [3], which can cause conformational changes in the S protein [4]. These cellular proteases (TMPRSS 2) are needed for the S protein priming, cleavage, and allow the fusion of viral and cellular membranes [2]. A prior study by Kuba and colleagues showed the first genetic proof that SARS-CoV needs ACE2 as a receptor in vivo [5]. Wrapp et al. have shown that on the cryoelectron microscopy, the S protein of the nCoV has 10- to 20-fold higher affinities to ACE2 compared to SARS-CoV [4].

Angiotensin-converting enzyme 2 (ACE2) is a zinc metalloprotease discovered in 2000 and has substantial homology with human angiotensin-converting enzymes (ACEs) [6]. The mRNA (messenger ribonucleic acid) of ACE2 is widely distributed in all human tissues, and the protein is widely expressed in the oral and nasal mucosa, nasopharynx, lung, gastrointestinal tract, kidney, and lymphoid tissue [7]. There is a high expression of ACE2 receptors on the epithelial cells of oral mucosa that plays a vital role in the transmission of COVID-19 [8]. Type II alveolar cells and the capillary endothelium express ACE2 receptors [7].

ACE2 is expressed in the proximal tubular cells significantly compared to other components in the kidney [9]. In kidney tubules, there is significant ACE2 expression on brush border and less expression in the cytoplasm [9]. The gene expression for ACE2 is 100-fold higher in kidney tissue compared to the lung [10]. There are significant proteinuria and hematuria in the patients infected with COVID-19 [10]. Of the patients who developed severe disease, a significant proportion of patients developed acute kidney injury and was associated with mortality [11].

Hypertension, diabetes, and cardiovascular disease are the common comorbidities associated with COVID-19 [11]. ACEI and ARB are the commonly used medications for the treatment of hypertension and kidney and heart diseases. Angiotensinogen is converted to angiotensin I by renin, which in turn is converted to angiotensin II (Ang II) by ACE. Angiotensin II activates angiotensin receptor type 1 (AT1R) and aldosterone and exerts vasoconstriction and sodium retention, resulting in hypertension. ACE2 converts angiotensin II to angiotensin (Ang)-(1–7), which exerts vasodilatory effects through the MAS receptor and thus negatively regulates the RAS system [12].

Angiotensin II causes inflammation, fibrosis, and edema through AT1R, and the absence of ACE2 causes the unrestricted activity of Ang II, which results in acute severe

Table 2: Clinical characteristics and outcome of the patients.

Patient	Age	Sex	Symptoms	Smoking	Comorbidities	ACEI or ARB	Diuretic use at home	Diuretic use in the hospital	Dialysis	Computed tomography with IV contrast	Outcome
1	49	Caucasian male	Fever, cough, SOB, chills, and body aches	Ex-smoker, 28-pack-year smoking history	Hypertension, diabetes, and dyslipidemia	Lisinopril 40 mg	HCTZ 25 mg	No	Yes	Yes	Died (DNR, comfort measures)
2	48	African American female	Dry cough and fever	Nonsmoker	Hypertension and dyslipidemia	Losartan 100 mg	HCTZ 25 mg	Yes	No	No	DNR, still remains critically ill and intubated
3	64	African American female	Cough, SOB, and fever	Nonsmoker	Hypertension, diabetes, and dyslipidemia	Azilsartan 80 mg	Spironolactone 25 mg	Yes	Yes	Yes	Died (patient made DNR)
4	77	African American male	Cough, SOB, and fever	Nonsmoker	Hypertension, dyslipidemia, and diabetes	Olmesartan 40 mg	No	No	No	No	Died (patient made DNR)

Table 3: Summary of serum creatinine trend during hospital stay.

Patient	Serum creatinine on presentation (mg/dl)	Serum creatinine values during hospital stay (mg/dl)	Serum creatinine level at outcome (mg/dl)
1	0.96	0.96 ⟶ 2.2 ⟶ 3.8 ⟶ 4.9	5.4
2	0.87	0.87 ⟶ 1.2 ⟶ 1.9 ⟶ 2.7	3.65
3	1.1	1.7 ⟶ 2.5 ⟶ 3.3 ⟶ 5.3	6.9
4	1.8	1.8 ⟶ 2.4 ⟶ 3.9 ⟶ 5.6	7.4

respiratory distress syndrome (ARDS). ACE2/Ang-(1–7)/Mas axis has an inhibitory effect on the signaling pathways of inflammation, fibrinogenesis, and cellular proliferation [12]. The net effect of ACE2 is anti-inflammatory, antifibrogenic, and antiproliferative [12]. A mice study showed that higher Ang II levels cause ACE2 to be internalized in the cell and undergo lysosomal degradation [13]. The internalization was prevented by losartan [13]. There is also speculation that the ACE2 and AT1R physically interact and form complexes on the cell membrane in the absence of Ang II, thus reducing the potential virus interaction with ACE2 [14].

Increased cardiac ACE2 gene expression and cardiac ACE2 activity were seen in Lewis rats after selective use of lisinopril or losartan, whereas the combination resulted in elevated cardiac ACE2 but not cardiac ACE2 mRNA [15]. In adult Sprague-Dawley rats, enalapril abated/mitigated the downregulation of ACE2 in the late phase of ventricular dysfunction of experimental myocardial infarction [16]. There was no increased cardiac ACE2 expression with ramipril or valsartan or in combination in the rat myocardial infarction model [17].

In a study of 79 patients that evaluated plasma ACE2 activity and long-term cardiovascular outcomes in patients with obstructive coronary artery disease (CAD), the ACE2 levels did not vary with age and the use of ACE1/ARBs did not alter the levels [18]. This study revealed that there were 83% of male patients in the high ACE2 level group [18]. In a study of 617 hypertensive patients that evaluated the urinary ACE2 level, only patients treated with olmesartan had increased levels [19]. The urinary ACE2 measured is soluble and is not membrane-bound [19].

Kuba et al., in a mouse model, showed that the RAS blockade attenuated the lung injury in SARS-CoV [5]. In a retrospective study of 1055 adult patients admitted with pneumonia, continued use of ACEI and statins resulted in lower rates of deaths and intubations [20]. Severe acute lung injury induced by influenza (H7N9) virus was observed in an experimental ACE2 knockout (KO) mouse model [21]. This study shows that ACE2 plays a critical role in pathogenesis; the blockade of AT1R resulted in the mitigation of acute lung injury [21].

Fang et al. hypothesized that the use of ACE2 modulation medications in hypertensive and diabetic patients increased the risk of developing severe COVID-19 infection [1]. This hypothesis has created widespread confusion in healthcare providers and was perpetuated by media channels and social media [22]. Many international societies have released statements on the continued use of the ACEIs/ARBs [14].

The understanding of COVID-19 and its pathogenesis sheds light on the potential targets for the treatment: development of spike subunit 1 protein-based vaccine, inhibiting viral spike protein priming proteases, through the serine protease inhibitor camostat mesylate, blocking ACE2 receptors to inhibit the viral interaction with ACE2 [23]; soluble ACE2 utilization to overwhelm the body membrane-bound ACE2 that can prevent the virus entry into the cell [24]; and baricitinib, which inhibits the endocytosis via G-associated kinase and AP2-associated protein kinase (AAK1), which is critical for virus entry [25].

There are currently few clinical trials underway to analyze ACE2 and RAAS blockade, a potential target for COVID-19: recombinant human angiotensin-converting enzyme 2 (rhACE2) as a treatment for patients with COVID-19 (NCT04287686) [26], losartan for patients with COVID-19 not requiring hospitalization (NCT04311177) [27], and losartan for patients with COVID-19 requiring hospitalization (NCT04312009) [27].

2.1. COVID-19 Infection and AKI. The incidence of AKI in patients infected with COVID-19 is around 3–15% as per recently published studies from China [11, 28]. The rates of AKI increased significantly to 14.5–50% in patients with severe COVID-19 infection requiring ICU admission [11, 29]. AKI in COVID-19 infection could be due to combination of cytokine-induced systemic inflammatory response and virus-induced direct cytotropic effect and acute tubular necrosis (ATN) due to multiorgan failure and shock. Other factors like volume depletion, drug toxicity, contrast exposure, and hypotension can result in AKI.

2.2. Acute Kidney Injury and Mortality with COVID-19 Infection. AKI is associated with increased mortality in patients infected with COVID-19. The incidence of AKI was 23% in 101 patients reported by Shi et al., who died from COVID-19 infection [30]. Elevated BUN, elevated baseline serum creatinine, peak serum creatinine >1.5, AKI stages 2 and 3, proteinuria, and hematuria are all associated with mortality as per Cheng et al., after adjusting for confounding factors [28]. Since AKI was associated with increased in-hospital mortality, the patients should be managed by providing hemodynamic support, avoiding nonsteroidal anti-inflammatory drugs (NSAIDs), nephrotoxins, and contrast along with early institution of continuous renal replacement therapy (CRRT).

3. Conclusion

In the above case series, all the patients developed acute kidney injury, but other factors were contributing to acute kidney injury like diuretics, iodinated contrast administration, hemodynamic instability apart from ACE inhibitors, and angiotensin receptor blockers. The ACE inhibitors and ARBs were stopped in these patients due to acute kidney injury.

There is no established evidence that suggests that the use of ACEIs/ARBs is associated with the COVID-19 or can potentiate the severe infection. Preclinical and clinical studies have shown beneficial evidence in viral pneumonia. The patients must follow the healthcare provider's advice before changing the medications. The medical professionals should follow the guidance of the national and international societies.

Consent

Consent was obtained from all the cases and from power of attorney where needed.

References

[1] L. Fang, K. George, and M. Roth, "Are patients with hypertension and diabetes mellitus at increased risk for COVID-19 infection?" *The Lancet Respiratory Medicine*, vol. 8, no. 4, 2020.

[2] M. Hoffmann, H. Kleine-Weber, S. Schroeder et al., "SARS-CoV-2 cell entry depends on ACE2 and TMPRSS2 and is blocked by a clinically proven protease inhibitor," *Cell*, vol. 181, no. 2, pp. 271–280.e8, 2020.

[3] W. Li, M. J. Moore, N. Vasilieva et al., "Angiotensin-converting enzyme 2 is a functional receptor for the SARS coronavirus," *Nature*, vol. 426, no. 6965, pp. 450–454, 2003.

[4] D. Wrapp, N. Wang, K. S. Corbett et al., "Cryo-EM structure of the 2019-nCoV spike in the prefusion conformation," *Science*, vol. 367, no. 6483, pp. 1260–1263, 2020.

[5] K. Kuba, Y. Imai, S. Rao et al., "A crucial role of angiotensin converting enzyme 2 (ACE2) in SARS coronavirus-induced lung injury," *Nature Medicine*, vol. 11, no. 8, pp. 875–879, 2005.

[6] S. R. Tipnis, N. M. Hooper, R. Hyde, E. Karran, G. Christie, and A. J. Turner, "A human homolog of angiotensin-converting enzyme," *Journal of Biological Chemistry*, vol. 275, no. 43, pp. 33238–33243, 2000.

[7] I. Hamming, W. Timens, M. Bulthuis, A. Lely, G. Navis, and H. van Goor, "Tissue distribution of ACE2 protein, the functional receptor for SARS coronavirus. A first step in understanding SARS pathogenesis," *The Journal of Pathology*, vol. 203, no. 2, pp. 631–637, 2004.

[8] H. Xu, L. Zhong, J. Deng et al., "High expression of ACE2 receptor of 2019-nCoV on the epithelial cells of oral mucosa," *International Journal of Oral Science*, vol. 12, no. 1, pp. 1–5, 2020.

[9] A. T. Lely, H. Inge, Harry van Goor, and G. J. Navis, "Renal ACE2 expression in human kidney disease," *The Journal of Pathology: A Journal of the Pathological Society of Great Britain and Ireland*, vol. 204, no. 5, pp. 587–593, 2004.

[10] Z. Li, M. Wu, J. Yao et al., "Caution on kidney dysfunctions of COVID-19 patients," *SSRN Electronic Journal*, 2020.

[11] F. Zhou, Yu Ting, R. Du et al., "Clinical course and risk factors for mortality of adult inpatients with COVID-19 in Wuhan, China: a retrospective cohort study," *The Lancet*, vol. 395, no. 10229, pp. 1054–1062, 2020.

[12] A. Simões e Silva, K. Silveira, A. Ferreira, and M. Teixeira, "ACE2, angiotensin-(1-7) and Mas receptor axis in inflammation and fibrosis," *British Journal of Pharmacology*, vol. 169, no. 3, pp. 477–492, 2013.

[13] M. R. Deshotels, H. Xia, S. Sriramula, E. Lazartigues, and C. M. Filipeanu, "Angiotensin II mediates angiotensin converting enzyme type 2 internalization and degradation through an angiotensin II type I receptor-dependent mechanism," *Hypertension*, vol. 64, no. 6, pp. 1368–1375, 2014.

[14] M. A. Sparks and S. Hiremath, "The coronavirus conundrum: ACE2 and hypertension edition," 2020, http://www.nephjc.com/news/covidace2.

[15] C. M. Ferrario, J. A Jessup, M. C. Chappell et al., "Effect of angiotensin-converting enzyme inhibition and angiotensin II receptor blockers on cardiac angiotensin-converting enzyme 2," *Circulation*, vol. 111, no. 20, pp. 2605–2610, 2005.

[16] M. P. Ocaranza, I. Godoy, J. E. Jalil et al., "Enalapril attenuates downregulation of angiotensin-converting enzyme 2 in the late phase of ventricular dysfunction in myocardial infarcted rat," *Hypertension*, vol. 48, no. 4, pp. 572–578, 2006.

[17] L. J. Burchill, E. Velkoska, R. G. Dean, K. Griggs, S. K. Patel, and L. M. Burrell, "Combination renin-angiotensin system blockade and angiotensin-converting enzyme 2 in experimental myocardial infarction: implications for future therapeutic directions," *Clinical Science*, vol. 123, no. 11, pp. 649–658, 2012.

[18] J. Ramchand, S. K. Patel, P. M. Srivastava, O. Farouque, and L. M. Burrell, "Elevated plasma angiotensin converting enzyme 2 activity is an independent predictor of major adverse cardiac events in patients with obstructive coronary artery disease," *PLoS One*, vol. 13, no. 6, Article ID e0198144, 2018.

[19] M. Furuhashi, N. Moniwa, T. Mita et al., "Urinary angiotensin-converting enzyme 2 in hypertensive patients may be increased by olmesartan, an angiotensin II receptor blocker," *American Journal of Hypertension*, vol. 28, no. 1, pp. 15–21, 2015.

[20] C. Henry, M. Zaizafoun, E. Stock, S. Ghamande, A. C. Arroliga, and H. D. White, "Impact of angiotensin-converting enzyme inhibitors and statins on viral pneumonia," *Baylor University Medical Center Proceedings*, vol. 31, no. 4, pp. 419–423, 2018.

[21] P. Yang, H. Gu, Z. Zhao et al., "Angiotensin-converting enzyme 2 (ACE2) mediates influenza H7N9 virus-induced acute lung injury," *Scientific Reports*, vol. 4, p. 7027, 2014.

[22] C. J. Tignanelli, E. Nicholas, M. A. S. Ingraham et al., "Antihypertensive drugs and risk of COVID-19?" *The Lancet Respiratory Medicine*, vol. 8, no. 5, p. e28, 2020.

[23] H. Zhang, J. M. Penninger, Y. Li, N. Zhong, and A. S. Slutsky, "Angiotensin-converting enzyme 2 (ACE2) as a SARS-CoV-2 receptor: molecular mechanisms and potential therapeutic target," *Intensive Care Medicine*, vol. 46, no. 4, pp. 586–590, 2020.

[24] D. Batlle, J. Wysocki, and K. Satchell, "Soluble angiotensin-converting enzyme 2: a potential approach for coronavirus infection therapy?" *Clinical Science*, vol. 134, no. 5, pp. 543–545, 2020.

[25] P. Richardson, I. Griffin, C. Tucker et al., "Baricitinib as potential treatment for 2019-nCoV acute respiratory disease," *The Lancet*, vol. 395, no. 10223, pp. e30–e31, 2020.

[26] L. I. Yimin, "A Randomized, open label, controlled clinical study to evaluate the recombinant human angiotensin-con-

verting enzyme 2 (rhace2) in adult patients with COVID-19," 2020.

[27] C. Tignanelli and M. Puskarich, "Randomized controlled trial of losartan for patients with COVID-19 not requiring hospitalization," 2020.

[28] Y. Cheng, R. Luo, K. Wang et al., "Kidney disease is associated with in-hospital death of COVID-19 patients," *Kidney International*, vol. 97, no. 5, pp. 829–838, 2020.

[29] G. Zhang, C. Hu, L. Luo et al., "Clinical features and short-term outcomes of 221 patients with COVID-19 in Wuhan, China," *Journal of Clinical Virology*, vol. 127, 2020.

[30] Q. Shi, K. Zhao, J. Yu et al., "Clinical characteristics of 101 COVID-19 nonsurvivors in Wuhan, China: a retrospective study," *medRxiv*, 2020.

First Case of COVID-19-Associated Collapsing Glomerulopathy in Sub-Saharan Africa

Yannick M. Nlandu,[1] Jean-Robert R. Makulo,[1] Nestor M. Pakasa,[2] Ernest K. Sumaili,[1] Clarisse N. Nkondi,[1] Justine B. Bukabau,[1] François K. Beya,[2] Nazaire M. Nseka,[1] and François B. Lepira[1]

[1]*Kinshasa University Hospital, Nephrology Unit, Kinshasa, Democratic Republic of the Congo*
[2]*Division of Uro-Nephropathology, Department of Pathology, Kinshasa, Democratic Republic of the Congo*

Correspondence should be addressed to Yannick M. Nlandu; yannicknlandu@yahoo.fr

Academic Editor: Raoul Bergner

Although the lungs remain the main target of SARS-CoV-2, other organs, such as kidneys, can be affected, which has a negative impact on the outcomes of COVID-19 patients. Although previous studies of kidney disease in COVID-19 reported mainly SARS-CoV-2-induced tubular and interstitial injury, there is growing evidence coming out of Africa of glomerular involvement, especially collapsing glomerulopathy seen particularly in people of African descent. We report a case of collapsing glomerulopathy revealed by acute kidney injury and a new onset of full blown nephrotic syndrome in a black Congolese patient coinfected with COVID-19 and malaria.

1. Introduction

The COVID-19 pandemic has caused unprecedented health, social, and economic crises worldwide [1, 2]. While the lungs are the organ primary target of SARS-CoV-2 and subsequent COVID-19, other organs, including kidneys, can be affected, and this is associated with increased mortality and morbidity [3, 4]. Previous autopsy reports from China and more recent reports from the USA have described mostly kidney tubular injury associated with SARS-CoV-2 [5, 6]. However, cumulating evidence from Europe and the USA yields collapsing glomerulopathy (CG), a variant of focal segmental glomerulosclerosis (FSGS) [7]. Interestingly, the patients reported in these early papers are of African descent, and the presence of two apolipoprotein L1 (*APOL1*) risk alleles likely contributes to the pathogenesis of the renal disease [7]. To date, there has been no similar report from continental Africa. We report the first COVID-19-associated CG from sub-Saharan Africa, in a Congolese patient infected with COVID-19, who presented with acute kidney injury (AKI) and de novo nephrotic syndrome.

2. Case Presentation

A 48-year-old African man presented to the Kinshasa University Hospital (KUH) for persistent fever since March 16, 2020, associated with dry cough, vomiting, myalgia, and generalized weakness. At home, he self-medicated with two antimalarial medications (artemether and lumefantrine) for three days. His symptoms persisted, and he visited a medical center on March 23, 2020. A blood smear demonstrated *Plasmodium falciparum* and was given intravenous Artesunate, another antimalarial drug, for five days combined with cefixime, a broad-spectrum, third generation cephalosporin.

Two weeks after his symptoms began, he experienced anuria and he visited the emergency unit of KUH on April 2, 2020. He stated that sixteen days previously he had been in contact with a person known to have COVID-19. His past

TABLE 1: Summary of laboratory evaluations and relevant trends during hospitalization.

Test	Reference	March 16, 2020	April 2, 2020	April 15, 2020	April 22, 2020	April 29, 2020	May 2, 2020	May 7, 2020
Blood urea (mg/dl)	11.3–40.3		222.4	108.3	99.1	198.8	138	195.9
Serum creatinine (mg/dl)	0.6–1.3		15.98	15.9	2	13	12	6.77
Potassium (mmol/l)	3.0–5.0		5.2	4.7		3.7		
Sodium (mmol/l)	135–145		135	135		133		
Bicarbonate (mmol/l)	18–24		14.1			22		
Ionized calcium (mmol/l)	1.18–1.32		0.92	1.07		0.72		
Hemoglobin (g/dl)	12.5–15		18.3			14.3	11.1	11.4
Hematocrit (%)	36–45		50.1			42	33	31.9
White blood cell count (elements/mm^3)	4,000–10,000		14,630					7,830
Lymphocyte count (%)	20–40		17.1					9.5
Platelets (elements/mm^3)	150,000–450,000		313,000					366,000
Albumin (g/dl)	35–45						2.3	
Total cholesterol(mg/dl)	<200			22.06			384	
HDL cholesterol (mg/dl)	>45			840			51	
LDL cholesterol (mg/dl)	<100						272	
Triglycerides (mg/dL)	<150						307	
Erythrocyte sedimentation rate (mm/h)	10–20		85					
CRP (mg/l)	<6	>16					<6	

medical history was remarkable for diabetes mellitus type II and hypertension for the past three years. His medications included the oral antidiabetic drug repaglinide and the antihypertensive drug amlodipine. His family history was notable in that his father had chronic kidney disease. Laboratory tests six months prior to admission included a serum creatinine of 0.72 mg/dL and urinalysis that showed no proteinuria.

On hospital admission, he was noted to be dyspneic, with a respiratory rate of 23 breaths per minute. His blood pressure was 152/84 mmHg and oxygen saturation was 93%. A nasopharyngeal swab sample was positive for COVID-19 mRNA by reverse transcriptase-PCR (RT-PCR). Kidney function tests revealed severe kidney dysfunction, with increased plasma level of urea (222 mg/dL) and creatinine (15.9 mg/dL). A kidney ultrasound excluded an obstructive uropathy; kidney echogenicity, length (13.2 cm), and resistive index (0.8) were increased. In the setting of anuria, no urinalysis was performed. Initial laboratory assessment and selected trends are depicted in Table 1.

A diagnosis of COVID-19 was made and the patient received chloroquine, azithromycin, and vitamin C, starting on day 1, according to the national COVID-19 management protocol (unpublished data). COVID-19 RT-PCR testing and *Plasmodium falciparum* blood smear performed on days 14 and 21 after his hospital admission were negative.

Assessment of kidney function included anuria, metabolic acidosis, hyperkalemia, and stage 3 AKI according to Kidney Disease Improving Global Outcomes (KDIGO) criteria. On April 2, the patient started hemodialysis three sessions per week. After five dialysis sessions, the patient progressively recovered renal function, with diuresis reaching 4 liters/day and a fall in serum creatinine levels (2 mg/dL). The clinical diagnosis was acute tubular necrosis.

One week after recovery of kidney function (admission day 27), he developed full blown nephrotic syndrome (NS), characterized by heavy proteinuria (18 g/d), hypoalbuminemia (serum albumin 2.3 g/dL), and dyslipidemia; microscopic urinalysis was normal. He experienced progressive increase in serum creatinine up to 13 mg/dL. There were no episodes of hypotension, and the patient received no nephrotoxic drugs. A kidney ultrasound excluded renal vein thrombosis. Serologic analyses for hepatitis B, hepatitis C, cytomegalovirus, and HIV were negative. A percutaneous kidney biopsy was performed on hospital day 30. The biopsy contained three cores, each of which contained with both renal cortex and medulla. They yielded a total of 17 glomeruli, none of which was globally sclerotic. All but one displayed segmental or global collapse, implosion of the glomerular capillary tuft, and enlargement of Bowman space (Figure 1).

Bowman space was occupied by hypertrophic and hyperplastic epithelial cells in 1–3 layers some of which showed cytoplasmic vacuolization and occasional protein droplets. Multiple early synechiae connecting glomeruli to Bowman capsule were seen. There was a severe tubular injury, with degenerative and regenerative changes. They included epithelial cell denudation loss and attenuation of the tubular brush border and cellular blebbing and mitoses. These changes in tubules were strongly Ki-67 positive, a molecular marker of cell proliferation (not shown) by immunohistochemistry.

Tubules showed microcystic dilatation and contained positive proteinaceous casts. Some proximal tubules also contained abundant PAS-positive resorption protein droplets. Tubulitis was not seen. The interstitium showed mild edema and patchy moderate fibrosis and patchy moderate to marked chronic inflammatory cell infiltrate.

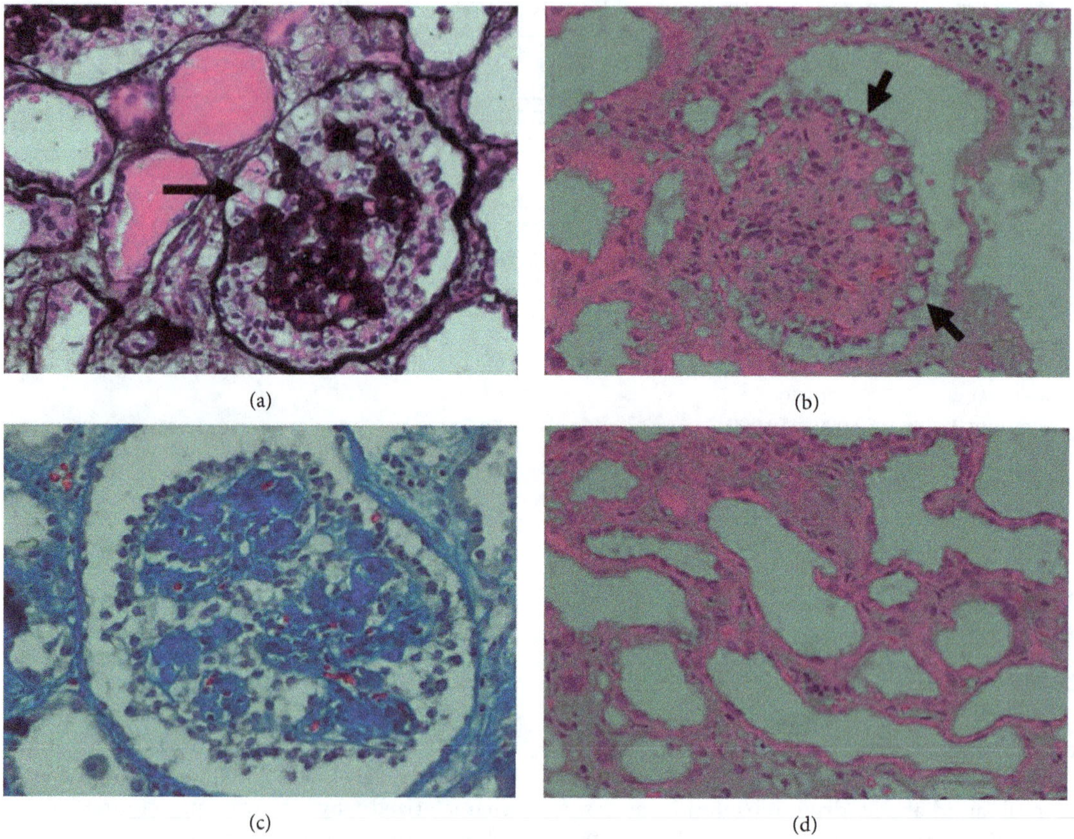

FIGURE 1: Kidney biopsy: representative light microscopy shows global collapse of the glomerular capillary loops accompanied by hyperplasia and hypertrophy of overlying glomerular epithelial cells (a–c) many of which contain scattered eosinophilic protein droplets (a, arrow) and numerous intracytoplasmic vacuoles (b, arrows). a: Jones methenamine silver stain; b: H&E stain; c: Masson's trichrome stain, ×400. Acute tubular injury is manifest in many cortical tubules, accompanied by interstitial edema and patchy interstitial mononuclear inflammatory infiltrates (d: H&E stain, ×400).

The arteries and arterioles showed no conspicuous changes. The biopsy findings were interpreted as being consistent with the collapsing variant of FSGS based on Columbia classification of FSGS, also known as collapsing glomerulopathy (CG) [8].

Shortly after the kidney biopsy, the patient began producing urine. The patient received pulse therapy with methyl prednisolone intravenously, 500 mg on days 1, 2, and 3, and cyclophosphamide intravenously, 500 mg day 1; despite this therapy, proteinuria remains still heavy (4 g per day). Figure 2 shows changes in serum creatinine and proteinuria with time. Although kidney function does not return to normal, serum creatinine levels decreased to 5.0 mg/dL after two weeks.

3. Discussion

Prior studies on kidney disease, based on postmortem autopsy specimens in COVID-19 patients, showed acute tubular injury without glomerular abnormalities [5]. The authors linked these observations to the fact that angiotensin converting enzyme type 2 (ACE2) and transmembrane protein serine type 2 (TMPRSS2), proteins required for SARS-CoV-2 entry and replication in host cells, are prominently expressed in epithelial cells of proximal convoluted tubes [9]. However, recent reports from COVID-19 patients demonstrated the glomerular injury mainly in the form of CG encountered particularly in people of African ancestry [7]. CG is an aggressive variant of FSGS exhibiting high rates of podocyte injury and depletion. Diseased podocytes exhibit a loss and gain of markers of differentiation and proliferation, respectively, and podocytes have been described to "transdifferentiate" toward a macrophage-like cell [10]. By light microscopy, CG is characterized by hyperplasic and hypertrophic visceral epithelial cells overlying segmentally or globally collapsed glomerular capillaries that are narrowed or obliterated by wrinkling and retraction of glomerular basement membranes [11]. The tubulointerstitial compartment often contains an infiltrate of mononuclear cells. Tubular epithelial cells typically display degenerative and regenerative changes and aberrant cellular proliferation and differentiation, leading to microcystic transformation. Tubular atrophy and interstitial fibrosis are common [11]. This histologic description corroborates the findings in the patient herein reported. Ancillary techniques such as electron microscopy (EM), immunofluorescence, in situ hybridization, and other sophisticated techniques have been used to identify pathogenic viral particles in biopsies from kidney structures in well-resourced settings, yielding so far no conclusive results besides podocyte changes related

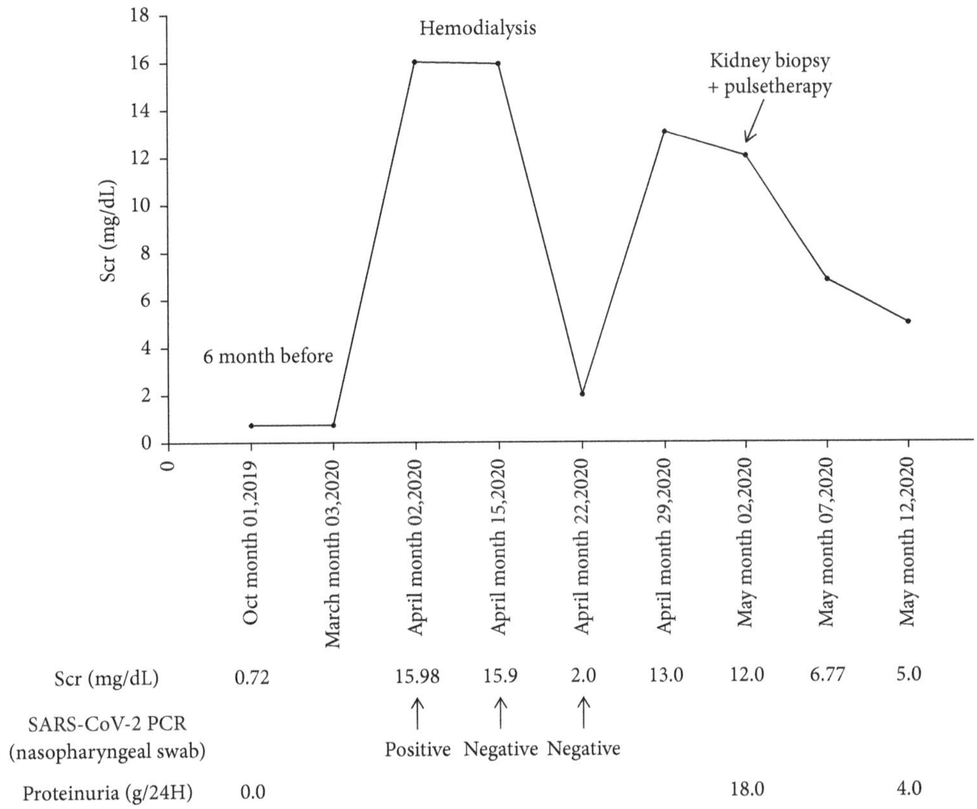

FIGURE 2: Changes in serum creatinine and proteinuria with time in a 48-year-old African male admitted for acute kidney injury with COVID-19.

to proteinuria [12–14], although a recent EM report of a necropsy claims ultrastructural evidence for the presence of virus in podocytes [15].

In the present case report, AKI and NS with a bland microscopic urinalysis were the clinical expression CG. This clinical presentation of CG in the context of COVID-19 illness has been recently reported [11-17]. CG can be of idiopathic origin or most commonly secondary to autoimmune diseases, interferon therapy, and viral illnesses, including HIV, cytomegalovirus, and parvovirus B19 [16]. Our previous experience also reported CG associated with filariasis [17]. As many of these secondary causes were ruled out in the present patient, COVID-19 and coinfection with malaria were retained as potential causes of CG and ensuing NS and AKI. To date, less than 30 cases of CG have been described worldwide in the context of COVID-19, while AKI alone occurs in 1.3% to 36.4% [18]. Although rare, some cases of CG associated with malaria have also been described; indeed, malaria can be associated with hemolytic uremic syndrome or hemophagocytic syndrome [19, 20].

Kidney involvement in COVID-19 is now believed to originate from a double hit mechanism thought to rely upon the interaction of environmental factors, mainly SARS-CoV-2, altered host immune response, and genetic susceptibility. Recent data indicate that kidney injury in COVID-19 could be initiated by viral cytotoxicity or cytokine storm related to sepsis or other associated comorbidities [21]. Direct infection of kidney resident cells is enabled by the high expression of ACE2 and TMPRSS2 in epithelial cells of proximal convoluted tubes and podocytes [9]. The virus likely gains access to the kidney via the bloodstream [21].

Reports from Europe and the United States of America on CG in COVID-19 patients have indicated a high susceptibility of people of African descent compared to other people [7]. This high susceptibility of black people to CG has been reported to be linked to the presence of high kidney risk genotypes of *APOL1* genes, well-known risk factors for the development of CG in HIV and non-HIV black patients [22]. Regardless of the associated disease, nearly 70% of these African-descent patients with CG are homozygous for *APOL1* risk alleles [23]. In the Democratic Republic of the Congo, G1 *APOL1* risk variants are frequent and are associated with hypertension-attributed nephropathy [24]. High-risk *APOL1* genotype may mediate podocyte damage via up regulation of *APOL1* through activation of a viral program in the podocyte, leading to dysregulated endosomal trafficking and autophagic flux, resulting in podocyte depletion and glomerular scarring [11].

In conclusion, this first report from African continent confirms that collapsing glomerulopathy now referred to as collapsing-associated nephropathy (COVAN) represents an emerging entity in the context of COVID-19 pandemic, particularly involving individual with sub-Saharan African ancestry.

Consent

Informed consent was obtained from the patient.

Acknowledgments

This case benefited from a second opinion by Dr. Vivette d'Agati MD, Columbia University, College of Physicians and Surgeons, New York, USA. The authors gratefully thank the staff of the Nephrology Unit and the histotechnologists of the Pathology Department, Kinshasa University Hospital, for their commitment to always provide the utmost care to our patients. The authors also thank Dr. Jeffrey Kopp MD (National Institute of Health, Bethesda, USA) who provided editorial assistance.

References

[1] World Health Organization, *Pneumonia of Unknown Cause—China*, World Health Organization, Geneva, Switzerland, 2020, https://www.who.int/csr/don/05-january-2020-pneumonia-of-unkown-cause-china/en/.

[2] M. Nicola, Z. Alsafi, C. Sohrabi et al., "The socio-economic implications of the coronavirus pandemic (COVID-19): a review," *International Journal of Surgery*, vol. 78, pp. 185–193, 2020.

[3] F. Zhou, T. Yu, R. Du et al., "Clinical course and risk factors for mortality of adult inpatients with COVID-19 in Wuhan, China: a retrospective cohort study," *The Lancet*, vol. 395, pp. 1054–1062, Article ID 10229, 2020.

[4] Y. Cheng, R. Luo, K. Wang et al., "Kidney disease is associated with in-hospital death of patients with COVID-19," *Kidney International*, vol. 97, no. 5, pp. 829–838, 2020.

[5] H. Su, M. Yang, C. Wan et al., "Renal histopathological analysis of 26 postmortem findings of patients with COVID-19 in China," *Kidney International*, vol. 98, no. 1, pp. 219–227, 2020.

[6] M. E. Sise, M. V. Baggett, J.-A. O. Shepard, J. S. Stevens, and E. P. Rhee, "Case 17-2020: a 68-year-old man with covid-19 and acute kidney injury," *New England Journal of Medicine*, vol. 382, no. 22, pp. 2147–2156, 2020.

[7] S. H. Nasr and J. B. Kopp, "COVID-19-associated collapsing glomerulopathy: an emerging entity," *Kidney International Reports*, vol. 5, no. 6, pp. 759–761, 2020.

[8] M. Albaqumi and L. Barisoni, "Current views on collapsing glomerulopathy," *Journal of the American Society of Nephrology*, vol. 19, no. 7, pp. 1276–1281, 2008.

[9] S. Mizuiri and Y. Ohashi, "ACE and ACE2 in kidney disease," *World Journal of Nephrology*, vol. 4, no. 1, pp. 74–82, 2015.

[10] J. A. Schwimmer, G. S. Markowitz, A. Valeri, and G. B. Appel, "Collapsing glomerulopathy," *Seminars in Nephrology*, vol. 23, no. 2, pp. 209–218, 2003.

[11] Y. Peleg, S. Kudose, V D'Agati et al., "Acute kidney injury due to collapsing glomerulopathy following COVID-19 infection," *Kidney International Reports*, vol. 5, no. 6, pp. 940–945, 2020.

[12] S. Kudose, I. Batal, D. Santoriello et al., "Kidney biopsy findings in patients with COVID-19," *Journal of the American Society of Nephrology*, vol. 31, no. 9, pp. 1959–1968, 2020.

[13] H. Wu, C. P. Larsen, C. F. Hernandez-Arroyo et al., "aki and collapsing glomerulopathy associated with COVID-19 and apol1 high-risk genotype," *Journal of the American Society of Nephrology*, vol. 31, no. 8, pp. 1688–1695, 2020.

[14] A. Couturier, S. Ferlicot, K. Chevalier et al., "Indirect effects of severe acute respiratory syndrome coronavirus 2 on the kidney in coronavirus disease patients," *Clinical Kidney Journal*, vol. 13, no. 3, pp. 347–353, 2020.

[15] M. Abbate, D. Rottoli, and A. Gianatti, "COVID-19 attacks the kidney: ultrastructural evidence for the presence of virus in the glomerular epithelium," *Nephron*, vol. 144, no. 7, pp. 341-342, 2020.

[16] L. Nicholas Cossey, C. P. Larsen, and H. Liapis, "Collapsing glomerulopathy: a 30-year perspective and single, large center experience," *Clinical Kidney Journal*, vol. 10, no. 4, pp. 443–449, 2017.

[17] N. M. Pakasa, N. M. Nseka, and L. M. Nyimi, "Secondary collapsing glomerulopathy associated with loa loa filariasis," *American Journal of Kidney Diseases*, vol. 30, no. 6, pp. 836–839, 1997.

[18] X. Yang, Y. Jin, R. Li, Z. Zhang, R. Sun, and D. Chen, "Prevalence and impact of acute renal impairment on COVID-19: a systematic review and meta-analysis," *Critical Care*, vol. 24, no. 1, 2020.

[19] V. B. Kute, H. L. Trivedi, A. V. Vanikar, P. R. Shah, M. R. Gumber, and K. V. Kanodia, "Collapsing glomerulopathy and hemolytic uremic syndrome associated with falciparum malaria: completely reversible acute kidney injury," *Journal of Parasitic Diseases*, vol. 37, no. 2, pp. 286–290, 2013.

[20] A. Niang, S. E. Niang, E. H. F. Ka, M. M. Ka, and B. Diouf, "Collapsing glomerulopathy and haemophagocytic syndrome related to malaria: a case report," *Nephrology Dialysis Transplantation*, vol. 23, no. 10, pp. 3359–3361, 2008.

[21] X.-W. Pan, D. Xu, H. Zhang, W. Zhou, L.-H. Wang, and X.-G. Cui, "Identification of a potential mechanism of acute kidney injury during the COVID-19 outbreak: a study based on single-cell transcriptome analysis," *Intensive Care Medicine*, vol. 46, no. 6, pp. 1114–1116, 2020.

[22] S. Kissling, S. Rotman, C. Gerber et al., "Collapsing glomerulopathy in a COVID-19 patient," *Kidney International*, vol. 98, no. 1, pp. 228–231, 2020.

[23] C. P. Larsen, T. D. Bourne, J. D. Wilson, O. Saqqa, and M. D. A. Sharshir, "Collapsing glomerulopathy in a patient with COVID-19," *Kidney International Reports*, vol. 5, no. 6, p. 935, 2020.

[24] E. K. Sumaili, R. Shemer, E. Kruzel-Davila et al., "G1 is the major APOL1 risk allele for hypertension-attributed nephropathy in Central Africa," *Clinical Kidney Journal*, vol. 12, no. 2, pp. 188–195, 2018.

39

Galactose-Deficient IgA1 Deposits in Clear Cell Renal Cell Carcinoma-Related Henoch–Schönlein Purpura Nephritis

Yuhong Zhao,[1] Youngki Kim,[2] Milind Junghare,[3] Viral Vakil,[3] Xuesong Su,[4] Faqian Li,[5] and Lihong Bu[5]

[1]*Department of Nephrology, Central Hospital Affiliated to Shenyang Medical College, Shenyang, Liaoning 110024, China*
[2]*Department of Pediatrics, Division of Pediatric Nephrology, University of Minnesota, Minneapolis, MN 55455, USA*
[3]*Department of Renal Disease and Hypertension, University of Minnesota, Minneapolis, MN 55455, USA*
[4]*Department of Nephrology, Shengjing Hospital of China Medical University, Shenyang, Liaoning 110004, China*
[5]*Department of Laboratory Medicine and Pathology, University of Minnesota, Minneapolis, MN 55455, USA*

Correspondence should be addressed to Lihong Bu; lbu@umn.edu

Academic Editor: Ze'ev Korzets

Recent studies suggest that galactose-deficient IgA1 (Gd-IgA1) plays a role in the pathogenesis of primary IgA nephropathy (IgAN) and Henoch–Schönlein purpura nephritis (HSPN). Furthermore, immunostaining of KM55, an antibody that identifies Gd-IgA1, may be helpful to differentiate primary IgAN and HSPN from secondary causes of glomerular IgA deposition. We report sequential kidney biopsies of a malignancy-associated HSPN, showing intense glomerular mesangial IgA deposition at the initial kidney biopsy and dramatic decrease in disappearance of glomerular deposits after tumor removal. We demonstrate that the glomerular IgA deposition contains Gd-IgA1, detected by immunostaining of KM55, with similar distribution and intensity to IgA. This suggests that renal Gd-IgA1 deposition may play a role in the pathogenesis of malignancy-associated HSPN.

1. Introduction

Henoch–Schönlein purpura (HSP), also referred as immunoglobulin A vasculitis (IgAV), is the most common systemic vasculitis involving the small blood vessels in pediatric population with kidney involvement present in 30–50% [1]. Similar to IgA nephropathy (IgAN), Henoch–Schönlein purpura nephritis (HSPN) is characterized by the deposition of IgA dominant or codominant immune complex in the glomerular mesangial and capillary wall regions. The glomerular IgA deposition in IgAN is predominantly of the IgA1 subclass [2]. Galactose-deficient IgA1 (Gd-IgA1) has been identified to be a key element in the pathogenesis of IgAN with glomerular deposition of autoantibodies recognizing overproduced, aberrantly glycosylated Gd-IgA1 [3]. KM55, a Gd-IgA1-specific monoclonal antibody generated by immunizing rats with the human Gd-IgA1 hinge region peptide, has been shown to recognize Gd-IgA1 in renal biopsy tissue on formalin-fixed paraffin-embedded sections [4, 5]. Recent study shows KM55 is specifically detected in primary IgAN and HSPN, but not in other examined renal diseases, such as lupus nephritis, cirrhosis, or hepatitis C-related glomerular disease [6]. These findings suggest IgAN and HSPN share a common feature involving Gd-IgA1 in pathogenesis [6]. However, the specificity of KM55 for primary IgAN and HSPN was questioned in a more recent study demonstrating KM55 staining in incidental IgA deposition, secondary IgAN, and staphylococcal infection-associated glomerulonephritis, albeit with weaker staining than in primary IgAN [7].

Unlike HSPN in children, clinical presentation of HSPN in adults is frequently severe [8] and associated with malignancies in up to 28% [9] of cases, including hematolymphoid neoplasm and solid tumor from primary organ of respiratory, digestive, neurologic, and urologic systems [10, 11]. The pathophysiology of malignancy-associated HSPN remains speculative. Proposed mechanisms include abnormal production of antibodies directed against tumor neoantigens leading to the formation of immune complexes and similarities between tumor antigens and endothelial cell antigens. It is unknown whether Gd-IgA1 plays a role in the pathogenesis of malignancy-associated HSPN.

Here, we report detailed clinical pathological findings and immunostaining of KM55 on sequential kidney biopsies of a 35-year-old man with a clear cell renal cell carcinoma-(CCRCC-) associated HSPN.

2. Case Presentation

2.1. Initial Clinical History, Laboratory Data, and Pathology Findings. A 35-year-old man with a past history of schizoaffective disorder controlled by medication was admitted with a bilateral, palpable, nontender rash on his legs, leg stiffness, and leg pain for 24–36 hours. The patient complained of nausea, constipation, and worsening abdominal pain. No fevers, chills, diarrhea, difficulty in urinating, shortness of breath, or cough were noted. There was no personal or family history of rheumatologic disease or hypertension. There was no history of recent ill contacts, travel, wilderness exposure, or tick bites. The pertinent laboratory results were as follows: serum creatinine, 0.75 mg/dL (Table 1) and serum albumin, 3.2 g/dL. Urinalysis (UA) revealed a protein albumin urine of 100 mg/dL and 7 RBCs/hpf. Serological testing was negative for antinuclear antibodies (ANAs), double-stranded DNA (dsDNA), and antineutrophil cytoplasmic antibodies (ANCA). Complement levels and rheumatoid factor were normal. Renal ultrasound showed a 6.0 cm complex lesion in the lower pole of the right kidney.

Two days after admission, a skin biopsy of the lower shin was performed, showing leukocytoclastic vasculitis (Figure 1) with intravascular deposition of IgA and C3 (not shown), consistent with HSP. The patient was started with oral prednisone at a dose of 60 mg daily with improvement of the rash, leg pain, and abdominal pain. In the next week, the patient's symptoms worsened with oliguria, rapid increase in serum creatinine (from 0.75 to 5.14 mg/dL) (Table 1), and nephrotic-range proteinuria (8.9 g/g Cr). UA showed 13 RBCs/hpf while on pulse methylprednisolone (500 mg) intravenously (IV) for 3 days (Table 1). Dialysis was initiated, and mycophenolate mofetil (MMF) (1 g twice daily by mouth) was added. A kidney biopsy showed diffuse global endocapillary and focal segmental mesangial proliferative glomerulonephritis with IgA-dominant mesangial and capillary wall deposition, consistent with active HSPN (Figure 2). With the consideration of paraneoplastic syndrome, an urgent partial nephrectomy was performed. A clear cell renal cell carcinoma (CCRCC) pT1b was diagnosed. A few crescentic lesions were identified in the nonneoplastic kidney of the partial nephrectomy specimen (Figure 3). Renal function improved, and dialysis was discontinued seven days following the nephrectomy. The patient was discharged on the postoperative day eight on a regimen of mycophenolate and prednisone.

2.2. Follow-Up and Sequential Kidney Biopsy Findings. Two weeks later, the patient was admitted for shortness of breath with an increase in creatinine (from 2.58 mg/dL to 4.76 mg/dL) (Table 1) and oliguria caused by a leak in his nephrectomy wound. A second renal biopsy was performed at three weeks after surgical removal of the kidney tumor. The biopsy revealed diffuse cellular and fibrocellular crescents and minimal IgA deposition along glomerular capillary wall (Table 1; Figures 4(a) and 4(b)). Therapeutic plasma exchange (PLEX) was performed every other day for a total of 2 weeks, along with IV cyclophosphamide at 15 mg/kg x1 and continuation of the prednisone and MMF. Several days after discharge, the patient had pancytopenia, hematochezia, and epistaxis. MMF was discontinued due to concern of side effect, while prednisone and cyclophosphamide were continued with PLEX. Over the next two weeks, there was no obvious improvement in renal function. Fluid retention was controlled by renal replacement therapy. The steroid was tapered, and cytoxan was given orally instead of intravenously. During the next 4 months, clinical manifestation and laboratory tests of the patient remained stable (Table 1).

To further clarify the kidney disease etiology, determine the level of chronic kidney damage, and assess disease activity while continuing to treat with cytotoxic therapies, a third renal biopsy was performed at five months after surgical resection of the kidney tumor. The renal biopsy showed only chronic changes with fibrous crescents and negligible IgA deposition in nonsclerotic glomeruli (Figures 4(c)–4(f)). Therefore, cytoxan was discontinued, and prednisone was tapered off over the next 21 days, with continued renal replacement therapy.

2.3. Gd-IgA1 Immunohistochemical Staining on Kidney Biopsies. Gd-IgA1 (anti-human Gd-IgA1 (KM55) rat IgG monoclonal antibody, Immuno-Biological Laboratories Co., Ltd, at a concentration of 50 μg/mL) was stained for all three kidney biopsies, one prior to partial nephrectomy and two after surgical removal of CCRCC. KM55 displayed similar staining pattern and intensity to IgA in all biopsies (Figure 5). Diffuse global granular capillary wall staining and segmental granular mesangial staining for Gd-IgA1, similar to IgA, were observed on the first biopsy, while dramatically decreased Gd-IgA1 and IgA staining along the capillary wall and in mesangium were seen on the follow-up kidney biopsies (Figure 5).

3. Discussion

Malignancy-associated HSPN usually affects patients older than 40 years of age (range from 29 to 79), with a male predominance [9]. The majority of the neoplasms (80%) are detected at the time of or within 1 year after the occurrence of HSP, and 67% of the malignancies are solid tumors [9]. The renal manifestations of HSPN can range from microscopic hematuria and proteinuria only to a rapidly progressive glomerulonephritis (RPGN). Of those who undergo a kidney biopsy, 95% show IgA deposition in the mesangial area [12–22]. The most frequent lesion in renal biopsies is proliferative endocapillary glomerular nephritis [11]. The outcome of HSPN in adults is relatively poor, and the most frequent cause of death was neoplasia (up to 27% of death)

Table 1: Laboratory results before each kidney biopsy and after tumor resection.

Variables	Baseline (at presentation)	Before the 1st kidney biopsy	Three weeks after tumor resection (before the 2nd kidney biopsy)	Five months after tumor resection (before the 3rd kidney biopsy)	Reference range
Sodium (mmol/L)	140	134	144	138	133–144
Potassium (mmol/L)	4.5	4.0	3.7	4.6	3.4–5.3
Chloride (mmol/L)	105	101	115	104	94–109
Carbon dioxide (mmol/L)	24	20	15	24	20–32
Calcium (mg/dL)	9.4	7.5	7.1	8.2	8.5–10.1
Phosphorus (mg/dL)	3.8	5.6	7.4	3.9	2.4–4.5
BUN (mg/dL)	12	62	58	32	7–30
Cr (mg/dL)	0.75	5.14	4.76	4.89	0.66–1.25
Protein, total (g/dL)	7.2	5.2	3.8	4.7	6.8–8.8
Albumin (g/dL)	3.6	1.6	1.0	1.4	3.4–5.0
Protein, total urine (g/gr Cr.)	–	8.91	9.19	16.99	0–0.2
Glucose (mg/dL)	98	84	80	101	70–99
WBC (10^9/L)	10.9	18.7	5.8	2.5	4.0–11.0
Hemoglobin (g/dL)	14.6	10.3	7.7	8.7	13.3–17.7
Platelets (10^9/L)	317	204	335	123	150–450
ANA	—	<1.0	—	—	<1.0
dsDNA (IU/mL)	—	2	—	—	<10
ANCA	—	<1 : 20	—	—	—
Cryoglobulin (%)	—	—	Neg	—	(NEG%)
C3 (mg/dL)	—	130	110	—	76–169
C4 (mg/dL)	—	15	23	—	15–50
IgA (mg/dL)	—	118	—	—	70–380
IgG (mg/dL)	—	479	—	—	695–1620
IgM (mg/dL)	—	25	—	—	60–265
Myeloperoxidase Ab, IgG (AI)	—	0.2	0.2	—	0.0–0.9
Proteinase 3Ab, IgG (AI)	—	0.2	0.2	—	0.0–0.9

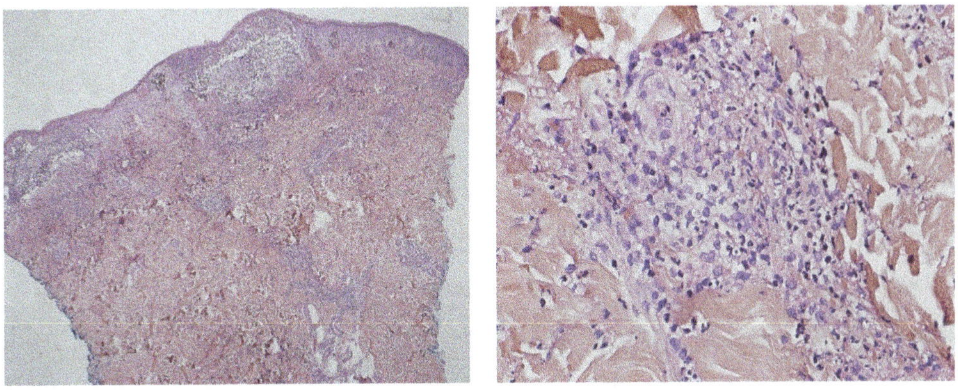

(a) (b)

Figure 1: A punch biopsy of skin involved by a brisk acute small vessel neutrophilic vasculitis that extends from the papillary to midreticular dermis. There is prominent associated fibrinoid necrosis of vessel wall, leukocytoclasis, purpura, and epidermal degeneration. Original magnification: 4X in (a) and 40X in (b).

[10–12, 14, 16, 18, 21] although significant improvement of renal function was reported in some cases with treatment of the cancer and corticosteroids for HSPN [13–15, 22]. The independent prognostic factors of renal outcome in patients with HSPN are proteinuria level, initial renal failure, and the histologic quantification of interstitial fibrosis and glomerular sclerosis [11].

Our patient's clinical characteristics and biopsy findings are in concordance with the reported cases in the literature. The disappearance of glomerular IgA deposits soon after

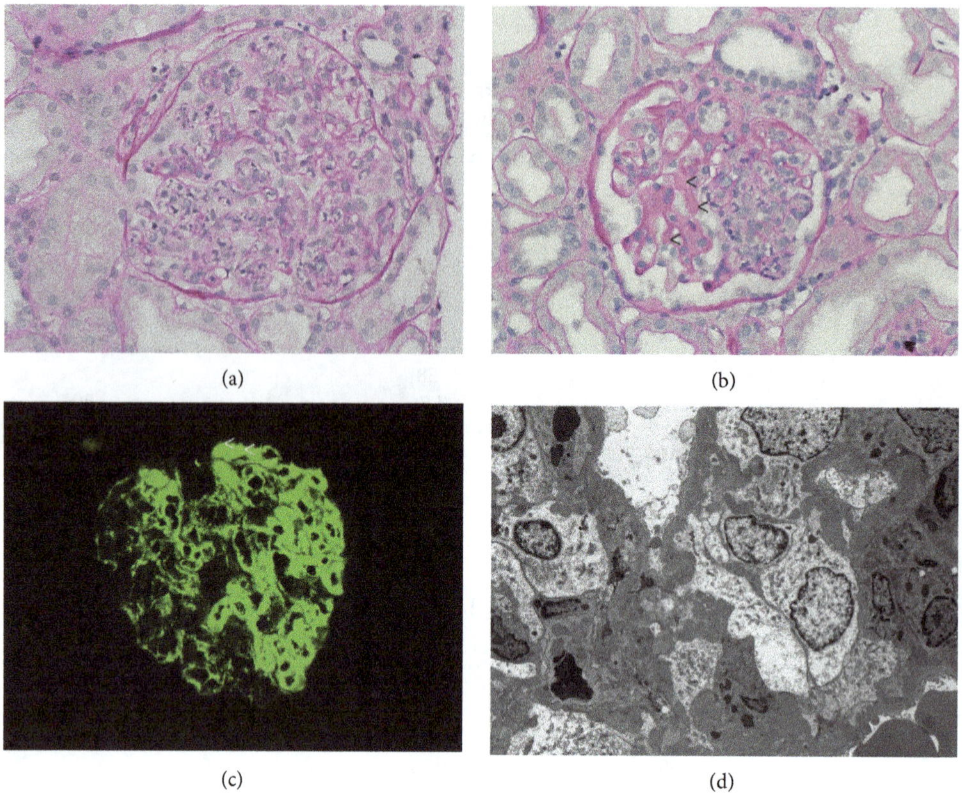

Figure 2: Findings of initial kidney biopsy: (a) a representative glomerulus with global endocapillary proliferation on periodic acid-Schiff stain; (b) a glomerulus with segmental mesangial and endocapillary proliferation (right side) and intracapillary pseudothrombi (<); (c) immunofluorescence staining of IgA shows global granular mesangial and capillary wall staining and a few intracapillary pseudothrombi (<); (d) electron microscopy shows many electron dense mesangial and subendothelial deposits with severe foot process effacement. Original magnification: 400X in (a–c) and 5000X in (d).

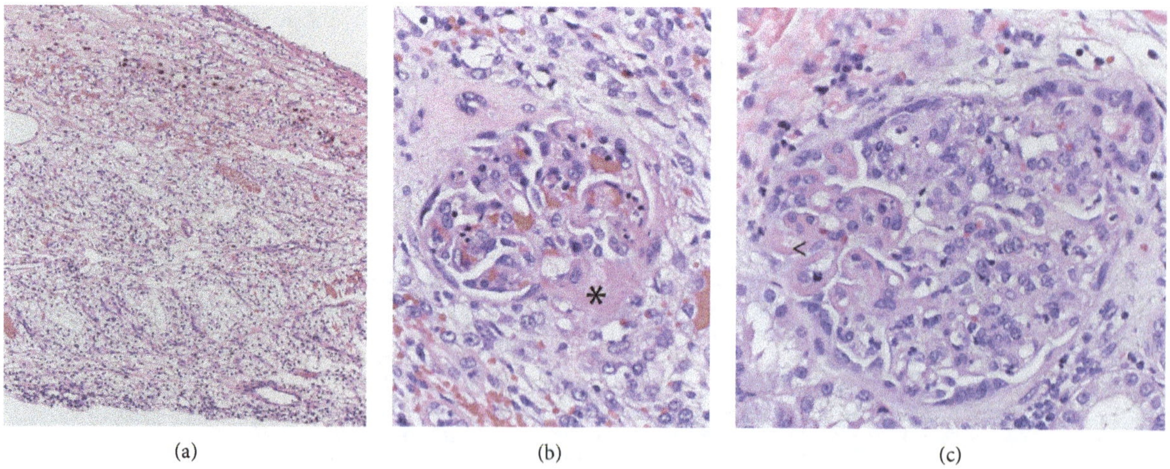

Figure 3: Clear cell renal cell carcinoma, low grade of partial nephrectomy (a). In adjacent nonneoplastic kidney, several glomeruli show segmental to global endocapillary proliferation with segmental necrotizing lesion (∗) in (b) and rare glomeruli show large glomerular deposits (<) in (c). Original magnification: 40X in (a) and 400X in (b) and (c).

tumor removal supports that the patient's HSPN is associated with the patient's concurrent kidney cancer. The disappearance of mesangial IgA deposits on repeat biopsies has been rarely reported in children [23] and adults [24]; however, the disappearance is observed after prolonged combination therapy, two years and 77 months on average for pediatric and adult patients, respectively. Despite tumor removal and immunosuppression treatment, our patient's renal function deteriorated and the patient was on maintenance dialysis, as reported in other cases [17, 21].

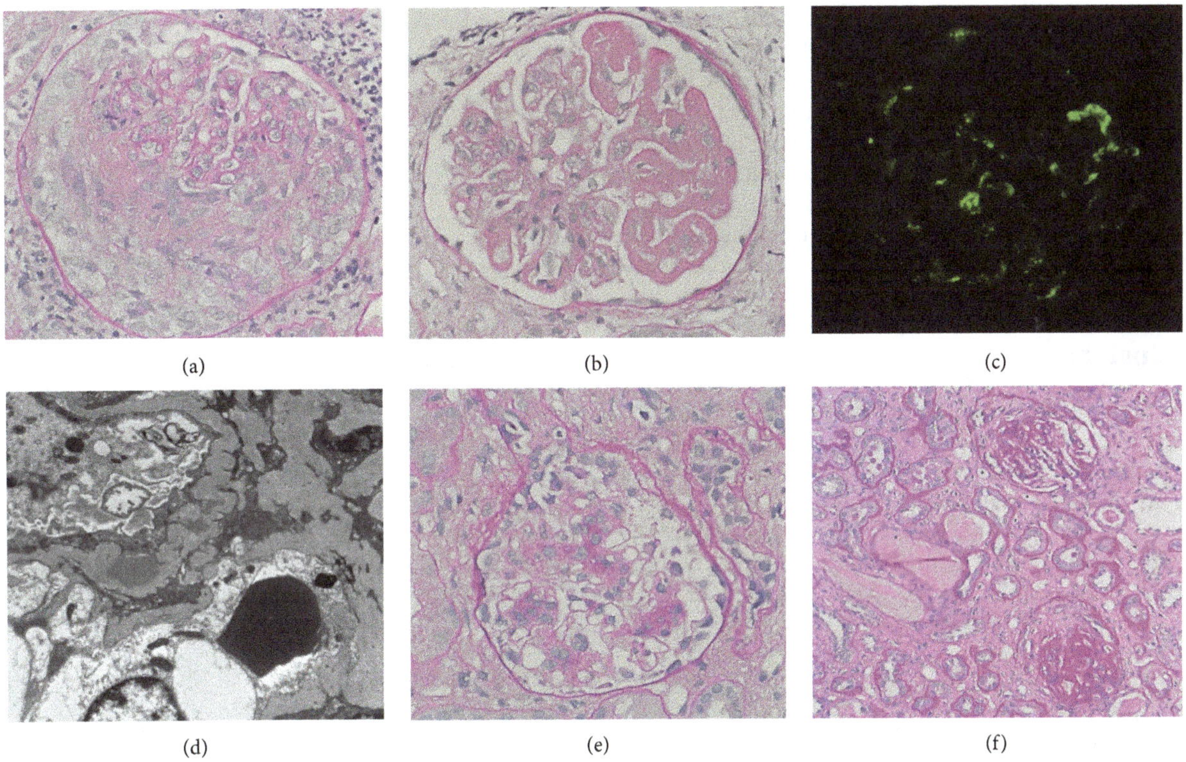

FIGURE 4: Findings of the second and third kidney biopsies, at three weeks (a, b) and five months (c–f) after surgical resection of clear cell renal cell carcinoma, respectively. Sequential biopsies demonstrate progression and transition from active lesions (a, b) to sclerosing lesions (e, f), and dramatic clearance of glomerular IgA deposits following tumor resection (c, d). (a) A representative glomerulus shows endocapillary hypercellularity and a nearly circumferential cellular crescent with necrosis. (b) Segmental large subendothelial deposits (right half of the glomerulus) are visible by light microscopy. (c) Immunofluorescence staining of IgA shows only modest glomerular mesangial and capillary wall IgA deposition. (d) Electron microscopy shows a small number of electron dense deposits mainly in mesangium. (e) Nonsclerosed glomeruli show only mild mesangial hypercellularity without endocapillary hypercellularity. (f) Representative glomeruli with fibrous crescents, one globally sclerotic (the lower glomerulus) and the other segmentally scarred (the upper glomerulus). The third biopsy shows significant chronic changes with approximately 35% global glomerulosclerosis and additional 35% glomeruli with fibrous crescents and segmental sclerosis. There is severe tubulointerstitial scarring. Original magnification: 400X in (a–c) and (e), 8000X in (d), and 200X in (f).

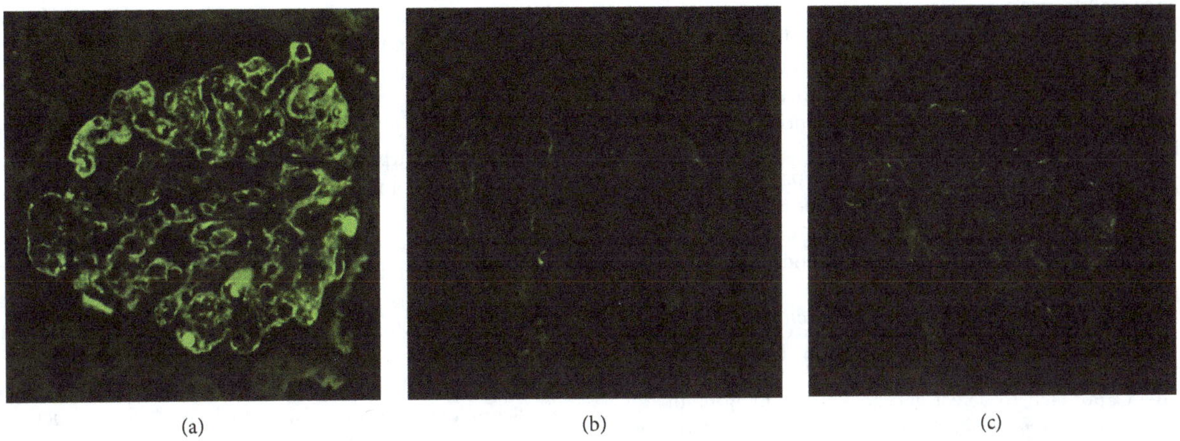

FIGURE 5: Immunofluorescence staining of KM55 shows global, granular, mesangial, and capillary wall as well as intracapillary pseudothrombi staining on initial kidney biopsy (a) and diminished/minimal glomerular capillary wall staining on sequential kidney biopsies three weeks (b) and five months (c) after surgical resection of clear cell renal cell carcinoma. Original magnification: 400X in all.

Gd-IgA1 plays an important role in the pathogenesis of IgAN. Gd-IgA1 is reported to increase in blood circulation and/or be deposited in renal mesangium in patients with primary IgAN and/or HSPN [25–28]. The data are sparse and controversial on whether immunostaining of KM-55, a Gd-IgA1-specific monoclonal antibody, is specific for patients with primary IgAN and HSPN, but not secondary form [6, 7, 29]. Here, we demonstrate glomerular KM55 staining with a similar pattern and intensity to IgA in this malignancy-associated HSPN, a secondary form of IgA deposition. These data show that KM55 staining may not be helpful in distinguishing primary from secondary HSPN. Furthermore, the KM55 staining in the sequential kidney biopsies suggests the production of autoantibodies against Gd-IgA1 molecules might be one of the pathophysiologies of malignancy-associated HSPN.

4. Conclusions

Here, we report KM55 staining on three sequential kidney biopsies from a 35-year-old man with HSPN and a concurrent kidney carcinoma. Positive glomerular staining of KM-55, an antibody that identifies Gd-IgA1, in this malignancy-associated HSPN was seen with a similar staining pattern and intensity to IgA on the initial kidney biopsy. Disappearance of glomerular mesangial IgA and Gd-IgA1 deposits was observed on two sequential kidney biopsies at three weeks and five months after surgical resection of the kidney tumor. The findings suggest Gd-IgA1, not specific to primary IgAN and HSPN, may play a role in the pathogenesis of malignancy-associated HSPN.

Acknowledgments

The authors would like to thank Dr. Patrick H. Nachman for reviewing the manuscript.

References

[1] M. H. Heineke, A. V. Ballering, A. Jamin, S. Ben Mkaddem, R. C. Monteiro, and M. Van Egmond, "New insights in the pathogenesis of immunoglobulin A vasculitis (Henoch-Schönlein purpura)," *Autoimmunity Reviews*, vol. 16, no. 12, pp. 1246–1253, 2017.

[2] M. E. Conley, M. D. Cooper, and A. F. Michael, "Selective deposition of immunoglobulin A1 in immunoglobulin A nephropathy, anaphylactoid purpura nephritis, and systemic lupus erythematosus," *Journal of Clinical Investigation*, vol. 66, no. 6, pp. 1432–1436, 1980.

[3] H. Suzuki, K. Kiryluk, J. Novak et al., "The pathophysiology of IgA nephropathy," *Journal of the American Society of Nephrology*, vol. 22, no. 10, pp. 1795–1803, 2011.

[4] R. Coppo, "A new monoclonal antibody for detecting degalactosylated IgA1 as serum biomarker of IgA nephropathy," *Nephrology Dialysis Transplantation*, vol. 30, no. 8, pp. 1234–1236, 2015.

[5] J. Yasutake, Y. Suzuki, H. Suzuki et al., "Novel lectin-independent approach to detect galactose-deficient IgA1 in IgA nephropathy," *Nephrology Dialysis Transplantation*, vol. 30, no. 8, pp. 1315–1321, 2015.

[6] H. Suzuki, J. Yasutake, Y. Makita et al., "IgA nephropathy and IgA vasculitis with nephritis have a shared feature involving galactose-deficient IgA1-oriented pathogenesis," *Kidney International*, vol. 93, no. 3, pp. 700–705, 2018.

[7] C. A. Cassol, C. Bott, G. M. Nadasdy et al., "Immunostaining for galactose-deficient immunoglobulin A is not specific for primary immunoglobulin A nephropathy," *Nephrology Dialysis Transplantation*, 2019.

[8] J.-C. Davin, "Henoch-Schönlein purpura nephritis: pathophysiology, treatment, and future strategy," *Clinical Journal of the American Society of Nephrology*, vol. 6, no. 3, pp. 679–689, 2011.

[9] E. Pertuiset, F. Lioté, E. Launay-Russ, F. Kemiche, I. Cerf-Payrastre, and A.-M. Chesneau, "Adult Henoch-Schönlein purpura associated with malignancy," *Seminars in Arthritis and Rheumatism*, vol. 29, no. 6, pp. 360–367, 2000.

[10] P. S. Kellerman, "Henoch-Schönlein purpura in adults," *American Journal of Kidney Diseases*, vol. 48, no. 6, pp. 1009–1016, 2006.

[11] E. Pillebout, E. Thervet, G. Hill et al., "Henoch-Schonlein purpura in adults: outcome and prognostic factors," *Journal of the American Society of Nephrology*, vol. 13, no. 5, pp. 1271–1278, 2002.

[12] R. K. Kim, A. R. Thomas, M. E. Card, D. Malhotra, and J. L. Holleck, "Four cancers and a rash: Henoch-Schönlein purpura," *The American Journal of Medicine*, vol. 130, no. 10, pp. 1158–1160, 2017.

[13] I. Mimura, A. Tojo, S. Kinugasa, T. Fujita, and H. Uozaki, "Renal cell carcinoma in association with IgA nephropathy in the elderly," *The American Journal of the Medical Sciences*, vol. 338, no. 5, pp. 431-432, 2009.

[14] J. M. Zurada, K. M. Ward, and M. E. Grossman, "Henoch-Schönlein purpura associated with malignancy in adults," *Journal of the American Academy of Dermatology*, vol. 55, no. 5, pp. S65–S70, 2006.

[15] N. Akizue, E. Suzuki, M. Yokoyama et al., "Henoch-Schönlein purpura complicated by Hepatocellular carcinoma," *Internal Medicine*, vol. 56, no. 22, pp. 3041–3045, 2017.

[16] J. Podjasek, D. Wetter, M. Pittelkow, and D. Wada, "Henoch-Schönlein purpura associated with solid-organ malignancies: three case reports and a literature review," *Acta Dermato Venereologica*, vol. 92, no. 4, pp. 388–392, 2012.

[17] P. Blanco, R. Denisi, P. Rispal et al., "Henoch-Schonlein purpura associated with segmental and focal proliferative glomerulonephritis in a patient with Hodgkin's disease," *Nephrology Dialysis Transplantation*, vol. 14, no. 1, pp. 179-180, 1999.

[18] P. Arrizabalaga, A. Saurina, M. Solé, and J. Bladé, "Henoch-Schönlein IgA glomerulonephritis complicating myeloma kidneys: case report," *Annals of Hematology*, vol. 82, no. 8, pp. 526–528, 2003.

[19] Y. H. Hong, "Renal cell carcinoma presenting as Henoch-Schönlein purpura with leukocytoclastic vasculitis, hematuria, proteinuria and abdominal pain," *Rheumatology International*, vol. 30, no. 10, pp. 1373–1376, 2010.

[20] T. Posas-Mendoza, D. Lucuab-Fegurgur, and J. Roberts, "Adult onset Henoch-Schonlein purpura associated with a metastatic malignancy of unknown primary origin," *Hawai'i Journal of Medicine & Public Health*, vol. 77, pp. 243–245, 2018.

[21] S. Joshi, S. Pillai, A. Chakera, and Y. C. G. Lee, "Henoch-Schonlein purpura in mesothelioma," *Respirology Case Reports*, vol. 2, no. 4, pp. 138–140, 2014.

[22] M. S. Y. Ng, L. Francis, E. Pillai et al., "Paraneoplastic immunoglobulin A nephropathy and associated focal segmental glomerulosclerosis in asymptomatic low volume B-cell lymphoma-a case report," *BMC Nephrology*, vol. 19, p. 224, 2018.

[23] Y. Shima, K. Nakanishi, K. Kamei et al., "Disappearance of glomerular IgA deposits in childhood IgA nephropathy showing diffuse mesangial proliferation after 2 years of

combination/prednisolone therapy," *Nephrology Dialysis Transplantation*, vol. 26, no. 1, pp. 163–169, 2011.

[24] O. Hotta, T. Furuta, S. Chiba, S. Tomioka, and Y. Taguma, "Regression of IgA nephropathy: a repeat biopsy study," *American Journal of Kidney Diseases*, vol. 39, no. 3, pp. 493–502, 2002.

[25] Z. Moldoveanu, R. J. Wyatt, J. Y. Lee et al., "Patients with IgA nephropathy have increased serum galactose-deficient IgA1 levels," *Kidney International*, vol. 71, no. 11, pp. 1148–1154, 2007.

[26] Y. Wada, K. Matsumoto, T. Suzuki et al., "Clinical significance of serum and mesangial galactose-deficient IgA1 in patients with IgA nephropathy," *PLoS One*, vol. 13, Article ID e0206865, 2018.

[27] W. J. Placzek, H. Yanagawa, Y. Makita et al., "Serum galactose-deficient-IgA1 and IgG autoantibodies correlate in patients with IgA nephropathy," *PLoS One*, vol. 13, Article ID e0190967, 2018.

[28] M. Mizerska-Wasiak, Ł. Gajewski, K. Cichoń-Kawa et al., "Serum GDIgA1 levels in children with IgA nephropathy and Henoch-Schönlein nephritis," *Central European Journal of Immunology*, vol. 43, no. 2, pp. 162–167, 2018.

[29] M. Wang, J. Lv, X. Zhang, P. Chen, M. Zhao, and H. Zhang, "Secondary IgA nephropathy shares the same immune features with primary IgA nephropathy," *Kidney International Reports*, vol. 5, no. 2, pp. 165–172, 2020.

40

Ischemic Stroke in a Young Patient with Nephrotic Syndrome and Antiphospholipid Syndrome

K. K. Neoh,[1] A. S. N. Tang,[1] I. Looi,[1,2] and B. M. Anita[1]

[1]*Department of Internal Medicine, Seberang Jaya Hospital, Penang, Malaysia*
[2]*Clinical Research Center (CRC), Seberang Jaya Hospital, Penang, Malaysia*

Correspondence should be addressed to K. K. Neoh; kkneoh@yahoo.com

Academic Editor: Hern N. Trimarchi

We report a case of a 21-year-old man with underlying nephrotic syndrome (NS) secondary to minimal change disease, who developed an ischemic stroke with left hemiparesis. He received intravenous thrombolysis followed by a mechanical thrombectomy. After mechanical thrombectomy, he developed acute kidney injury which subsequently required haemodialysis. Further workup revealed that he had concomitant antiphospholipid syndrome (APS) and NS. He was started on vitamin K antagonist anticoagulant. This case report illustrates the importance of workup in identifying causes of ischemic stroke in a young patient.

1. Background

Acute ischemic stroke in young adults are uncommon as compared to the elderly. It accounts for about 10% of all stroke cases. Physical disability caused by stroke in young adults can lead to huge economic loss to patients and their families. In addition, these groups of patients have longer life expectancies at poststroke, which in turn impose greater burden to healthcare systems.

2. Case Presentation

We describe a case of a 21-year-old obese Chinese man with underlying nephrotic syndrome (NS) secondary to renal biopsy-proven minimal change disease who suffered from a right middle cerebral artery territory infarct.

He was initially admitted to our hospital six months prior to stroke, with a complaint of generalized body swelling and shortness of breath for one month. Twenty months prior to the weakness of limbs, he received treatment in a private clinic, but subsequently defaulted. Clinical examination revealed anasarca.

His initial workup for NS revealed that his urea was 10.7 mmol/L, serum creatinine was 134 μmol/L, and serum albumin was 7 g/L. His urinalysis results showed protein 4+ and blood 2+. His 24-hour urine protein was 32.3 g/24 hours. Both kidneys were normal in size and echogenic, with preserved cortical thickness on ultrasound. The bipolar length of the right kidney was 10.3 cm and that of the left kidney was 10.4 cm. Ultrasound Doppler of bilateral kidneys showed no evidence of renal vein thrombosis. Autoimmune workup including ANA, Jo-1, La, Ro, U1RNP, Scl, and SM was negative. He had no history of illicit drug abuse or smoking. His hepatitis B, hepatitis C, and HIV serology were negative. Renal biopsy was planned upon improving his edematous state.

He required temporary haemodialysis alternate with ultrafiltration for 6-week duration due to fluid overload and worsening of kidney function (creatinine up to 282 μmol/L and urea of 17.3 mmol/L). He was started on prednisolone 80 mg per day, furosemide 80 mg three times per day, and cyclosporine 25 mg twice per day.

At the second month of treatment, his kidney function improved with the creatinine level of 97 μmol/L and urea of 9.9 mmol/L. He had weight reduction from 120 kg (BMI: 41.5 kg/m^2) to 100 kg (BMI: 34.6 kg/m^2). His haemodialysis was withheld. Renal biopsy was performed and was highly suggestive of minimal change disease. His medications were changed to furosemide 40 mg once per day, prednisolone tapering dose to 20 mg once per day, and cyclosporine 50 mg twice per day.

At the fourth month of treatment, his kidney function further deteriorated with the serum creatinine level of 264 μmol/L and urea of 9.0 mmol/L. His albumin was 12 g/L, and 24-hour urine protein was 19.8 g/24 hours. His weight increased to 115 kg (BMI: 39.8 kg/m^2). The patient was admitted and reassessed. He was not responding to intravenous steroids and diuretics. His immunosuppressive medication was switched from cyclosporin to mycophenolate mofetil (MMF) 500 mg twice per day due to deterioration of renal function.

He visited us in the clinic at the fifth month of treatment, and he was unable to tolerate MMF due to nausea. He was started on tacrolimus 1 g twice per day. His albumin was 10 g/L, serum creatinine was 278 μmol/L, and 24-hour urine protein was 26.4 g/24 hours. Weight remained the same.

At the sixth month of treatment, he presented to the hospital with left hemiparesis. He was afebrile, vital signs were stable, Glasgow Coma Scale of 15/15, blood glucose was 6.0 mmol/L, and NIHSS score of 12 (left facial palsy: 2 marks, left upper limb: 4 marks, left lower limb: 3 marks, left side sensory: 1 mark, dysarthria: 1 mark, and inattention: 1 mark). Muscle power of the left upper limb was graded 0/5 and that of the left lower limb was 2/5, with reduced sensation over the left upper and lower limbs.

Blood investigation revealed: hemoglobin, 8.8 g/dL (normochromic and normocytic); platelet, $580 \times 10^3/\mu L$; WBC, $13.9 \times 10^3/\mu L$; urea, 6.0 mmol/L; creatinine, 316 μmol/L; INR, 1.2; PT, 15.8 sec; and aPTT, 15.8 sec. Venous blood gas revealed metabolic acidosis, with a pH of 7.25 and HCO_3 of 13.7 mmol/L. Toxicology screening was not done.

Plain CT brain at 210 minutes poststroke onset showed a normal CT brain (Figure 1), and he was given intravenous thrombolysis with alteplase of a dose of 0.9 mg/kg.

MRI and MRA brain scan at 375 minutes poststroke onset and 135 minutes post-rTPA thrombolysis revealed that he had a right middle cerebral artery territory infarct and stenosis at distal M1 segment of the right middle cerebral artery (Figures 2–4). Mechanical thrombectomy was carried out with partial recanalization of M2 segment of the right middle cerebral artery.

His kidney function deteriorated further postcontrast when serum creatinine peaked at 528 μmol/L. He was intubated for respiratory distress as he developed fluid overload. After intubation, he was nursed in intensive care unit and required haemodialysis via a temporary femoral catheter. He also required a tracheostomy to sustain his airway.

He was further evaluated. He had normal C3 and C4 levels, and cANCA and pANCA were negative. Echocardiogram, electrocardiogram, and Doppler ultrasound of carotid arteries were normal. However, his repeated lupus anticoagulant (LA) titre was detected. Hence, the diagnosis of concomitant APS with NS was made. He was subsequently started on vitamin K antagonist (VKA) anticoagulant.

3. Outcome and Follow-Up

At three-month poststroke review, he still required regular haemodialysis. It was then decided that he required long-term renal replacement therapy as his kidney function continued to deteriorate.

His Modified Rankin Scale (MRS) after stroke three months was 3. He was able to walk without assistance, but was unable to carry out any other activities. His left upper limb power improved to 2/5, and left lower limb power was 4/5. He further improved at six months after stroke. He still experienced slight disability, but was able to walk independently, and his left upper and lower limbs power improved to 4/5.

4. Discussion

Stroke was previously thought as a disease of the elderly, more common in adults aged above 50 years. The incidence of arterial ischemic stroke in young adults less than 45 years of age ranged from 3.4–11.3/100000 people per year, and the common causes were vasculopathy, cardiac defects, pregnancy, hypercoagulable state, smoking, illicit drug use, premature atherosclerosis, young hypertension, low physical activity, and metabolic disease [1].

Ji R's study that recruited 215 young subjects aged between 18–45 years with ischemic stroke or transient ischemic attack showed that the mean age of attack was 37.5 years, and 51% of those diagnosed were males. This group of subjects has a higher incidence rate of traditional vascular risk factors such as hypertension (20%), diabetes mellitus (11%), dyslipidemia (38%), and smoking (34%) [2].

Our patient had NS diagnosed 6 months prior to the onset of stroke, at the age of 20 years. NS was associated with an annual incidence of 9.85% venous thrombosis and 5.5% arterial thrombosis within the first six months of diagnosis [3].

Our patient had proteinuria of 32 g/day, and his albumin level was 0.6 g/dL upon admission. Each 1 g/dL reduction in serum albumin was associated with a 2.13-fold of increased risk of venous thromboembolism, and albumin level of <2.8 g/dL is the most significant independent predictor of venous thrombotic risk [4]. However, the pathogenesis of hypercoagulable state in NS was not well understood, and it was postulated to be due to loss of natural anticoagulants such as antithrombin III, plasminogen, and protein C and S in urine [5].

Arterial thromboembolic event in NS is lesser compared to venous thromboembolism, and there were limited studies addressing this issue. Bakhtawar and colleagues revealed that neither the degree of proteinuria nor serum albumin level was related to arterial thromboembolism [3]. However, sex, age, hypertension, diabetes, smoking, prior history of arterial thromboembolism, and estimated glomerular filtration are parameters of prediction for arterial thromboembolism.

Obesity is another risk factor for stroke in our patient. Obesity-driven chronic inflammation and impaired fibrinolysis are major effector mechanisms of thrombosis in obesity. These mechanisms will trigger endothelial

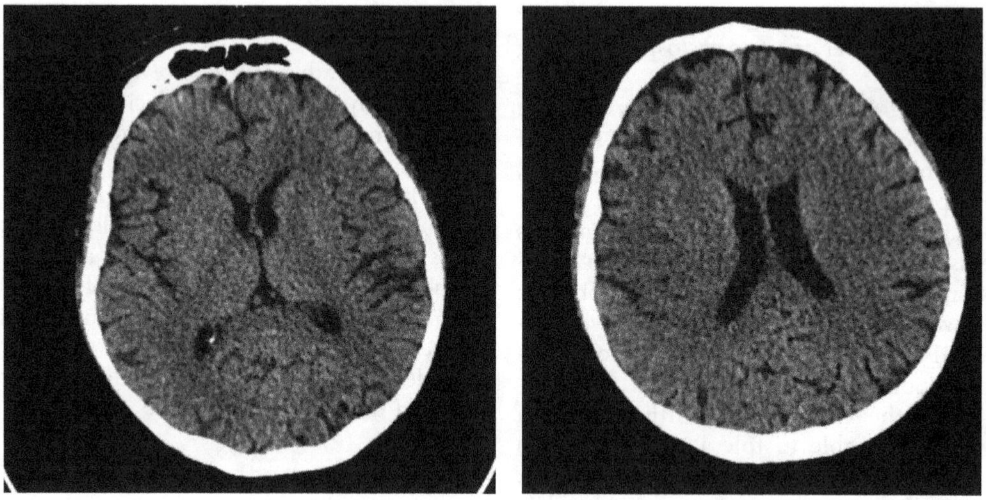

(a) (b)

FIGURE 1: Plain CT brain: normal.

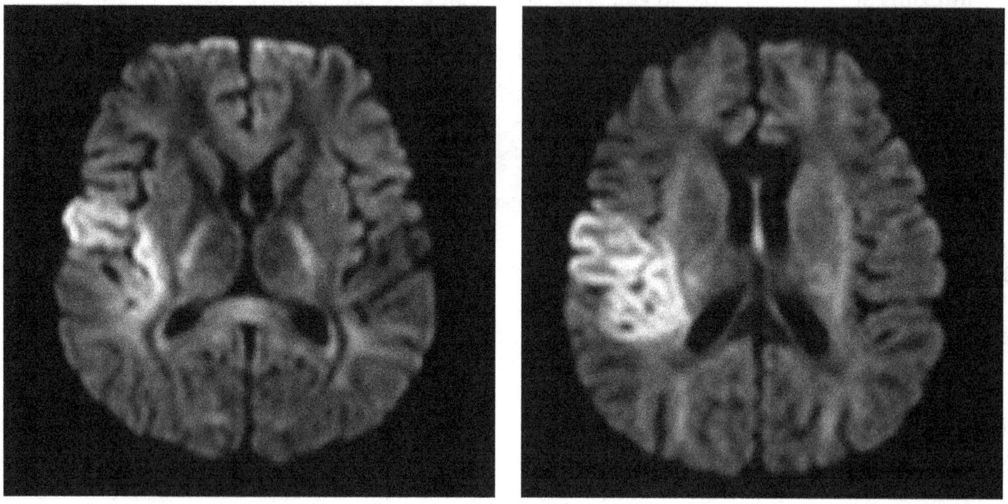

(a) (b)

FIGURE 2: DWI: hyperintensity over right temporal lobe and insular region.

dysfunction, plaque rupture, and platelet activation and end up with arterial thrombosis event [6].

Cyclosporin and tacrolimus are calcineurin inhibitors, and they suppress the immune response by downregulating the transcription of various cytokine genes, particularly interleukin-2 (IL-2), which serves as the major activation factor for T cells. They also have antiproteinuric action through an effect on glomerular permeability [7]. Patients treated with calcineurin inhibitors are at risk of developing acute or chronic kidney injury, and the proposed mechanisms were tubular dysfunction, and rarely thombotic microangiopathy [8]. There were a number of reports on increased risk of thromboembolic events in postrenal transplant patients, and studies suggested that the increase of thromboembolic events was due to multifactorial causes, such as prolonged hospitalization, nephrotic syndrome, proteinuria, steroid usage, and also immunosuppression drugs [9]. Calcineurin inhibitors are associated with a hypercoagulable state in vitro but not in vivo. However, these findings were based on retrospective small sample size studies. More studies are needed to establish the relationship between calcineurin inhibitors and thromboembolic risks [10].

Mycophenolate mofetil (MMF) is an inhibitor of inosine-5′-monophosphate dehydrogenase, and it depletes guanosine nucleotides preferentially in T and B lymphocytes and thus inhibits their proliferation. Studies have shown that MMF is capable of decreasing the in vitro aggregation of platelets in normal subjects [11, 12]. However, the relationship between MMF and thromboembolic events had not yet been established.

APS was diagnosed in our patient where he had positive lupus anticoagulant titre and with a clinical manifestation of

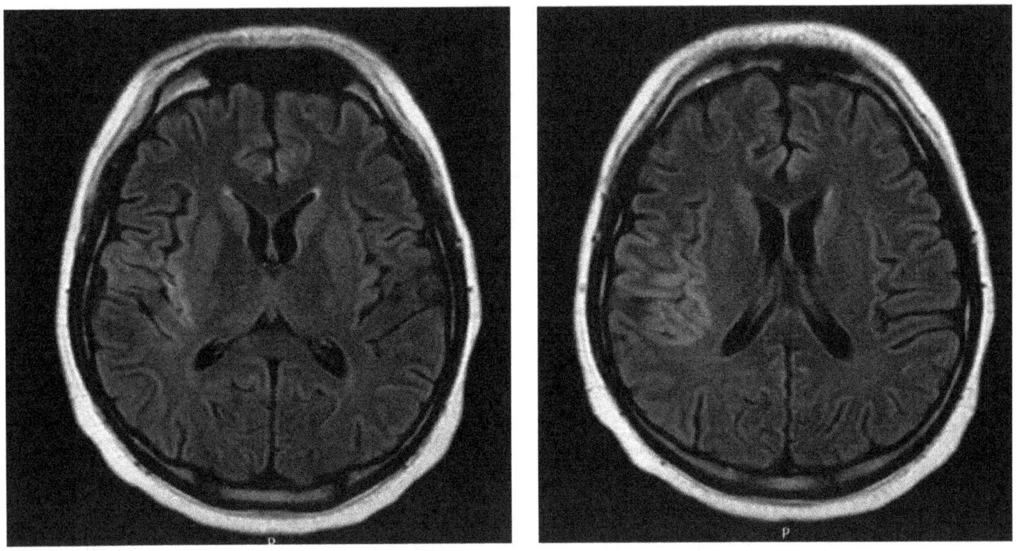

(a) (b)

Figure 3: FLAIR: hyperintensity over right temporal lobe and insular region.

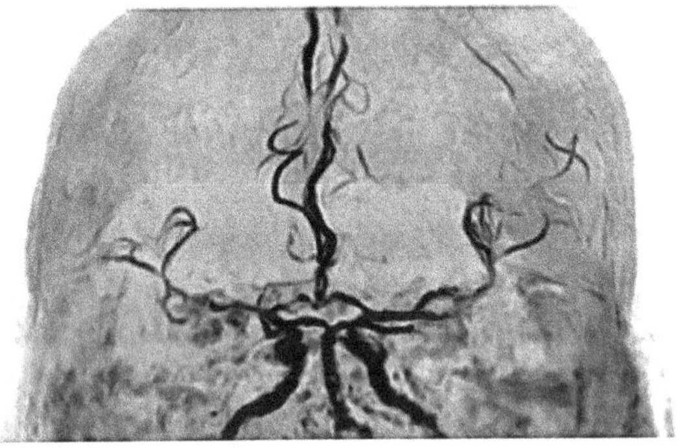

Figure 4: MRA: stenosis at distal M1 segment of the right middle cerebral artery.

arterial thrombosis. APS is an autoimmune multisystem disease with a group of autoantibodies targeting phospholipid binding protein. A critical review of literature done by Androli et al. showed that antiphospholipid frequency was estimated as 6% for pregnancy morbidity, 13.5% for stroke, 11% for myocardial infarct, and 9.5% for deep vein thrombosis [13].

The revised Sapporo diagnosis of APS requires one clinical criteria of vascular thrombosis or pregnancy morbidity and laboratory criteria of presence of either one of the antiphospholipid antibodies (anticardiolipin, anti-beta 2-glycoprotein, or lupus anticoagulant) to be present for at least 2 occasions with 12 weeks apart [14].

APS can lead to kidney damage, either as primary or systemic lupus erythematous- (SLE-) associated APS. Kidney involvement in APS involves a variety of manifestations, such as renal artery thrombosis or stenosis, renal vein thrombosis, allograft loss due to thrombosis after kidney transplantation, and injury to the renal microvasculature [15].

There were limited studies looking into the association of APS and minimal change disease. In Fakhouri et al.'s study of 29 renal biopsies performed in patients with antiphospholipid syndrome, 20 cases showed characteristic features of APS nephropathy, 3 cases were membranous nephropathy, 3 cases were minimal change disease/focal segmental glomerulosclerosis, 2 cases were mesangial C3 nephropathy, and 1 case was pauci-immune crescentic glomerulonephritis [16].

As for the prevention of thromboembolism, anticoagulant (vitamin K antagonist or low-weight molecular heparin) is recommended for all patients with NS who do not have a contraindication.

Antithrombotic medication is generally not recommended for primary thrombosis prevention in patients with APS previously (patients with laboratory criteria but no clinical criteria of APS) as there was lack of high-quality evidence. However, EULAR guideline 2019 recommended low-dose aspirin for asymptomatic APS patients, patients with systemic lupus erythematous (SLE) and APS without prior thrombosis event, nonpregnant woman with a history of obstetric APS, and patients with high title of antiphospholipid antibody [17].

All patients with APS who had a previous thrombotic event are recommended for long-term anticoagulant, either vitamin K antagonist or low-weight molecular heparin [18].

The use of direct oral anticoagulants in NS or APS is controversial, and it is not generally recommended as previous trials were associated with more vascular events compared to that of warfarin, and with limited evidence, further studies are warranted [19–21].

4.1. *Learning Points*

(i) Young patients with thrombotic events require extensive workup to look for underlying causes of thromboembolism.

(ii) The use of direct oral anticoagulants in NS or APS was not proven well. Current recommendation still favors the use of vitamin K antagonist in these groups.

Consent

Informed consent was obtained from the study subject in this article.

Acknowledgments

The authors would like to thank the Director General of Health, Malaysia for his permission to publish this article.

References

[1] M. Giroud, M. Lemesle, J.-B. Gouyon, J.-L. Nivelon, C. Milan, and R. Dumas, "Cerebrovascular disease in children under 16 years of age in the city of Dijon, France: a study of incidence and clinical features from 1985 to 1993," *Journal of Clinical Epidemiology*, vol. 48, no. 11, p. 1343, 1995.

[2] R. Ji, L. H. Schwamm, M. A. Pervez, and A. B. Singhal, "Ischemic stroke and transient ischemic attack in young adults," *Journal of the American Medical Association Neurology*, vol. 70, no. 1, pp. 51–57, 2013.

[3] B. K. Mahmoodi, M. K. Ten Kate, F. Waanders et al., "High absolute risks and predictors of venous and arterial thromboembolic events in patients with nephrotic syndrome," *Circulation*, vol. 117, no. 2, p. 224, 2008.

[4] S. Lionaki, V. K. Derebail, S. L. Hogan et al., "Venous thromboembolism in patients with membranous nephropathy," *Clinical Journal of the American Society of Nephrology*, vol. 7, no. 1, p. 43, 2012.

[5] B. A. Kerlin, R. Ayoob, and W. E. Smoyer, "Epidemiology and pathophysiology of nephrotic syndrome-associated thromboembolic disease," *Clinical Journal of the American Society of Nephrology*, vol. 7, no. 3, pp. 513–520, 2012.

[6] O. B. Ilya and R. L. Steven, "Mechanism of thrombosis in obesity," *Current Opinion in Hematology*, vol. 20, no. 5, pp. 437–444, 2013.

[7] D. C. Cattran, E. Alexopoulos, P. Heering et al., "Cyclosporin in idiopathic glomerular disease associated with the nephrotic syndrome: workshop recommendations," *Kidney International*, vol. 72, no. 12, pp. 1429–1447, 2007.

[8] M.-C. Fortin, M.-A. Raymond, F. Madore et al., "Increased risk of thrombotic microangiopathy in patients receiving a cyclosporin-sirolimus combination," *American Journal of Transplantation*, vol. 4, no. 6, p. 946, 2004.

[9] J. C. Verhave, V. Tagalakis, S. Suissa, F. Madore, M. H. Hébert, and H. Cardinal, "The risk of thromboembolic events in kidney transplant patients," *Kidney International*, vol. 85, no. 6, pp. 1454–1460, 2014.

[10] R. M. Langer and B. D. Kahan, "Sirolimus does not increase the risk for postoperative thromboembolic events among renal transplant recipients1," *Transplantation*, vol. 76, no. 2, pp. 318–323, 2003.

[11] A. Kazory and D. Ducloux, "Acquired hypercoagulable state in renal transplant recipients," *Thrombosis and Haemostasis*, vol. 91, no. 4, pp. 646–654, 2004.

[12] A. C. Allison, "Mechanisms of action of mycophenolate mofetil," *Lupus*, vol. 14, no. Suppl 1, pp. s2–s8, 2005.

[13] L. Andreoli, C. B. Chighizola, A. Banzato, G. J. Pons-Estel, G. R. De Jesus, and D. Erkan, "Estimated frequency of antiphospholipid antibodies in patients with pregnancy morbidity, stroke, myocardial infarction, and deep vein thrombosis: a critical review of the literature," *Arthritis Care & Research*, vol. 65, no. 11, pp. 1869–1873, 2013.

[14] S. Miyakis, M. D. Lockshin, T. Atsumi et al., "International consensus statement on an update of the classification criteria for definite antiphospholipid syndrome (APS)," *Journal of Thrombosis and Haemostasis*, vol. 4, no. 2, pp. 295–306, 2006.

[15] G. Maria, "Tektonidou. Antiphospholipid syndrome nephropathy: from pathogenesis to treatment," *Frontiers in Immunology*, vol. 9, p. 1181, 2018.

[16] F. Fakhouri, L.-H. Noël, J. Zuber et al., "The expanding spectrum of renal diseases associated with antiphospholipid syndrome," *American Journal of Kidney Diseases*, vol. 41, no. 6, pp. 1205–1211, 2003.

[17] M. G. Tektonidou, L. Andreoli, M. Limper et al., "EULAR recommendations for the management of antiphospholipid syndrome in adults," *Annals of the Rheumatic Diseases*, vol. 78, no. 10, p. 1296, 2019.

[18] G. Ruiz-Irastorza, M. Cuadrado, I. Ruiz-Arruza et al., "Evidence-based recommendations for the prevention and long-term management of thrombosis in antiphospholipid antibody-positive patients: report of a task force at the 13th International Congress on antiphospholipid antibodies," *Lupus*, vol. 20, no. 2, p. 206, 2011.

[19] V. Dufrost, J. Risse, S. Zuily, and D. Wahl, "Direct oral anticoagulants use in antiphospholipid syndrome: are these drugs an effective and safe alternative to warfarin? A systematic review of the literature," *Current Rheumatology Reports*, vol. 18, no. 12, p. 74, 2016.

[20] V. Pengo, G. Denas, G. Zoppellaro et al., "Rivaroxaban vs. warfarin in high-risk patients with antiphospholipid syndrome," *Blood*, vol. 132, no. 13, p. 1365, 2018.

[21] D. J. Sexton, D. G. de Freitas, M. A. Little et al., "Direct-acting oral anticoagulants as prophylaxis against thromboembolism in the nephrotic syndrome," *Kidney International Reports*, vol. 3, no. 4, p. 784, 2018.

41

Tocilizumab Use in a Chronic Hemodialysis Patient for the Management of COVID-19-Associated Pneumonia and Acute Respiratory Distress Syndrome

Sudeendra Gupta,[1] Rakesh Madhyastha,[1] Fadi Hamed,[2] Maher Balkis,[1] Wasim El Nekidy,[3] and Nizar Attallah[1]

[1]*Medical Sub-specialities Institute, Cleveland Clinic Abu Dhabi, Abu Dhabi, UAE*
[2]*Critical Care Institute, Cleveland Clinic Abu Dhabi, Abu Dhabi, UAE*
[3]*Department of Pharmacy, Cleveland Clinic Abu Dhabi, Abu Dhabi, UAE*

Correspondence should be addressed to Nizar Attallah; attalln@clevelandclinicabudhabi.ae

Academic Editor: Rumeyza Kazancioglu

Novel coronavirus disease 2019 (COVID-19) is a highly infectious, rapidly spreading viral disease. As of writing this article, there are over 4.4 million people affected by COVID-19, and unfortunately, 300,000 have succumbed to the infection. In this article, we address a particularly more susceptible group of the population of end-stage renal disease (ESRD) patients on dialysis who may potentially benefit from being treated with tocilizumab. The use of tocilizumab has not been reported widely in ESRD patients on dialysis to treat COVID-19. In this case report, we describe a patient with ESRD on hemodialysis who was admitted to the intensive care unit, with severe pneumonia secondary to COVID-19 infection. This patient was treated with tocilizumab 400 mg intravenous and had a favorable outcome with no apparent adverse events.

1. Introduction

Coronaviruses are RNA viruses and typically cause symptoms similar to the common cold. But two coronaviruses—severe acute respiratory syndrome coronavirus (SARS-CoV-2) and Middle East respiratory syndrome coronavirus (MERS-CoV)—have been associated with severe pneumonia, acute respiratory failure, and death [1, 2]. In late 2019, deadly infections related to a novel coronavirus (SARS-CoV-2) appeared in China and has been rapidly spreading worldwide [3].

An epidemiological survey shows that patients with underlying conditions such as diabetes mellitus, hypertension, and cardiovascular disease or the elderly are more susceptible to acquire COVID-19 infection [2]. Hemodialysis (HD) patients are particularly vulnerable to infection and may exhibit greater variations in clinical symptoms and infectivity [3]. Patients with end-stage renal disease (ESRD) on HD are susceptible to infection mainly because of more exposure to the healthcare system and personnel on top of having multiple comorbidities [3–5].

In the absence of quality evidence, several agents that showed previous activity against SARS-CoV-1 and MERS-CoV have emerged. Hydroxychloroquine, an antimalaria drug commonly used to treat chronic inflammatory diseases, has shown in vitro activity against SARS-CoV-2, but that benefit has not been consistently demonstrated across large clinical trials and recently lost its approval [6, 7]. Lopinavir/ritonavir showed in vitro activity, and few case reports demonstrated success but without support from clinical trials [8]. Interferon-α and -β were used in China to treat SARS-CoV-2 [8]. Remdesivir showed activity against SARS-CoV-2 in recent clinical trials and received FDA approval for that [9, 10]. Favipiravir, another antiviral, used to treat influenza in Japan, showed activity against SARS-CoV-2 [6]. Finally, anticytokines immunomodulators such as tocilizumab antagonizes the interleukin-6 (IL-6) receptors and consequently inhibits the cytokine storm. In a small clinical trial from China, patients with severe SARS-CoV-2 infection significantly improved with tocilizumab and were successfully discharged [6, 11]. The drug can cause elevation of liver enzymes and uric acid; however, little is known about the use of this drug in patients on renal replacement therapy.

We report a patient with ESRD on HD who was admitted to the intensive care unit (ICU), with severe pneumonia secondary to COVID-19 infection. This patient was treated with tocilizumab and had a favorable outcome with no apparent adverse events.

2. Case Report

Our patient was a 39-year-old male with a history of ESRD (of unknown underlying cause) treated with maintenance HD twice a week for the past 4.5 years. The patient presented to the emergency department (ED) with a 4-day history of fever and cough and a 1-day history of breathlessness. The patient was admitted to the ICU from the emergency department due to acute hypoxic respiratory failure secondary to severe pneumonia. He was having breathlessness (normal jugular venous pressure) with no peripheral edema; however, he had extensive crackles bilaterally. The O_2 saturation was 70% on room air. He was tachypneic and in respiratory distress.

Furthermore, investigations revealed severe azotemia and lymphopenia with normal leucocyte counts. His arterial blood gas (ABG) was indicative of acute respiratory distress syndrome (ARDS) with $PaO_2/FiO_2 < 200$. Chest X-ray showed bilateral perihilar and basal infiltrates which rapidly worsened over the following 48 hrs with an increase in density and extensively involved the bilateral mid and upper zones.

The nasopharyngeal swab was positive for SARS-CoV-2 by real-time polymerase chain reaction (PCR). His inflammatory markers such as *C*-reactive protein (CRP), IL-6, and ferritin were significantly elevated (Figure 1). He was diagnosed with COVID-19-related bilateral pneumonia and ARDS. Noninvasive ventilation (NIV) was started. Hydroxychloroquine and regular HD with adequate ultrafiltration were initiated. On day 2 of admission, tocilizumab (IL-6 receptor antagonist) 400 mg IV one dose was given. On day 4, significant improvement occurred as shown by decreased breathlessness, decreased support of NIV and O_2 requirements, and improvement in the bilateral chest infiltrates as demonstrated by chest X-ray (Figure 2). By day 7, the patient was transferred to the isolation ward (dedicated to patients with COVID-19) with minimal oxygen requirement (nasal cannula). He was then discharged home after finishing 14 days of isolation in a stable condition.

3. Discussion

We report this unique case as we expect several dialysis patients to have a more severe form of the infection. The IL-6 receptors were proven to play a key role in the cytokine storm, and blocking these receptors might potentially help patients with severe COVID-19 infections [12].

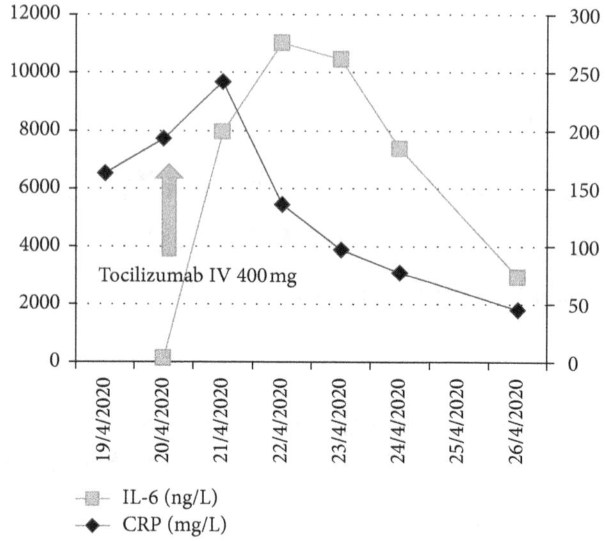

Figure 1: Effect of tocilizumab on inflammatory markers. IL-6, interleukin-6; CRP, *C*-reactive protein.

Several studies show that only 5% of COVID-19 patients have critical illness [13–15]. The mortality rate for ARDS patients with COVID-19 remains unclear but has relatively high variance as shown by an Italian study indicating critical care mortality up to 26% [14], while in the US the mortality was shown to be around 21% in the same population [15].

Management of patients with ARDS secondary to COVID-19 remains mainly supportive, although since the start of the pandemic, many other proposed treatments using antiviral medications, antimalarials, and anticytokine immunomodulators, such as the interleukin-6 (IL-6) receptor antagonist tocilizumab, have been utilized. Convalescent plasma has been used successfully in some instances [16].

Reports of using tocilizumab in an ESRD patient are scarce [15]. Tocilizumab is being used in patients to treat rheumatoid arthritis, but ESRD patients were excluded from the main studies [17, 18]. At the moment, the treatment of this infection in dialysis patients is supportive only. Unfortunately, the clinical trial of remedesivir, which is considered to be a novel agent against COVID-19, has excluded dialysis patients [9, 10, 19]. The risk profile for severe presentations of COVID-19 is reported to be concentrated in patients with comorbidities. Patients with ESRD are known to have multiple comorbidities. Unfortunately, most of those patients are excluded from the clinical trials, and we are left with no option but to use these medications to save this population' lives.

In a retrospective analysis of 21 patients used to treat COVID-19, tocilizumab effectively improved clinical symptoms and repressed deterioration of critically ill patients with COVID-19 [20]. Our patient was on chronic dialysis and was severely hypoxic on admission, with a rapidly deteriorating clinical condition for 48 hours before admission. After receiving tocilizumab, the

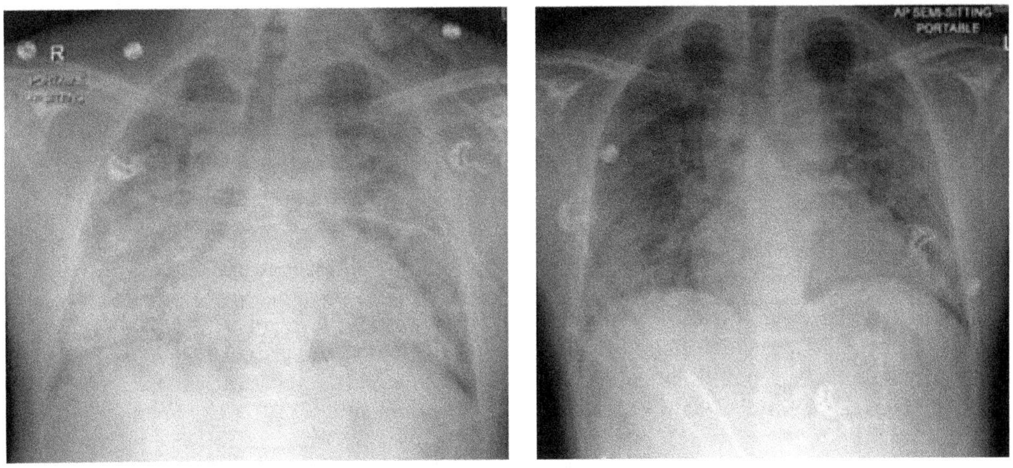

(a) (b)

FIGURE 2: Chest X-ray AP view showing extensive bilateral perihilar and basal opacities on day 2 (a), which has improved significantly by day 4 as shown in (b).

TABLE 1: Investigations.

	Day 1	Day 2	Day 3	Day 4	Day 5	Day 6	Day 7	Day 8	Day 9
BUN (mmol/L)	7.1	10.1	8.2	14.0	11.2	18.7	24.9	12.2	16.8
Creatinine (μmol/L)	624	820	604	789	674	926	1121	710	931
Sodium (mmol/L)	135	132	137	133	136	131	129	134	133
Potassium (mmol/L)	3.9	4.7	4.9	5.1	4.2	4.1	4.3	4.3	4.6
Chloride (mmol/L)	92	91	93	92	93	89	87	92	90
Calcium (mmol/L)	2.21	1.95	2.05	2.06	2.11	2.27	2.26	2.27	2.32
Phosphorous (mmol/L)		0.77	2.1	2.16	1.73	1.98	2.07	1.79	2.12
Total bilirubin (μmol/L)	3.6	4.3	5.0	3.6	3.7	4.4	3.6	4.0	3.3
Total protein/albumin (g/L)	69/38	68/36	66/34	64/32	64/34	67/35	66/33	67/35	65/35
AST (U/L)	87	111	125	69	115	133	61	46	34
ALT (U/L)	60	81	102	72	87	120	81	61	47
ALP (IU/L)	145	143	145	141	162	168	157	156	150
CRP (mg L)	163	193	242	136	97.5	77.9	57.9	45	30.2
IL 6 (ng/L)			7946	11024	10453	7360		2938	
Pro calcitonin (mcg/L)		18.9	30.1	28.28					
Ferritin (mcg/L)		6508	>8000	6656	5507	5152			
Hemoglobin (g/L)	90	90	91	81	81	80	82	85	85
Hematocrit	0.27	0.27	0.28	0.25	0.25	0.24	0.24	0.26	0.26
WBC ($\times 10^9$L)	2.68	3.22	3.42	4.0	4.0	4.63	5.56	5.62	6.46
Neutrophil/lymphocyte (%)	84/12.9	68/27	62/26	70/16.8	66/16	65/18.6	66/18	63/20	60/20
Platelets ($\times 10^9$/L)	117	118	110	116	126	124	137	161	174

	Day 1	Day 2	Day 3	Day 4	Day 5	Day 6	Day 7
pH	7.4	7.49	7.40	7.42	7.43	7.43	7.44
$PaCO_2$ (kPA)	4.7	4.8	5.43	4.43	5.48	4.72	4.29
PaO_2 (kPA)	12.93	6.95	9.64	7.40	12.75	10.95	11.11
HCO_3 (mmol/L)	25	27	24	21	27	23	22

picture completely inverted illustrating the role of this drug in the management of cytokine storm demonstrated by the reduction in all inflammatory markers (Figure 1 and Table 1) and improvement in patient's clinical picture.

IL-6 is a pleiotropic proinflammatory cytokine produced by a variety of cell types including T and B cells, lymphocytes, monocytes, and fibroblasts [21]. The overproduction of early response proinflammatory cytokines results in what has been described as a cytokine storm, leading to an increased risk of vascular hyperpermeability, multiorgan failure, and eventually death when the high cytokine concentrations are unabated over time [22]. IL-6 may play a key role in driving the inflammatory response that leads to morbidity and mortality and patients with COVID-19 who develop ARDS [22].

Tocilizumab is a recombinant humanized anti-human IL-6 receptor monoclonal antibody which inhibits IL-6-mediated signaling. The drug is recommended at a dose of

8 mg/kg intravenous either alone or in combination with corticosteroids. Our protocol recommends an intravenous dose of 4–8 mg/kg, up to a maximum of 400 mg in 250 ml of normal saline in one hour. The dose may be repeated in 12 hours. The maximum dose should not exceed 800 mg. The drug should not be administered to patients with tuberculosis or gastrointestinal perforation [23]. The drug, however, should not be initiated in a patient with severe neutropenia, thrombocytopenia, or elevated liver enzymes [11, 23, 24].

The pharmacokinetics of the drug reveals a volume of distribution of 6.4 L. The drug is known to have biphasic elimination from the circulation (nonrenal/nonhepatic). The drug has a long half-life between 11 and 13 days depending on the dose (4 mg/kg or 8 mg/kg, respectively). No formal study of the effect of renal impairment on the pharmacokinetics of tocilizumab was conducted. However, the drug manufacturer recommends no dose adjustment in patients with mild to moderate renal impairment. However, there is a lack of studies in patients with severe renal impairment or patients utilizing renal replacement therapies [23].

4. Conclusion

COVID-19 infection is affecting patients with different risk factors. Patients with ESRD are at higher risk for that mainly due to higher exposure to the healthcare system and have multiple comorbidities. Tocilizumab can be considered to treat sick patients with ESRD in the ICU with COVID-19 infection to combat the cytokine storm. It needs to be tested formally in a randomized controlled study.

Consent

No written consent has been obtained from the patients as there is no patient identifiable data included in this case report.

References

[1] C. I. Paules, H. D. Marston, and A. S. Fauci, "Coronavirus infections-more than just the common cold," *The Journal of the American Medical Association*, vol. 323, no. 8, pp. 707-708, 2020.

[2] T. Rajesh, J. B. Lynch, and C. D. Rio, "Mild or Moderate Covid-19," *The New England Journal of Medicine*, vol. 383, pp. 1757–1766, 2020.

[3] B. Meijers, P. Messa, and C. Ronco, "Safeguarding the maintenance hemodialysis patient population during the coronavirus disease 19 pandemic," *Blood Purification*, vol. 49, no. 3, pp. 259–264, 2020.

[4] K. Su, Y. Ma, Y. Wang et al., "How we mitigated and contained the COVID-19 outbreak in a hemodialysis center: lessons and experience," *Infection Control & Hospital Epidemiology*, vol. 41, no. 10, pp. 1240–1242, 2020.

[5] Y. Ma, B. Diao, X. Lv et al., "2019 novel coronavirus disease in hemodialysis (HD) patients: report from one HD center in Wuhan,China," *MedRxiv*, vol. 2, Article ID 20027201, 24 pages, 2020.

[6] J. M. Sanders, M. L. Monogue, T. Z. Jodlowski, and J. B. Cutrell, "Pharmacologic treatments for coronavirus disease 2019 (COVID-19)," *The Journal of the American Medical Association*, vol. 13, p. 2020, 2020.

[7] A. V. Hernandez, Y. M. Roman, V. Pasupuleti, J. J. Barboza, and C. M. White, "Hydroxychloroquine or chloroquine for treatment or prophylaxis of COVID-19," *Annals of Internal Medicine*, vol. 173, no. 4, p. 287, 2020.

[8] B. Cao, Y. Wang, D. Wen et al., "A trial of lopinavir-ritonavir in adults hospitalized with severe covid-19," *New England Journal of Medicine*, vol. 382, no. 19, pp. 1787–1799, 2020.

[9] J. Grein, N. Ohmagari, D. Shin et al., "Compassionate use of remdesivir for patients with severe covid-19," *New England Journal of Medicine*, vol. 382, no. 24, p. 2327, 2020.

[10] J. Beigel, K. Tomashek, L. Dodd et al., "Remdesivir for the treatment of COVID-19—preliminary report," *New England Journal of Medicine*, vol. 383, pp. 1813–1826, 2020.

[11] P. Luo, Y. Liu, L. Qiu, X. Liu, D. Liu, and J. Li, "Tocilizumab treatment in COVID-19: a single center experience," *Journal of Medical Virology*, vol. 92, no. 7, p. 814, 2020.

[12] B. Fu, X. Xu, and H. Wei, "Why tocilizumab could be an effective treatment for severe COVID-19?" *Journal of Translational Medicine*, vol. 18, p. 164, 2020.

[13] Z. Wu and J. M. McGoogan, "Characteristics of and important lessons from the coronavirus disease 2019 (COVID-19) outbreak in China: summary of a report of 72 314 cases from the Chinese Center for Disease Control and Prevention," *The Journal of the American Medical Association*, vol. 323, no. 13, pp. 1239–1242, 2020.

[14] Z. A. Grasselli, A. Zanella, M. Antonelli et al., "Baseline characteristics and outcomes of 1591 patients infected with SARS-CoV-2 admitted to ICUs of the Lombardy region," *The Journal of the American Medical Association*, vol. 323, no. 16, pp. 1574–1581, 2020.

[15] S. Richardson, J. S. Hirsch, M. Narasimhan et al., "Presenting characteristics, comorbidities, and outcomes among 5700 patients hospitalized with COVID-19 in the New York city area," *The Journal of the American Medical Association*, vol. 323, no. 20, p. 2052, 2020.

[16] E. Bloch, S. Shoham, A. Casadevall et al., "Deployment of convalescent plasma for the prevention and treatment of COVID-19," *Journal of Clinical Investigation*, vol. 130, no. 6, pp. 2757–2765, 2020.

[17] M. Iwamoto, S. Honma, Y. Asano, and S. Minota, "Effective and safe administration of tocilizumab to a patient with rheumatoid arthritis on haemodialysis," *Rheumatology International*, vol. 31, no. 4, pp. 559-560, 2011.

[18] S. P. P. Campos, T. T. A. Santana, K. V. M. Campos, A. S. Braz, and E. A. M. Freire, "Use of tocilizumab in hemodialysis patients as treatment of Rheumatoid arthritis: case report," in *Anais do 36° Congresso Brasileiro de Reumatologia*vol. 1, p. 305, Blucher, São Paulo, Brazil, 2019.

[19] A. J. Ferrey, G. Choi, R. M. Hanna, and Y. Chang, "A case of novel coronavirus disease 19 in a chronic hemodialysis patient presenting with gastroenteritis and developing severe pulmonary disease," *Journal of the American Society of Nephrology*, vol. 51, no. 5, pp. 337–342, 2020.

[20] C. Zhanga, Z. Wu, J. W. Li, H. Zhao, and G. Q. Wang, "The cytokine release syndrome (CRS) of severe COVID-19 and Interleukin-6 receptor (IL-6R) antagonist Tocilizumab may be the key to reduce the mortality," *International Journal of Antimicrobial Agents*, vol. 55, no. 5, Article ID 105954, 2020.

[21] S. Rose-John, K. Winthrop, and L. Calabrese, "The role of IL-6 in host defence against infections: immunobiology and

clinical implications," *Nature Reviews Rheumatology*, vol. 13, no. 7, pp. 399–409, 2017.

[22] R. Jose and A. Manuel, "COVID-19 cytokine storm: the interplay between inflammation and coagulation," *The Lancet Respiratory Medicine*, vol. 8, no. 6, pp. e46–e47, 2020.

[23] FDA, *Actemra (Tocilizumab)*, Genentech, Inc., San Francisco, CA, USA, 2019.

[24] C. Kotch, D. Barrett, and D. T. Teachey, "Tocilizumab for the treatment of chimeric antigen receptor T cell-induced cytokine release syndrome," *Expert Review of Clinical Immunology*, vol. 15, no. 8, pp. 813–822, 2019.

Permissions

All chapters in this book were first published by Hindawi Publishing Corporation; hereby published with permission under the Creative Commons Attribution License or equivalent. Every chapter published in this book has been scrutinized by our experts. Their significance has been extensively debated. The topics covered herein carry significant findings which will fuel the growth of the discipline. They may even be implemented as practical applications or may be referred to as a beginning point for another development.

The contributors of this book come from diverse backgrounds, making this book a truly international effort. This book will bring forth new frontiers with its revolutionizing research information and detailed analysis of the nascent developments around the world.

We would like to thank all the contributing authors for lending their expertise to make the book truly unique. They have played a crucial role in the development of this book. Without their invaluable contributions this book wouldn't have been possible. They have made vital efforts to compile up to date information on the varied aspects of this subject to make this book a valuable addition to the collection of many professionals and students.

This book was conceptualized with the vision of imparting up-to-date information and advanced data in this field. To ensure the same, a matchless editorial board was set up. Every individual on the board went through rigorous rounds of assessment to prove their worth. After which they invested a large part of their time researching and compiling the most relevant data for our readers.

The editorial board has been involved in producing this book since its inception. They have spent rigorous hours researching and exploring the diverse topics which have resulted in the successful publishing of this book. They have passed on their knowledge of decades through this book. To expedite this challenging task, the publisher supported the team at every step. A small team of assistant editors was also appointed to further simplify the editing procedure and attain best results for the readers.

Apart from the editorial board, the designing team has also invested a significant amount of their time in understanding the subject and creating the most relevant covers. They scrutinized every image to scout for the most suitable representation of the subject and create an appropriate cover for the book.

The publishing team has been an ardent support to the editorial, designing and production team. Their endless efforts to recruit the best for this project, has resulted in the accomplishment of this book. They are a veteran in the field of academics and their pool of knowledge is as vast as their experience in printing. Their expertise and guidance has proved useful at every step. Their uncompromising quality standards have made this book an exceptional effort. Their encouragement from time to time has been an inspiration for everyone.

The publisher and the editorial board hope that this book will prove to be a valuable piece of knowledge for researchers, students, practitioners and scholars across the globe.

List of Contributors

Chinmay Patel
University of Pikeville, Kentucky College of Osteopathic Medicine, Division of Nephrology, Pikeville Medical Center, USA

Caitlin P. Wilson
Family Practice Residency Program, Pikeville Medical Center, USA

Naveed Ahmed
Neurology Program, University of Pikeville, Kentucky College of Osteopathic Medicine, Pikeville Medical Center, USA

Yousef Hattab
Division of Pulmonary and Critical Care Medicine, Pikeville Medical Center, USA

Ernie Yap, Tahir Ahmad, A. Sanusi and Anthony Joseph
State University of New York, Downstate Medical Center, Brooklyn, NY 11203, USA

Moro Salifu and Mary Mallappallil
State University of New York, Downstate Medical Center, Brooklyn, NY 11203, USA
Division of Nephrology, Department of Medicine, SUNY Downstate Health Sciences University, Brooklyn, NY, USA
Division of Nephrology, Department of Medicine, Kings County Hospital Center, Brooklyn, NY, USA

Akshay Athavale, Kate R Wyburn, Paul L Snelling and Steven J Chadban
Department of Renal Medicine, Royal Prince Alfred Hospital, Sydney, New South Wales, Australia
Central Clinical School, Faculty of Medicine and Health, University of Sydney, Sydney, New South Wales, Australia

Amaresh Vanga and Harlan Rust
Nephrology, Eastern Virginia Medical School, 855WBrambelton Ave, Norfolk, VA 23510, USA

Amna Z. Rana
Eastern Virginia Medical School, Norfolk, VA, USA

Jolanta Kowalewska
Pathology, Eastern Virginia Medical School, 855WBrambelton Ave, Norfolk, VA 23510, USA

Michael Andrew Yu
Emory University, Department of Internal Medicine, USA

Ramzi Mulki and Julia Massaad
Emory University, Division of Digestive Diseases, USA

Shin Teshirogi, Jun Muratsu, Hidenori Kasahara, Ken Terashima, Sho Miki, Tomohiro Minami, Yujiro Okute, Suguru Yoneda, Atsuyuki Morishima and Katsuhiko Sakaguchi
Department of Nephrology and Hypertension, Sumitomo Hospital, 5-3-20 Nakanoshima, Kita-ku, Osaka 530-0005, Japan

Shinji Kunishima
Department of Advanced Diagnosis, Clinical Research Center, National Hospital Organization Nagoya Medical Center, Nagoya, Japan

Saeid Mirzai, Aron Tidrick, Qitan Huang and Justin Hale
Alabama College of Osteopathic Medicine, 445 Health Sciences Blvd, Dothan, AL 36303, USA

Ahmad Oussama Rifai
The Virtual Nephrologist, INC., Lynn Haven, FL 32444, USA

Ulrich Jehn, Stefan Reuter, Hermann Pavenstädt and Britta George
Department of Medicine D, Division of General Internal Medicine, Nephrology and Rheumatology, University Hospital of Münster, Münster 48149, Germany

Cornelie Müller-Hofstede
Institute of Human Genetics, University Hospital of Münster, Münster 48149, Germany

Barbara Heitplatz and Veerle Van Marck
Gerhard Domagk Institute of Pathology, University Hospital Münster, Münster 48149, Germany

F. A. K. Lodhi, T. Akcan and J. N. Mojarrab
Department of Internal Medicine, Marshfield Clinic Health System, Marshfield, WI, USA

S. Sajjad
Department of Pathology, Marshfield Clinic Health System, Marshfield WI, USA

R. Blonsky
Department of Nephrology, Marshfield Clinic Health System, Marshfield, WI, USA

Satyanand Sathi, Anil Kumar Garg, Manoj Kumar Singh, Virendra Singh Saini and Devinder Vohra
Department of Medicine, S.M.M.H. Government Medical College, Saharanpur, Uttar Pradesh, India

José C. De La Flor, Cristina Albarracín, Elisa Ruiz and Miguel Rodeles
Department of Nephrology, Central Defense Gomez Ulla Hospital, Madrid, Spain

Francisco Valga
Department of Nephrology, Doctor Negrín University Hospital, Las Palmas de Gran Canaria, Spain

Alexander Marschall
Department of Cardiology, Central Defense Gomez Ulla Hospital, Madrid, Spain

Tania Monzon
Department of Hemodialysis, Avericum S.L., Las Palmas de Gran Canaria, Spain

Mariana Leone, Anwar Iqbal, J. R. Hugo Bonatti, Samina Anwar and Catherine Feaga
Meritus Health, Hagerstown, MD, USA

Javier Reque, Rosa Arlandis, Maria José Pascual and Alejandro Perez-Alba
Nephrology Department, Hospital General Universitario de Castellón, Castellón de la Plana, Spain

Nayara Panizo
Nephrology Department, Hospital Clínico Universitario Valencia, Valencia, Spain

Christine Persaud, Victor Hoang, Joshua Tate, Wayne Latack and David Dado
Department of Medicine, Keesler Medical Center, Biloxi 39534, MS, USA

Uttsav Sandesara
Department of Medicine, University of Mississippi Medical Center, Jackson 39216, MS, USA

Kullaya Takkavatakarn and Pisut Katavetin
Division of Nephrology, Department of Medicine, King Chulalongkorn Memorial Hospital, Faculty of Medicine, Chulalongkorn University, Bangkok, Thailand

Hansamon Poparn
Department of Pediatric Hematology and Oncology, Department of Pediatrics, Faculty of Medicine, Chulalongkorn University, Bangkok, Thailand
Integrative and Innovative Hematology/Oncology Research Unit, Faculty of Medicine, Chulalongkorn University, Bangkok, Thailand

Tsuyoshi Tsukada and Atsushi Ueda
Department of Nephrology, Hitachi General Hospital, 2-1-1 Jonan-Cho, Hitachi, Ibaraki 317-0077, Japan
Department of Nephrology, Faculty of Medicine, University of Tsukuba, 1-1-1 Tennodai, Tsukuba, Ibaraki 305-8575, Japan

Akiko Sakata
Department of Pathology, Hitachi General Hospital, 2-1-1 Jonan-Cho, Hitachi, Ibaraki 317-0077, Japan

Kei Nagai
Department of Nephrology, Hitachi General Hospital, 2-1-1 Jonan-Cho, Hitachi, Ibaraki 317-0077, Japan
Department of Nephrology, Faculty of Medicine, University of Tsukuba, 1-1-1 Tennodai, Tsukuba, Ibaraki 305-8575, Japan

John Odhiambo and Fazal Yakub
Internal Medicine, The Aga Khan University Hospital, Nairobi, Kenya

Hanika Patel
Radiology, The Aga Khan University Hospital, Nairobi, Kenya

Anderson Mutuiri and Ahmed Sokwala
The Aga Khan University Hospital, Nairobi, Kenya

Lalani De Silva, Dinesha Jayasinghe and Priyani Amarathunga
Department of Pathology, Faculty of Medicine, University of Colombo, Colombo, Sri Lanka

Akbar Hamid, Jacob Sabu, Omar Elhawary and Isha Puri
Division of Nephrology, Department of Medicine, SUNY Downstate Health Sciences University, Brooklyn, NY, USA
Division of Nephrology, Department of Medicine, Kings County Hospital Center, Brooklyn, NY, USA

Man Oh
Division of Nephrology, Department of Medicine, SUNY Downstate Health Sciences University, Brooklyn, NY, USA

Sapna A. Mehta, Bonnie E. Lonze and Nicole M. Ali
New York University Grossman School of Medicine, New York, NY, USA
New York University Langone Transplant Institute, New York, NY, USA

Maya C. Graves
New York University Grossman School of Medicine, New York, NY, USA

Antonio Faieta
Department of Internal Medicine, Beaumont Health System, Royal Oak, MI, USA

Tavis Dancik
Department of Nephrology, Beaumont Health System, Royal Oak, MI, USA

Benjamin T. Burdorf
Northeast Ohio Medical University, Rootstown, OH 44272, USA

Au Cheuk, William Lee, Ka-Fai Yim, Clara Poon, Ivy Wong, Bosco Lam, Hon-Lok Tang and Samuel K. Fung
Princess Margaret Hospital, Hong Kong

Carlos E. Duran, Juan Guillermo Posada and Johanna Schweineberg
Department of Nephrology, Fundacion Valle del Lili, Cali, Colombia

Mayra Estacio
Health Sciences Faculty, Universidad CES, Cali, Colombia

Fredy Lozano
Health Sciences Faculty, Universidad del Valle, Cali, Colombia

Esteban Echeverri and Maria Juliana Riascos
Health Sciences Faculty, Universidad ICESI, Cali, Colombia

Ho-Kwan Sin, Ping-Nam Wong, Kin-Yee Lo, Man-Wai Lo, Shuk-Fan Chan, Kwok-Chi Lo, Yuk-Yi Wong, Lo-Yi Ho, Wing-Tung Kwok, Kai-Chun Chan, Andrew Kui-Man Wong and Siu-Ka Mak
Department of Medicine and Geriatrics, Kwong Wah Hospital, 25 Waterloo Road, Kowloon, Hong Kong

Tawfeeq I. Sangey
TMJ Super Specialized Polyclinic, Dar Es Salaam, Tanzania

Hamim Abdul Rusheke
School of Medicine and Dentistry, University of Dodoma, Dodoma, Tanzania

Ansaar I. Sangey and Advera Ngaiza
Muhimbili National Hospital, Dar Es Salaam, Tanzania

Nimishkumar Chaya
TMJ Hospital, Dar Es Salaam, Tanzania

Nand K. Wadhwa
Nephrology Division, NY Health, Stony Brook, NY, USA

Jason A. Kline
Cooper Medical School of Rowan University, Camden, NJ, USA

Sreedhar R. Adapa
The Nephrology Group, Inc., Visalia, CA, USA

Hideyuki Hayasaka, Masaya Kofuji, Takayuki Uchida and Naoki Momose
Department of Clinical Engineering, Saitama Medical Center, Jichi Medical University, Saitama, Japan

Kiyonori Ito, Susumu Ookawara, Haruhisa Miyazawa, Yuichiro Ueda, Keiji Hirai and Yoshiyuki Morishita
Division of Nephrology, First Department of Integrated Medicine, Saitama Medical Center, Jichi Medical University, Saitama, Japan

Shunto Kawamura, Ayumi Gomyo, Shun-ichi Kimura and Shinichi Kako
Division of Hematology, First Department of Integrated Medicine, Saitama Medical Center, Jichi Medical University, Saitama, Japan

Joelle Suillot and Eric Descombes
Service of Nephrology, HFR Cantonal Hospital Fribourg, Fribourg, Switzerland
University of Fribourg, Fribourg, Switzerland

Jürg Bollmann
Service of Urology, HFR Cantonal Hospital Fribourg, Fribourg, Switzerland

Samuel Rotman
Service of Clinical Pathology, Lausanne University Hospital, University of Lausanne, Lausanne, Switzerland

Virin Ramoutar
Nephrologist & Infectious Disease Specialist, Cumberland Kidney Specialists, Cookeville, TN, USA

Raafat Makary
Pathology Department, University of Florida, Jacksonville, FL, USA

Malleswari Ravi
Division of Infectious Disease, University of Florida, Jacksonville, FL, USA

Leighton James
Division of Nephrology, Medical College of Georgia, Augusta University, Augusta, GA, USA

Charles Heilig
Division of Nephrology, University of Florida, Jacksonville, FL, USA

Kevin John, Ajay Kumar Mishra, Karthik Gunasekaran and Ramya Iyyadurai
Department of Medicine, Christian Medical College, Vellore, India

Sophia Lionaki, Kalliope Vallianou and Ioannis Boletis
Nephrology Department and Transplantation Unit, Laiko Hospital, National & Kapodistrian University of Athens, Faculty of Medicine, Athens, Greece

George Liapis
Pathology Department, Laiko Hospital, Athens, Greece

Chrysovalantis Vergadis
Radiology Department, Laiko Hospital, Athens, Greece

Eri Kasama, Jun Ino, Fumika Iemura, Saeko Kumon, Mio Kodama, Keitaro Sato and Hitoshi Eizumi
Department of Nephrology, Kidney Center, Toda Central General Hospital, 1-19-3 Hon-cho, Toda City, Saitama 335-0023, Japan

Kosaku Nitta and Junichi Hoshino
Department of Nephrology, Tokyo Women's Medical University, 8-1 Kawada-cho, Shinjyuku-ku, Tokyo 162-0054, Japan

Nur Ezzaty Mohammad Kazmin
Medical Department, National University of Malaysia Medical Centre, Kuala Lumpur, Malaysia

Lydia Kamaruzaman, Voon Ken Fong, Rozita Mohd and Ruslinda Mustafar
Nephrology Unit, Medical Department, National University of Malaysia Medical Centre, Kuala Lumpur, Malaysia

Zhiqin Wong
Gastroenterology Unit, Medical Department, National University of Malaysia Medical Centre, Kuala Lumpur, Malaysia

C. M. H. Hilton
Department of Cardiology, Nephrology and Endocrinology, Nordsjællands Hospital-Hillerød, 3400 Hillerød, Denmark
Department of Otorhinolaryngology, Nordsjællands Hospital-Hillerød, 3400 Hillerød, Denmark

L. Boesby and K. E. Nelveg-Kristensen
Department of Cardiology, Nephrology and Endocrinology, Nordsjællands Hospital-Hillerød, 3400 Hillerød, Denmark

Nidrit Bohra, Abigayle Sullivan and Haseeb Chaudhary
Internal Medicine Department, Reading Hospital, West Reading, PA, USA

Trudy Demko
Nephrology Department, Reading Hospital, West Reading, PA, USA

Avantika Chenna
Department of Internal Medicine, Division of Nephrology, Phobe Putney Memorial Hospital, Medical College of Georgia, 417 W 3rd Avenue, Albany 31701, GA, USA

Venu Madhav Konala
Department of Internal Medicine, Division of Medical Oncology, Ashland Bellefonte Cancer Center, 122 St Christopher Dr, Ashland 41169, KY, USA

Subhasish Bose and Sasmit Roy
Lynchburg Nephrology Physicians, Lynchburg, VA, USA

Bhaskar Reddy Madhira
Fellow in Hematology and Oncology, Sunny Upstate Medical University, Syracuse, NY, USA

Vijay Gayam
Department of Medicine, Interfaith Medical Center, Brooklyn, NY, USA

Srikanth Naramala
Department of Internal Medicine, Division of Rheumatology, Adventist Medical Center, Hanford 93230, CA, USA

Sreedhar Adapa
Department of Internal Medicine, Division of Nephrology, Adventist Medical Center, Hanford 93230, CA, USA

Yannick M. Nlandu, Jean-Robert R. Makulo, Ernest K. Sumaili, Clarisse N. Nkondi, Justine B. Bukabau, Nazaire M. Nseka and François B. Lepira
Kinshasa University Hospital, Nephrology Unit, Kinshasa, Democratic Republic of the Congo

Nestor M. Pakasa and François K. Beya
Division of Uro-Nephropathology, Department of Pathology, Kinshasa, Democratic Republic of the Congo

Yuhong Zhao
Department of Nephrology, Central Hospital Affiliated to Shenyang Medical College, Shenyang, Liaoning 110024, China

Youngki Kim
Department of Pediatrics, Division of Pediatric Nephrology, University of Minnesota, Minneapolis, MN 55455, USA

Milind Junghare and Viral Vakil
Department of Renal Disease and Hypertension, University of Minnesota, Minneapolis, MN 55455, USA

Xuesong Su
Department of Nephrology, Shengjing Hospital of China Medical University, Shenyang, Liaoning 110004, China

Faqian and Lihong Bu
Department of Laboratory Medicine and Pathology, University of Minnesota, Minneapolis, MN 55455, USA

K. K. Neoh, A. S. N. Tang and B. M. Anita
Department of Internal Medicine, Seberang Jaya Hospital, Penang, Malaysia

I. Looi
Department of Internal Medicine, Seberang Jaya Hospital, Penang, Malaysia
Clinical Research Center (CRC), Seberang Jaya Hospital, Penang, Malaysia

Sudeendra Gupta, Rakesh Madhyastha, Maher Balkis and Nizar Attallah
Medical Sub-specialities Institute, Cleveland Clinic Abu Dhabi, Abu Dhabi, UAE

Fadi Hamed
Critical Care Institute, Cleveland Clinic Abu Dhabi, Abu Dhabi, UAE

Wasim El Nekidy
Department of Pharmacy, Cleveland Clinic Abu Dhabi, Abu Dhabi, UAE

Index